Introducing
Dental Implants

Commissioning Editor: Michael Parkinson
Project Development Manager: Janice Urquhart
Project Manager: Frances Affleck
Designer: Judith Wright
Illustrator: Robert Britton

Introducing
Dental Implants

John A. Hobkirk PhD, BDS, FDSRCSEd, FDSRCSEng, DrMedHC

Professor of Prosthetic Dentistry, Eastman Dental Institute for Oral Health Care Sciences, University College London, University of London, UK

Roger M. Watson MDS, BDS, FDSRCSEng

Emeritus Professor of Prosthetic Dentistry, Guy's King's and St Thomas's Dental Institute, King's College London, University of London, UK

Lloyd J. J. Searson BDS, MSc Michigan, FDSRCSEng

Consultant in Restorative Dentistry, Eastman Dental Hospital, London, UK

Foreword by

George A. Zarb BChD (Malta) DDS MS (Michigan) MS (Ohio) FRCD(C) DrOdont LLD MD
Professor and Head of Prosthodontics, Faculty of Dentistry, University of Toronto, Canada

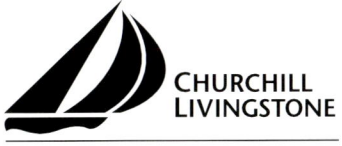
CHURCHILL
LIVINGSTONE

EDINBURGH LONDON NEW YORK OXFORD PHILADELPHIA ST LOUIS SYDNEY TORONTO 2003

CHURCHILL LIVINGSTONE
An imprint of Elsevier Science Limited

First published 2003

ISBN 0 443 07185 3

British Library Cataloguing in Publication Data
A catalogue record for this book is available from the British Library

Library of Congress Cataloging in Publication Data
A catalog record for this book is available from the Library of Congress

Notice
Medical knowledge is constantly changing. Standard safety precautions must be followed, but as new research and clinical experience broaden our knowledge, changes in treatment and drug therapy may become necessary or appropriate. Readers are advised to check the most current product information provided by the manufacturer of each drug to be administered to verify the recommended dose, the method and duration of administration, and contraindications. It is the responsibility of the practitioner, relying on experience and knowledge of the patient, to determine dosages and the best treatment for each individual patient. Neither the Publisher nor the authors assume any liability for any injury and/or damage to persons or property arising from this publication.
The Publisher

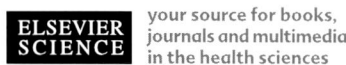

ELSEVIER SCIENCE your source for books, journals and multimedia in the health sciences

www.elsevierhealth.com

The publisher's policy is to use paper manufactured from sustainable forests

Printed in China

Foreword

Today's miracle medicine scenario of genetic engineering and regenerative medicine is a timely reminder of dentistry's relatively small yet indispensable, role in advancing health care. The dental profession has been in the body 'spare parts' business for a very long time, but without the anguish inherent in the tricky ethical questions associated with organ transplantation. Dentistry's term for hard and soft tissue analog replacement – prosthodontics – remains a tongue twister. It also conjures up memories of frustrating dental school pre-clinical experiences. Yet our profession's long-standing tradition of readily endorsing evidence-based, applied replacement bio-technology has served us well, as we sought to replicate artificially what has been lost in the oral cavity. Hence the commitment of leading clinical educators, particularly the authors of this very lucid and intelligent text, to use applied dental implant research to enhance the life quality of prosthodontic patients.

Brånemark's seminal research in osseointegration enabled the surgically related and prosthodontic disciplines exciting scope to enlarge and fulfil all three remits of dental scholarship – education, service and research. As a result, the prescription of dental implants has gradually eclipsed traditional techniques of pre-prosthetic surgery and offered predictable and even optimal treatment outcome alternatives to routine fixed and removable prostheses. In the past 20 years numerous fine publications have sought to articulate a strong case for inclusion of dental implant techniques in the dentist's routine clinical repertoire. However, this is the first text which I have been privileged to read which addresses the topic in a manner so comprehensive, and yet so superbly organized, that it may very well qualify not only as the finest book for the novice in the field, but also as a landmark publication. The authors have distilled their own considerable and internationally recognized scholarship into 10 very well balanced and rationally argued chapters. They are to be congratulated for raising the standard of communication in the fascinating field of dental implants. As a result, all of us in the profession – dentists, dental specialists and above all prosthodontic patients – will be the beneficiaries of the authors' outstanding contribution.

Professor George A. Zarb   Toronto, Canada

Preface

It is now seven years since our *Color Atlas and Text of Dental and Maxillo-Facial Implantology* was published, a period during which osseointegration has remained the basis of this form of treatment. While the fundamental principles may have remained largely unchanged the range and volume of research, clinical applications and manufacturers' products have all continued to expand. This has been reflected in the range of textbooks on the subject, although the novice to the field has been less well catered for. We hope that this book will be helpful to this group of colleagues.

We should like to thank the many who have helped with this project, including those whose skills are reflected in the illustrations. Geoffrey Forman, Hardev Coonar, Hind Abdel-Latif, Margaret Whateley, Vladimir Nikitin, Trevor Coward, Cameron Malton, David Davis, and Nadin Kurban have all helped the project in various ways, for which we are most grateful. Our biggest thanks are however due to our wives and families, who have cheerfully supported us during many evenings and weekends of very personal computing.

John A. Hobkirk   London 2003
Roger M. Watson
Lloyd J. J. Searson

Contents

1 Using this book

INTRODUCTION

This book is intended principally for undergraduate dental students in their final year and dentists taking postgraduate courses. It should also be of interest to professionals complementary to dentistry, seeking an introduction to the subject. The text is not intended to develop skills to the specialist level, but rather to help in preparing for examinations or clinical situations in which basic knowledge of the topic is required.

The text has been arranged in an ordered sequence from an introduction to the subject, through to completion of treatment using implant-stabilized prostheses and the all-important management of problems. Since there are a number of clinical situations where it may be advantageous to use dental implants, several of the chapters describe procedures that could be used in different circumstances.

The text is not primarily intended to be read from cover to cover, but rather as a series of discrete chapters, although many build on knowledge acquired in earlier sections. Readers may therefore find it helpful to select particular chapters when seeking information on one aspect of implant therapy. Consequently, many chapters contain brief résumés of information covered earlier in the book to avoid needless cross-referencing.

The information has been arranged in three ways. Firstly, there is the body text, which covers each topic in the intended detail; secondly there are supplementary photographs and diagrams; and finally there are a number of summary lists which are intended to be used by the reader as an aid when preparing for an examination or wishing to use the material in a clinical setting.

IMPLANT TREATMENT

Treatment with dental implants has evolved from earlier much-derided procedures to a mainstream clinical activity. However, its potential benefits and high success rates have led to the procedure sometimes being incorrectly used, with unfortunate outcomes.

A wide range of components is now available from many different manufacturers, and the technique is developing its own jargon, which is a mixture of traditional dental terminology, new terms and manufacturers' catalogue descriptions. This can be confusing for the novice. The introductory chapter is intended to explain the essential aspects of the subject and introduce the terminology that is in current use.

GENERAL TREATMENT DECISIONS

Treatment with dental implants has considerably extended the range of care that we can offer our patients; however, despite its applications in new areas such as maxillofacial prosthodontics, the anchoring of hearing aids and in orthodontic therapy, it is principally used for prosthodontic rehabilitation. If the potential benefits of such uses are to be maximized, then it is essential that implant treatment be selected on a logical basis, and placed within the context of the full range of treatment modalities available in restorative dentistry.

GATHERING INFORMATION AND TREATMENT PLANNING

Treatment should not be based on hope, be it in the mind of the dentist or the patient, but rather on accurate information, an understanding of the patient's problems, recognition of suitable treatment alternatives and the agreed selection of the one most appropriate to their needs. This may not necessarily be the most complex procedure or involve the use of dental implants. Their use is most likely to succeed where it has been selected on a sound basis.

IMPLANT SURGERY

The correct insertion of dental implants is essential for their optimal utilization and involves far more than merely the surgical creation of an intra-bony defect and insertion of the implant body. The technique must involve appropriate planning and consultation by the dental team, even where the surgeon and prosthodontist are the same individual. While an integrated dental implant is essential for success, it is of little use if it is inappropriately located.

THE EDENTULOUS CASE

While the number of edentulous individuals is falling in many countries, those that remain are often oral cripples. It was for this reason that treatment of such patients was one of the priorities for the early pioneers of dental implantology. The procedure can bring enormous benefits to such patients but must be set against a background of prosthodontic knowledge; an inadequate prosthesis does not become ideal merely because it is implant stabilized. The nature of these issues and the associated treatment procedures are considered in this chapter.

THE PARTIALLY DENTATE CASE

The great benefits achievable with implant treatment in the edentulous patient were soon translated into the resolution of specific problems in the partially dentate patient, where they have been shown to be highly effective in appropriate cases. The situation is, however, more complex than in the edentulous case, since there are often several treatment modalities that could be used, while the status of the existing teeth and their supporting structures are additional complications. Dental implants are not an alternative to inadequate oral hygiene or poor treatment planning, and if inserted inappropriately in the partially dentate patient can present a major problem when further teeth are lost. This chapter is concerned with the selection of appropriate patients and the treatment procedures that may be employed.

THE SINGLE-TOOTH SCENARIO

Missing single teeth, especially due to trauma, are a not uncommon problem, which in many cases can be easily solved using traditional restorative techniques. However, there are some situations where this is not technically feasible or produces an inferior result. Recognizing these cases, planning and carrying out appropriate implant-based treatment are discussed in this chapter.

OTHER APPLICATIONS

The ability of osseointegrated interfaces to develop in many locations has led to a wide range of potential applications for dental and skull implants, which are briefly considered in this chapter.

PROBLEMS

Treatment with dental implants can be a very complex procedure in terms of planning, execution and management of the subsequent problems. Despite the high success rate of the technique, these are not unknown and are best managed by avoidance rather than correction after the event. This chapter places great emphasis on this approach from the initial consultation onwards, while covering the various techniques that may need to be employed when difficulties arise.

2 Implants: an introduction

MANAGEMENT OF MISSING TEETH

Teeth are commonly absent from the dental arch either congenitally or as a result of disease, of which caries and periodontal breakdown are the most common. While it is not axiomatic that a missing tooth should always be replaced, there are many occasions where this is desirable to improve appearance, masticatory function or speech, or sometimes to prevent harmful changes in the dental arches, such as the overeruption or tilting/drifting of teeth. Tooth loss is also followed by resorption of the alveolar bone, which exacerbates the resultant tissue deficit.

In most countries with an oral care service a considerable component of the work of the dental team is directed towards prevention of tooth loss, repair of damaged teeth, and the replacement of those which are missing together with their supporting tissues. Where patients are edentulous, treatment for tooth loss has largely been restricted to the use of complete dentures; however, in the partially dentate, the potential treatments are more numerous, since a variety of techniques may be used to stabilize prostheses by linking them to the natural teeth. Removable partial dentures (RPDs) are widely employed because of their versatility and can give effective long-term results in suitable circumstances. They do, however, suffer from being relatively bulky, frequently need metal components, which may be difficult to disguise, are patient removable, and are inherently less stable than a fixed bridge that is secured permanently to one or more teeth. These may be based either on traditional designs involving extensive preparation of the abutment teeth, or more modern and less destructive adhesive techniques. In general, RPDs are used to manage extensive tooth loss or significant alveolar resorption and where there are advantages in their relative simplicity of fabrication and replacement. Fixed restorations are typically less versatile and more expensive to provide, but have advantages related to their stability and reduced bulk.

Clinicians have long sought to provide their patients with an artificial analogue of the natural teeth and a wide variety of materials and techniques have been used for this. However, it has not been possible to replicate the periodontal tissues and alternative strategies have therefore been adopted. These have been based on the principles of creating and maintaining an interface between the implant and the surrounding bone, which is capable of load transmission, associated with healthy adjacent tissues, predictable in outcome and with a high success rate. This outcome proved elusive until the discovery of the phenomenon of osseointegration.

OSSEOINTEGRATION

Extensive work by the Swedish orthopaedic surgeon P.-I. Brånemark led to the discovery that commercially pure titanium (CPTi), when placed in a suitably prepared site in the bone, could become fixed in place due to a close bond that developed between the two (Fig. 2.1), a phenomenon that he later described as osseointegration (OI). This state has anatomical and functional dimensions, as it requires both a close contact between the implant and surrounding healthy bone and the ability to transmit functional loads over an extended period without deleterious effects either systemically or in the adjacent tissues. OI is not defined in terms of the extent of the bone–implant contact, provided that functional requirements are met and the tissues are healthy. Many of the factors that predispose to the development of OI are now known, and where these exist a successful outcome will probably follow the placing of a suitable implant. Similarly, failure is more likely where factors known to predispose to an unsuccessful outcome exist. Occasionally, implants fail for no apparent reason, sometimes in groups in one patient – the so-called 'cluster

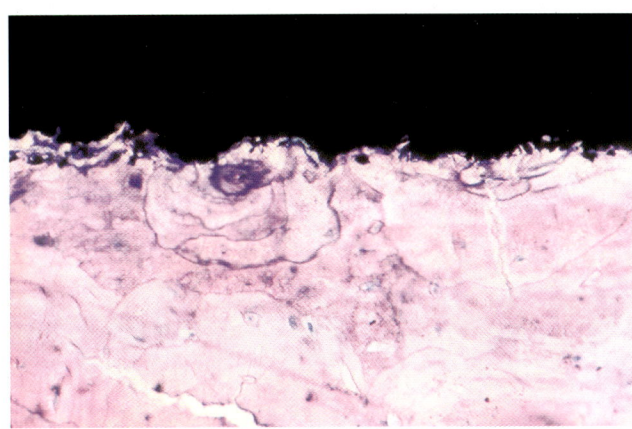

Fig. 2.1 Close physical approximation between the surface of a dental implant and vital bone is a key structural characteristic of osseointegration, which also has important functional parameters.

phenomenon'. It is therefore important to advise patients that a satisfactory outcome cannot be guaranteed.

OI is currently viewed as the optimum implant–bone interface, without which success cannot be obtained, and great emphasis has been placed on its production and maintenance. Nevertheless, it is only one component of successful dental implant treatment and does not in itself prevent that treatment from failing. While the absence of OI is equated with treatment failure, its achievement does not guarantee success, which is dependent on the design and performance of the final prosthesis. This may be precluded by an inappropriately placed implant, even if it is integrated.

While the osseointegrated interface and associated soft-tissue cuff where the implant penetrates the oral mucosa are often thought of as dental analogues, they have a number of important differences. In particular, the interface is more rigid and less displaceable than the periodontal ligament, and behaves essentially elastically as opposed to the viscoelasticity of the periodontal ligament. The stability of the interface also precludes implant repositioning by orthodontic manoeuvres, but may permit dental implants to be used as anchorage for fixed orthodontic appliances. The osseointegrated interface is also associated with a slow rate of loss of crestal alveolar bone, typically less than 0.1 mm per annum after the first year of implantation. As a result, most implants can be expected to be functional throughout adult life.

Inflammation of the tissues around an endosseous implant is sometimes observed; it is described as peri-implant mucositis when it involves only the soft tissues and peri-implantitis where loss of the bone interface occurs. While the microorganisms associated with these lesions are similar to those seen in periodontal disease, it is currently unclear whether they cause the lesion or colonize the region subsequently.

Factors influencing OI

A number of systemic and local factors have been identified as being associated with the production of an osseointegrated interface. Fewer systemic factors are now thought to be of significance than was once believed, and are considered below. Local factors are as follows.

Material

Osseointegration was originally believed to be unique to high-purity titanium (commercially pure or CPTi, 99.75%) and this material still forms the basis of the technique; however, it is known that a range of other materials can also form intimate bonds with bone. These include zirconium and some ceramics, particularly hydroxyapatite; however, they have not been as extensively researched as CPTi for dental implant applications.

Surface composition and structure

It is thought that CPTi owes its ability to form an osseointegrated interface to the tough and relatively inert oxide layer, which forms very rapidly on its surface. This surface has been described as osseoconductive, that is, conducive to bone formation. Other substrates also have this property and may also stimulate bone formation, a property known as osseoinduction. While the initial bone–implant contact with such a material can be more extensive and occur sooner than around CPTi, the long-term benefits are less evident. Nevertheless, there is considerable clinical and research interest in modifying the composition of implant surfaces for the purpose of obtaining more rapid OI and/or a mechanically and clinically superior host/implant interface (Fig. 2.2). This can take the form of surface coatings (such as hydroxyapatite), changes in the composition of the implant material by selective surface coping with small quantities of other elements, or the local use of biochemical molecules involved naturally in mediating bone formation, such as bone morphogenic protein (BMP).

Implant surface structure is also known to influence cellular behaviour, and a range of microstructured surfaces has been shown to modify cell spreading and orientation on the implant, benefiting initial anchorage in bone. The influence of these factors on OI in the long term, however, is not known.

Heat

Heating of bone to a temperature in excess of 47°C during implant surgery can result in cell death and denaturation of collagen. As a result, OI may not occur; instead the implant becomes surrounded by a fibrous capsule and the shear strength of the implant–host interface is significantly reduced. For these reasons great care has to be taken when preparing implant sites to control thermal trauma. This is related to drill speed, drill design, amount of bone being removed at

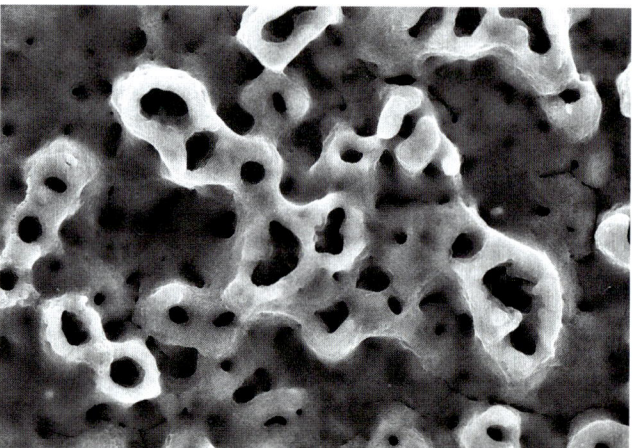

Fig. 2.2 Manufacturers have modified the surfaces of their dental implants with the intention of improving tissue responses so as to enhance osseointegration. This picture shows the TiUnite™ surface utilized by Nobel Biocare. (Courtesy Prof. N. Meredith)

one pass, bone density and use of coolants. In general, slow drill speeds and the use of copious amounts of coolant are recommended.

Contamination

Contamination of the implant site by organic and inorganic debris can prejudice the achievement of OI. Material such as necrotic tissue, bacteria, chemical reagents and debris from drills can all be harmful in this respect.

Initial stability

It is known that where an implant fits tightly into its osteotomy site then OI is more likely to occur. This is often referred to as primary stability, and where an implant body has this attribute when first placed failure is less probable. This property is related to the quality of fit of the implant, its shape, and bone morphology and density. Thus screw-shaped implants will be more readily stable than those with little variation in their surface contour. Soft bone with large marrow spaces and sparse cortices provides a less favourable site for primary stability to be achieved. Some manufacturers produce 'oversized' and self-tapping screw designs to help overcome these problems.

Bone quality

This bone property is well recognized by clinicians but is more difficult to measure scientifically. It is a function of bone density, anatomy and volume, and has been described using a number of indices. The classifications of Lekholm and Zarb and of Cawood and Howell are widely used to describe bone quality and quantity (Figs 2.3, 2.4). The former relates to the thickness and density of cortical and cancellous bone, and the latter to the amount of bone resorption. Bone volume does not by itself influence OI, but is an important determinant of implant placement. Where

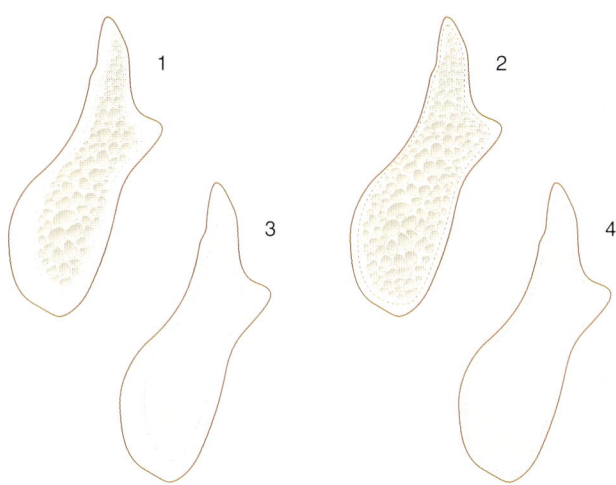

Fig. 2.3 A scheme for classifying patterns of bone in the edentulous jaw: (1) thick cortex and plentiful cancellous bone; (2) thin cortex and plentiful cancellous bone; (3) dense cortex with minimal cancellous bone; and (4) sparse cancellous bone and a thin cortex. All can provide effective support for a dental implant; however, there is an increased risk of thermal trauma in types 1 and 3, and problems are often encountered obtaining good primary fixation in types 2 and 4.

bone bulk is lacking, then small implants may need to be used, with the consequent risk of mechanical overload and implant failure.

Epithelial downgrowth

Early implant designs were often associated with downgrowth of oral epithelium, which eventually exteriorized the device. When the newer generation of CPTi devices was introduced great care was taken to prevent this by initially covering the implant body with oral mucosa while OI occurred. The implant body was then exposed and a superstructure added, since it was known that the osseointegrated interface was resistant to epithelial downgrowth. More recently, there has been a growing interest in using an implant

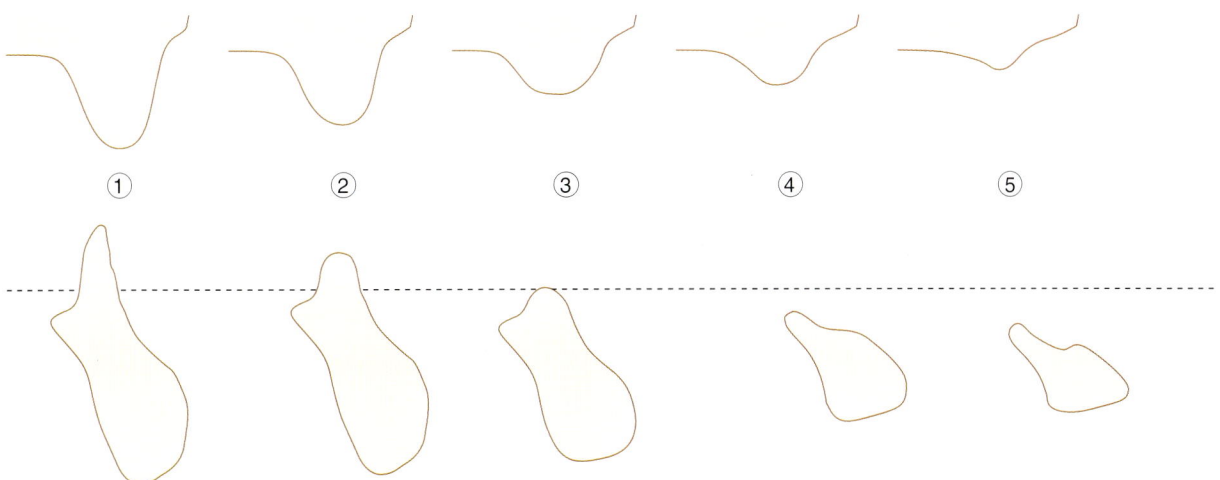

Fig. 2.4 A scheme for classifying the extent of bone resorption in the edentulous maxilla and mandible based on that proposed by Cawood and Howell in 1988.

design, which penetrates the mucosa from the time of placement. While this technique has no long-term data to rival that of the earlier methods, it does appear on the basis of preliminary findings to be effective and successful in suitable patients and locations. A recent development of this has been the introduction of a technique for placing a prefabricated superstructure on dental implants, which permits their use within hours of placement.

Early loading

There is good research evidence that high initial loads on an implant immediately following placement result in the formation of a fibrous capsule rather than OI. Nevertheless there is evidence from clinical studies that where the implant has good primary stability, early loading does not apparently preclude OI, below an ill-defined threshold.

Late loading

It has been shown that excessive mechanical loads on an osseointegrated implant can result in breakdown of the interface with resultant implant failure, and it is generally considered that overload is therefore to be avoided. This could arise as a result of bruxism, in patients who habitually use high occlusal forces, and as a result of superstructure designs in which the use of excessive cantilevering causes high forces on the implants. The research evidence for a link between occlusal loads and loss of OI is, however, not extensive, and there are currently no clinical guidelines as to its determination in a particular patient other than by general principles. Since bone is a strain-sensitive material, the modelling and remodelling of which is influenced by deformation, it is thought that there is probably a range of strains that are associated with bone formation and could thus be of therapeutic value.

IMPLANT COMPONENTS

There is a wide range of terms used to describe the various components employed in implant treatment, and attempts to standardize terminology have proved unhelpful. Some common descriptions are included here, under the heading of the term used in this book.

Box 2.1 Local factors that may influence osseointegration

- Material
- Surface composition and structure
- Heat
- Contamination
- Initial stability
- Bone quality
- Epithelial downgrowth
- Loading

Dental implant body

This term describes the component placed in the bone, which is sometimes also referred to as an implant, fixture or implant fixture. Occasionally the term is used colloquially to describe both the endosseous component and those parts placed immediately on top. The preferred term for the endosseous component is 'dental implant body', or 'implant body' where its application is clear from the context (Fig. 2.5).

The majority of dental implants are designed to be placed into holes drilled in the bone and are thus axisymmetric. Many are screw shaped, since this aids in primary stability, and are inserted into tapped holes. Where bone has a low density this may result in poor stability and thus some designs incorporate self-tapping features to overcome this problem. Others are made with a tapering design, which creates a wedging effect as the implant body is seated.

In addition to screw threads, other surface features may be included with the intention of enhancing OI. Typical of these are macro surface irregularities, and porous metallic and ceramic coatings, typically of hydroxyapatite. These features usually also enhance retention, which is important since an osseointegrated smooth titanium surface has a low shear strength.

The implant may either be of a multi-part design, which is intended to be buried while OI occurs, or a single-part design, which will penetrate the mucosa from the time of placement. Multi-part designs incorporate various mechanical linkages to facilitate the joining of the different components and the mechanical integrity of the joint (Fig. 2.6). These usually include a hexagonal socket on one component to provide resistance to rotation, or a tapered joint to provide both this and a seal. The joint is commonly held closed by a screw, although some manufacturers employ cement fixation. Following placement of a buried implant it is usual to insert a cover screw in its central

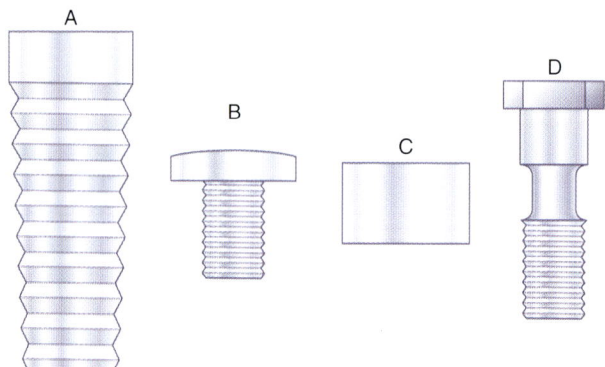

Fig. 2.5 Components used in dental implantology: (a) a threaded tapered implant body; (b) cover screw, used to cover the top of the implant; (c) parallel-sided transmucosal abutment; and (d) an abutment screw; this is used to secure the abutment to the implant body.

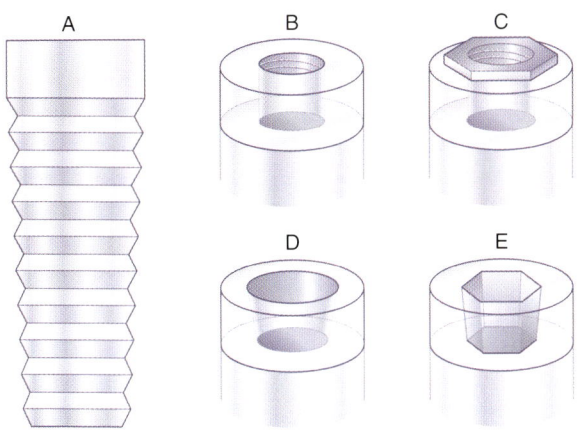

Fig. 2.6 Examples of the principles of some of the methods used by manufacturers to link implant abutments to the implant itself. The top of the implant body (a) may incorporate a threaded hole in combination with a butt joint, which will provide limited resistance to rotation (b), an external hexagonal feature that will provide resistance to rotation (c), an internal tapered recess that can provide a strong linkage with an enhanced sealing effect (d) and an internal hexagonal recess which provides good resistance to rotation (e).

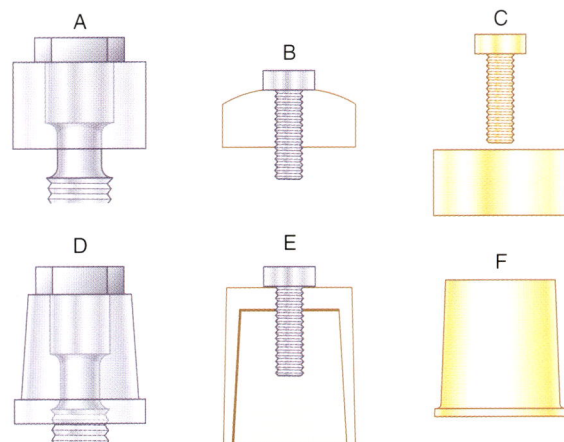

Fig. 2.7 Implant components. A standard abutment complete with screw (a), and the associated healing cap (b) and gold cylinder (c). When using tapered abutments (d) a special tapered healing cap (e) should be employed, while a pre-manufactured gold cylinder (f) is incorporated into the prosthesis to provide a precise and secure linkage with the underlying implant.

hole to prevent tissue ingress and bone growth over the top of the implant body.

Cover screw

This is placed at the time of first-stage surgery, and removed when locating the abutments. Where the implant body is not internally threaded the description 'screw' is inappropriate. Although the term 'dental implant obturator' has been proposed the name 'cover screw' is in wide use (Fig. 2.5).

Transmucosal abutment (TMA)

This is used to link the implant body to the prosthesis, and may also be referred to as an implant abutment. The proposed standard term is 'dental implant connecting component'. These parts have evolved from a simple cylindrical device into a family of components basically of four types: cylindrical, shouldered, angled and customizable. They are usually, but not exclusively, made of CPTi, and are provided in a range of lengths and, in the case of the shouldered design, shoulder heights (Figs 2.7, 2.8).

The cylindrical designs are employed where the mucosal aspect of the prosthesis is to be placed some distance above the oral mucosa to aid cleaning, the so-called 'oil rig' design. While this gap can prove troublesome to some patients, it is not normally evident where the adjacent lip is long, and can undoubtedly aid cleaning.

Shouldered designs permit the prosthesis to finish at or below the 'gingival margins', providing a more natural-appearing emergence profile for the super-structure. They are shaped so as to have a stylistically

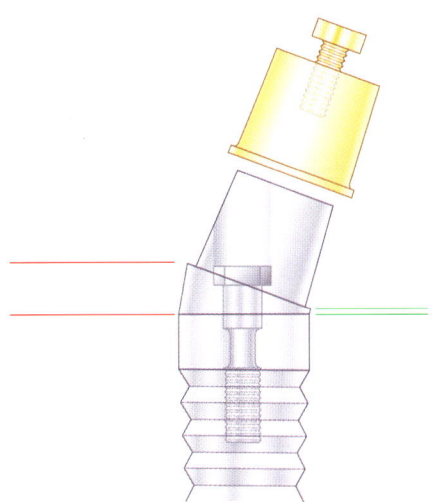

Fig. 2.8 An angled abutment with gold cylinder. This device enables the implant body and crown to have divergent long axes. Note that the shoulder of the abutment is higher on one side than the other as a result of its angulation. This can create problems when designing a restoration.

similar configuration to a crown preparation on a natural tooth, with a narrow shoulder surmounted by a largely tapered profile. As the components are pre-manufactured, some constraints are placed on their applications; in particular, the shoulder is often the same height around the abutment. Most manufacturers provide a range of lengths and shoulder heights to cater for different clinical situations.

Since the bony anatomy places constraints on the location and orientation of a dental implant, there are situations where the crown on the superstructure is required to have a long axis markedly divergent from that of the implant. This can be managed with an angulated abutment in which the long axes of the two linking surfaces, to the implant and the crown, are divergent. Some designs appear less suited to use with single teeth, as they are vulnerable to rotation under occlusal loads. In addition, the divergence imposes a minimum shoulder height on the external aspect (Fig. 2.8).

The customized abutment is pre-manufactured to fit the implant but has excess bulk, permitting its modification to a particular situation after the fashion of preparing a conventional crown. These abutments may be made in a dense ceramic, CPTi or gold alloy, and may be supplied as a gold core onto which a crown may be bonded using traditional techniques. While they allow considerable flexibility in crown design and placement, their ability to correct for incorrect implant location and angulation is limited. All are difficult to trim and this is best accomplished in the laboratory.

Healing abutment

This is a temporary implant-connecting part placed on the implant body to create a channel through the mucosa while the adjacent soft tissues heal.

They are normally wider than the corresponding regular abutment to compensate for some tissue collapse into the space when placing the regular abutment. They also allow for a period of resolution of tissue swelling before selecting the final abutment so as to ensure its optimum height. This is particularly important since soft-tissue contours can often change significantly in the period following placement of the abutments. This therefore greatly aids abutment selection, which is particularly important when using abutments that are intended to replicate a natural emergence profile, requiring the metal shoulder to be submucosal.

Impression coping

This is also described as a dental implant impression cap, and is used to transfer the position of the implant body or the abutment to the working cast.

Gold cylinder

This pre-manufactured component is used to link the superstructure to the abutment, and is usually screw retained. It can be provided in a range of shapes depending on the abutment design and may be intended for soldering to a gold bar for use with an overdenture, incorporation in a cast superstructure as the basis of a fixed bridge or as part of a single crown. Where it forms the basis of a single crown it is normal for it to incorporate an anti-rotation feature, such as an internal hexagon, a feature that may be present for other applications.

Healing caps

Most manufacturers provide temporary polymeric covers for their abutments to prevent damage and fouling of the screw retainer when the patient has to be without the superstructure during its fabrication or repair. Some of these are of a larger diameter than the abutment and are intended to retain a surgical pack immediately after its placement, typically at second-stage surgery.

Joints

There are two methods of joining implant superstructures to the abutments: screwed and cemented joints. The latter use standard dental cements, sometimes reformulated by the manufacturer for this application.

Screwed joints

A screwed joint functions by virtue of its components being held tightly together by the tension in the screw, acting after the fashion of a spring. Provided that

---

Box 2.2 Dental implant components

IMPLANT BODY
Often referred to as an implant

COVER SCREW
Prevents bone ingress in the implant head

TRANSMUCOSAL ABUTMENT (TMA)
Links the implant body to the mouth. May be pre-manufactured or custom formed

HEALING ABUTMENT
Placed temporarily on the implant body to maintain patency of the mucosal penetration

TEMPORARY COMPONENTS
Pre-manufactured components used to make temporary crowns and bridges for fitting on dental implants and abutments

IMPRESSION COPING
Used to transfer the location of the implant body or abutment to a dental cast

LABORATORY ANALOGUE
A base metal replica of the implant body, or a pre-manufactured abutment

GOLD CYLINDER
Pre-manufactured to fit an abutment and form part of a prosthesis

HEALING CAPS
Temporary covers for abutments

the loads on the joint do not exceed the tension in the screwed joint (pre-tension) then it will remain closed; however, once the pre-tension force is exceeded the joint will open and the screw will be subject to unfavourable bending moments. When securing the joint it is important to produce the maximum pre-tension without causing permanent distortion of the screw. There will nevertheless subsequently be some loss of pre-tension. This can occur due to deformation of the screw and joined components, counter-rotation of the screw or plastic deformation of the surfaces of the screwed joint in a process known as embedment relaxation. Many manufacturers therefore recommend routine checking of screw tightness after a short period of service.

Advantages

Retrievability

A major advantage of the screwed joint is its retrievability, which greatly aids the checking of the various connecting components and abutments and the surrounding soft tissues, the replacement of failed components such as abutments and abutment screws, and the superstructure itself. This may also be conveniently remounted on a dental cast for analysis and modification in the laboratory, including replacement of any plastic components.

Control of gap

If constructed correctly a screw-retained implant superstructure can fit the implants closely and consistently around the dental arch. There is considerable evidence of the difficulty of achieving this, and it is generally accepted that a truly passive fit of the superstructure is rarely achieved in clinical practice. Nevertheless, the repeatability of location has advantages in terms of the ability to remove and replace the prosthesis for servicing. In addition occlusal adjustments made in the laboratory are less likely to be rendered inaccurate as can occur with a cementation process. There are also advantages in the minimization of soft-tissue irritation due to gaps adjacent to the gingival cuff, or as a result of cement accretions.

Predictable failure

Screwed joints can be designed to be the weakest part of a linkage and thus fail preferentially. This can protect other components from mechanical overload, such as screws, which are difficult to retrieve if fractured, the bone–implant interface and the superstructure.

Disadvantages

Mechanical failure

Where mechanical failure of a screw occurs it can be difficult, and sometimes impossible, to retrieve the broken component, for example where it is within an implant body. A cementation procedure, in contrast, can usually be repeated.

Access holes

A screw joint requires access, which can sometimes be difficult if the gape is restricted, or if the implant is unfavourably angled or positioned in the posterior molar region. In addition, the hole must be concentric with the long axis of the implant body or angled abutment, if used. The access hole may therefore penetrate the prosthesis at an aesthetically unfavourable site or compromise the occlusion.

Contamination

Screwed joints can provide a pathway for bacteria to colonize the interfaces between the components, and act as a potential source of infection or track into the deeper tissues. Some screwed joints incorporate a tapered design, which provides a seal between the components, while others may include a synthetic rubber O-ring to reduce the risk of oral bacteria infecting deeper tissues.

Angulation problems

Due to the axisymmetric design of most dental implants the orientation of the long axis of the fixture determines the angulation of the superstructure,

---

Box 2.3 What local factors should be considered when contemplating possible implant treatment?

ACCESS
Room to insert the implants?

PROSTHETIC SPACE
Room to place a restoration?

DYNAMIC SPACE TO RESTORE THE IMPLANT
Do occlusal interferences preclude superstructure placement?

SIZE OF SPACES
How many implants?

BONE VOLUME
Will it house a suitable implant?

BONE CONTOUR
Will the implant penetrate a concavity?

BONE ORIENTATION
Can the implant be oriented correctly?

PROGNOSIS OF REMAINING TEETH?
Restore the mouth in its entirety

STATUS OF EXISTING PROSTHESES
Could they be improved upon? With implants?

unless an angled abutment is used. However, in some patterns these are unsuited to single-tooth applications because of the risks of rotation.

Cemented joints

Advantages

Simplicity

The cemented joint is inherently simple and uses well-established restorative techniques. It can thus be readily used without additional training or the equipment necessary to ensure that the screws are correctly tightened.

Passivity

If the joint is correctly cemented then the technique can in theory minimize the effects of errors in the fit of the superstructure.

Angulation

The cemented joint requires no access hole and can therefore be used where the projection of the long axis of the implant body would penetrate the labial or buccal aspect of the restoration.

Disadvantages

Retrievability

Cemented joints are not readily retrieved. As a result, where they overlay a screwed joint that has loosened the restoration may have to be destroyed to remove the prosthesis. Similarly, it can be impossible to retrieve a larger prosthesis intact for the purpose of checking or servicing an individual implant.

Cement excess

It is very difficult to prevent the flow of excess cement into the space adjacent to a dental implant, which can then cause irritation and inflammation of the adjacent tissues. Attempts to remove excess cement have often been shown to be ineffective and can also damage the implant surface.

Dimensions

It is evident that accurate control of cement thickness is very difficult and as a result the occlusion of the finally placed prosthesis may not be correct.

SYSTEMIC AND LOCAL FACTORS AFFECTING IMPLANT TREATMENT

Implant treatment is but one of a range of procedures available to the restorative dentist to help the partially dentate or totally edentulous patient. Its use must be set within a comprehensive assessment of patients' needs and the most suitable method of helping them. Treatment with dental implants does not in itself negate the need for care in patient assessment, treatment planning and provision, and cannot overcome

---

Box 2.4 Screwed joints

ADVANTAGES?
- Retrievability. Easy to remove
- Control of gap. This can be precise
- Predictable failure. Can be designed as a weak point in the system

DISADVANTAGES?
- Mechanical failure. Can be problematical
- Access holes. Necessary for screw placement
- Contamination. Can permit ingress of material and microorganisms from the mouth
- Angulation problems. May be very difficult to manage where long axis of crown diverges markedly from that of the implant body

---

neglect of basic principles or the use of inferior techniques. It is subject to the normal constraints on restorative and minor surgical procedures imposed by systemic conditions. In addition, there is a range of conditions that are associated with or thought to be associated with increased risk of implant failure.

Systemic factors having known links with implant failure

- Tobacco smoking. This has been shown to increase the risk of implant failure.

Systemic factors having possible association with implant failure:

- Active chemotherapy.
- Disphosphonate therapy.
- Ectodermal dysplasia.
- Erosive lichen planus.
- Type 2 (late-onset) diabetes: This is especially the case where this is not well controlled.
- Treatment by an operator with limited surgical experience.

Local factors having strong associations with implant failure

- The placement of implants in severely resorbed maxillae.
- A history of irradiation of the implant site.
- The use of implants of a press-fit cylindrical design.

Matters less strongly associated with a risk of implant failure

- The placement of implants in infected extraction sites.

- The use of small numbers of implants in the posterior maxillae.
- The use of short as opposed to long implants.

Is tooth replacement necessary?

The loss or absence of a tooth should always prompt some consideration as to the appropriateness of replacing it. There are many situations where it is not necessary to replace every missing tooth in the dental arch. A decision to do so will be based on the impact of the missing tooth or teeth on the patient's lifestyle, as determined by the patient, and a professional assessment as to the potential harm that may arise from failure to replace the unit. Patients tend to complain most about teeth missing from the front of the mouth, which has a negative impact on their appearance and speech, and where sufficient posterior teeth have been lost to make mastication difficult. A professional decision to replace missing teeth may also be dependent upon the potential for drifting and overeruption of the remaining teeth, although this does not inevitably follow tooth loss.

Of considerable importance also are the techniques that are potentially available to replace the missing tooth, and in many cases the tissues that previously supported it. All will have implications for the patient in terms of morbidity and cost, which may make the replacement ill matched to the patient's best interests.

Does tooth replacement need to be with an implant?

Where it has been decided to replace missing teeth, the use of an implant-stabilized prosthesis is merely one of a range of techniques that may be potentially available to the dentist. All will carry various benefits and disadvantages, and an evidence-based decision should be taken where possible as the most appropriate technique in a particular situation. In some cases implant treatment will be feasible and appropriate; however, there are many situations where this is not the case and a patient is best served by other forms of treatment. Table 2.1 shows a comparison of the relative advantages and disadvantages of some of the various techniques for tooth replacement in the partially dentate and edentulous patient.

Prognosis of the other remaining teeth

It is widely considered that dental implants have the potential to provide stability for prostheses for the remainder of a patient's life, although inevitably some will fail. This situation does not always pertain for the natural teeth, and consequently the partially dentate patient with few teeth missing who is treated with implants may in due course become edentulous or almost edentulous, while retaining implants that are ill suited to the new circumstances. It is therefore important to take a long-term view when planning implant treatment. Optimum results are often obtained by planning initially for the loss of teeth with a doubtful prognosis.

Is there room to insert dental implants?

The use of dental implants requires that there be adequate space in the jawbone to insert the device. Implants are typically 10–20 mm long and 3.5–4.0 mm wide, and must be placed with a margin of at least 1 mm of bone all round, thus defining the surgical space envelope. While shorter implants are available, their reported failure rates tend to be higher than those of longer devices, particularly in more unfavourable situations, for example where the bone is of poor quality. The space envelope is defined not only by the outline of the bone, but also by internal structures that must be avoided when preparing the implant site. These include tooth roots, the air sinuses and nose, and neurovascular bundles such as the mandibular canal.

Access

Successful placement and restoration of dental implants require there to be space, especially occlusally, to insert the necessary instrumentation and to manipulate the various components required for implant placement and restoration. This will vary with the technique and system used. Nevertheless there is a minimum requirement based on the length of the implant body, and the height of the instruments used for its insertion. Similarly the restorative phase of treatment has its own restrictions based on access and the dimensions of the necessary instrumentation and pre-manufactured components. Posteriorly it may not always be possible to place and restore an implant body, especially if there are overerupted opposing teeth.

Is there room to restore the implants?

The principal purpose in placing a dental implant is to provide a patient with a stable prosthesis, and it is on the quality of this outcome that the success of the treatment will largely be judged. Just as the implant must lie within a defined envelope, so must the superstructure. Vertically this is determined by the level of the occlusal plane (Fig. 2.13), mesially and distally by the positions of the adjacent teeth, whether they be natural or artificial, and labiopalatally by the adjacent dental arch and denture or prosthesis space. This is determined by soft-tissue anatomy and function, occlusal relationships and aesthetic considerations.

Oral hygiene

It had been widely accepted that implant treatment should only be carried out in patients with good oral

Table 2.1 This table summarizes the comparisons between various restorative treatment modalities for the edentulous and partially dentate patient. It should initially be read in conjunction with the text, as there can be large differences in the variables described, depending upon clinical circumstances

	Complete denture	RPD	Adhesive bridge	Conventional bridge	Implant-fixed prosthesis	Implant overdenture
Dentist's skill level	Competent/ advanced	Competent/ advanced	Competent/ advanced	Competent/ advanced	Advanced	Advanced
Technical support	Competent/ advanced	Competent/ advanced	Competent/ advanced	Advanced	Advanced	Advanced
Maintenance	High	High	Low	Low	Low	High
Duration of treatment	Moderate	Moderate	Short	Short/moderate	Long	Long
May preserve bone	No	No	No	No	Yes	Yes
Replaces soft tissues	Yes	Yes	No	No	No	Yes
Mucosal support	Yes	Partial	No	No	No	Yes, minimal
Tooth preparation	No	Yes, minimal	Yes, minimal	Yes	No	No
Subjective prosthesis security	Least	Usually acceptable	Very high	Very high	Very high	High
Aesthetic potential	Good	Good (retainers?)	Good	Good	Good (orientation?)	Good
Bulk	Considerable	Moderate/ considerable	Minimal	Minimal	Minimal	Considerable
Initial cost	Moderate	Low/moderate/ high	Moderate/ high	Moderate/high/ very high	High/ very high	High/ very high
Recurrent cost	Moderate	Moderate	Low	Low	Low	Moderate/high
Functional life	Moderate	Moderate	Good	Very good	Prosthesis very good. Implants extremely good	Prosthesis moderate. Implants extremely good
Modification of prosthesis	Straightforward	Straightforward/ impossible	Very difficult/ impossible	Very difficult/ impossible	Bridge difficult. Implants impossible	Denture straightforward. Implants impossible

Box 2.5 Cemented joints

ADVANTAGES?

- Simplicity. A familiar and relatively simple technology
- Passivity. A passive fit is theoretically possible
- Angulation. Less of a problem than with screws, no access hole

DISADVANTAGES?

- Retrievability. Difficult or impossible to remove without damaging superstructure
- Cement excess. Difficult to avoid, detect and remove

hygiene, since it was at one time thought that plaque accumulation led inevitably to loss of OI. The evidence for this is currently not compelling; however, it is strongly recommended that good oral hygiene be established prior to implant treatment.

WHAT MAY IMPLANTS BE USED FOR?

Treatment with dental implants is but one of a range of procedures that may be employed to help the partially dentate or edentulous individual. All potentially available procedures have both advantages and disadvantages, and it should not be assumed that implant therapy is inherently superior in all situations. The current endosseous designs were originally used principally to help the edentulous patient and it was only later that they began to be more widely employed for the partially dentate.

The edentulous patient

While many edentulous patients are satisfied with the performance of conventional complete dentures, there is a significant number for whom that is not the case. Problems reflect patients' expectations, their oral manipulative skills, quality of denture design and fabrication, and oral status. Thus a level of performance acceptable to one patient may not be so to another. Where a patient is dissatisfied with denture performance and the dentist considers that improvements can be produced by constructing new prostheses, or management of predisposing oral problems such as excessively displaceable tissue, then that treatment should be carried out prior to implant therapy. There is rarely justification for attempting to manage a prosthetic problem solely with implant treatment where other, often simpler procedures may produce a worthwhile improvement. Where it is believed that as good a result as feasible has been achieved by conventional prosthetic treatment, then consideration should be given to implant therapy.

It should be noted that while implant-stabilized prostheses can provide security, and may have reduced bulk, palatal coverage and minimal loading of the oral mucosa compared with conventional dentures, their appearance is in no way inherently superior.

In the edentulous patient implants can be used to stabilize both removable and fixed prostheses. In general these my be used in either or both jaws; however, treatment with dental implants in the upper jaw is often more complex and less certain of outcome due to mechanical problems, restrictions on implant placement and jaw resorption, which can make prosthesis design difficult.

Removable prostheses are essentially similar to conventional overdentures, except that they are linked to the underlying implants. Normally two or more implants are used, although in general fewer are required than for a fixed prosthesis. They are linked to individual implants with mechanical retainers, usually of a ball- and -socket design, or clipped on to a gold alloy bar that links the implants (Figs 2.9–2.13). Construction is similar to that for an overdenture. Chapter 6 compares the relative advantages and disadvantages of the two techniques.

Fixed prostheses are essentially a denture arch form, with as much supporting material as is necessary for a pleasing appearance and obturation of dead space within the limitations of maintaining good oral hygiene around the implant abutments (Fig. 2.14). Table 2.1 indicates the relative advantages and disadvantages of fixed and removable prostheses in the edentulous patient.

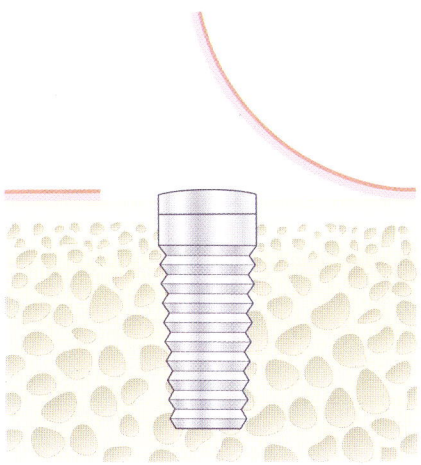

Fig. 2.9 Stage-one surgery for implant treatment. A mucoperiosteal flap has been raised, the surgical site prepared, an implant body inserted and a cover screw placed. The mucoperiosteal flap is about to be repositioned and secured.

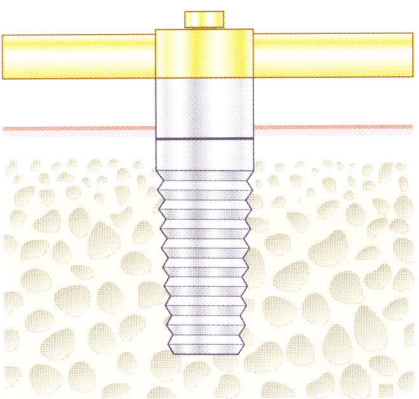

Fig. 2.10 Treatment with an implant-stabilized overdenture. Following stage two surgery and the placement of a transmucosal abutment, a gold bar soldered to the gold cylinder has been placed and secured with a gold screw. The bar acts as a retention device in conjunction with clips placed inside a recess in the overdenture.

The partially dentate patient

The partially dentate patient can present a wide range of clinical problems depending on systemic factors, the pattern of tooth loss and status of the remaining teeth. Treatment options include observation, where it is felt that no active therapy is required, orthodontic management, especially in the young, and treatment with conventional and adhesive fixed bridges and removable partial dentures. All have their roles; however, dental implant therapy can reduce the rate of alveolar bone resorption, provide a stable prosthesis

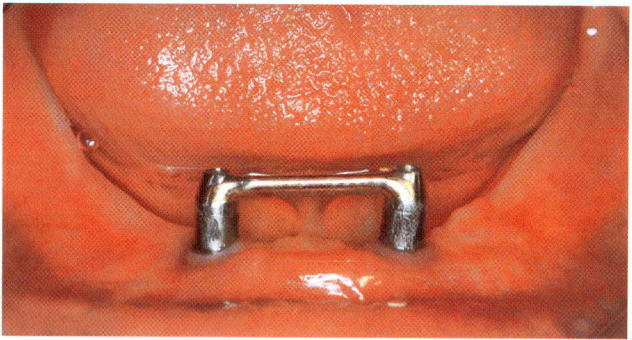

Fig. 2.11 A simple stabilizing system for a complete mandibular denture, utilizing a retention bar soldered to two gold cylinders secured on two implant abutments. This design is relatively straightforward to construct, but has little resistance to rotation of the prosthesis around the bar. This problem can be reduced with an increased number of appropriately sited implants or in some cases short distantly cantilevered bars.

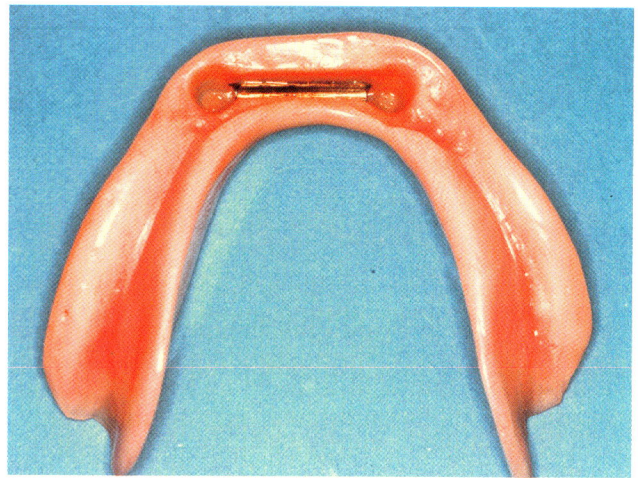

Fig. 2.12 The complete mandibular overdenture which has been used to treat the patient shown in Figure 2.11. The retention clip can be seen in a recess in the incisal region of the prosthesis.

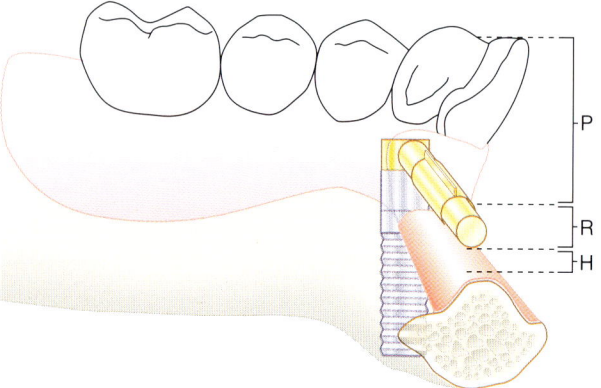

Fig. 2.13 A diagram depicting an implant-stabilized complete mandibular denture retained by a clip and bar system. It is important to ensure that there is adequate vertical space for the prosthesis (P), the retention system (R) as well as the necessary room below the bar for oral hygiene purposes (H).

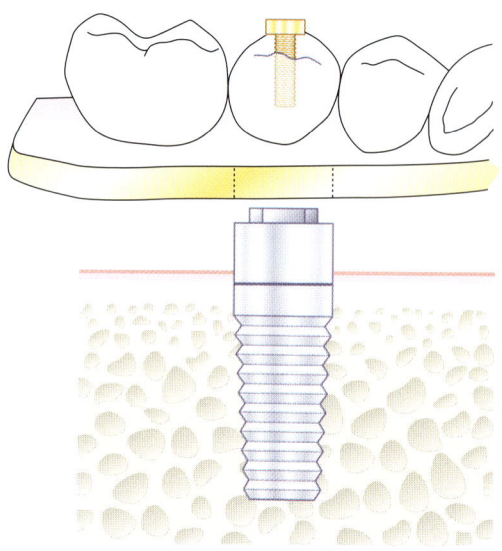

Fig. 2.14 A diagram of a fixed implant superstructure with a cast gold framework incorporating gold cylinders. This is secured to standard implant abutments using gold screws.

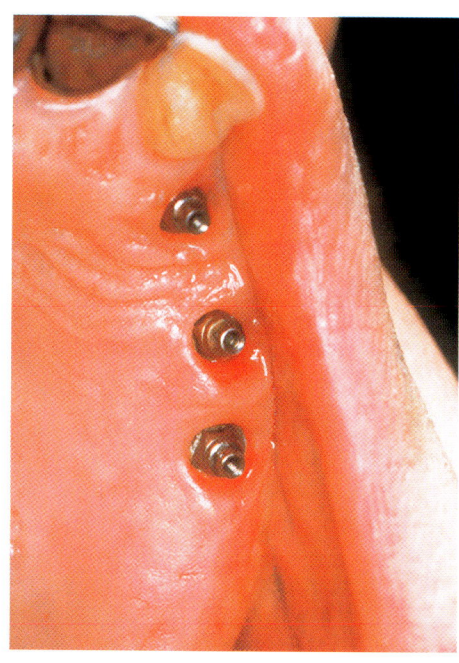

Fig. 2.15 This free-end edentulous area has been treated using an implant-stabilized prosthesis secured on three endosseous implants. Tapered abutments have been used to permit a more natural-appearing emergence profile, and to manage the reduced vertical space that is available between the top of the implant body and the opposing occlusal surfaces.

and avoid the need for tooth preparation. It is particularly valuable in some situations where a single missing tooth is to be replaced and in the management of the distal extension prosthesis (Figs 2.15 and 2.16). It rarely provides a denture that has a significantly superior appearance, and indeed the conflicting requirements of implant placement and prosthesis design can sometimes compromise appearance. In the majority of cases treatment with a fixed prosthesis is used; however, where a larger prosthesis is needed or

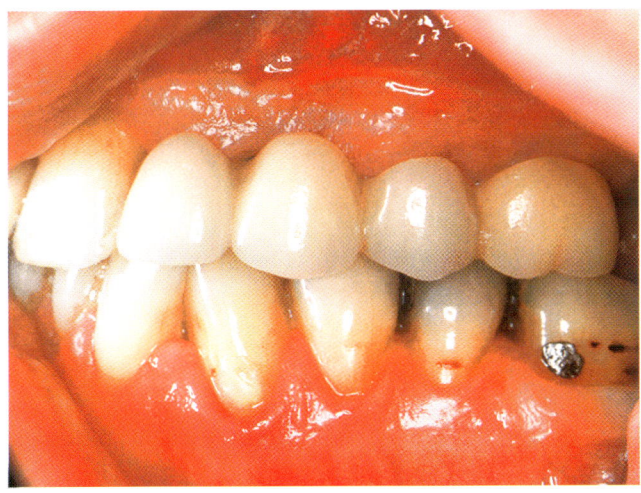

Fig. 2.16 The completed bridge in position.

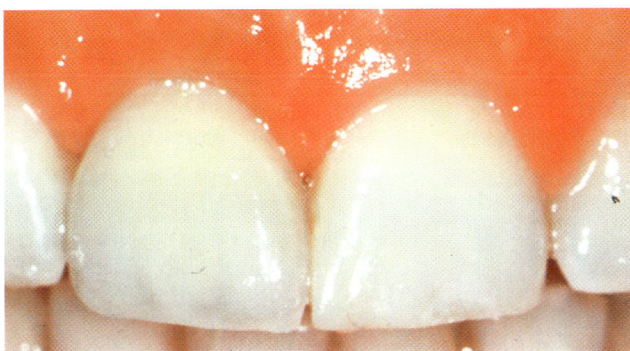

Fig. 2.17 A single-tooth implant replacing 11.

implant numbers are restricted by resources or lack of available sites, a removable prosthesis may be employed.

BASIC TREATMENT SEQUENCE

The treatment sequence for using implant-stabilized prostheses is outlined here and expanded in Chapters 6–8.

History

As with any clinical situation it is essential to commence by obtaining a history from the patient and confirming their complaints and perceptions with regard to treatment procedures and outcomes. This will help in reaching a diagnosis and formulating a treatment plan that will best meet their needs. It is common for patients to request implant treatment with little or no knowledge of the procedures and potential advantages and disadvantages, often on the basis of articles in the popular press or a belief that modern and complex procedures are inherently beneficial and infallible. The first contact with the patient is an important opportunity to educate them concerning these matters.

The history should include a dental history, which will partly reflect the patient's levels of dental disease, commitment to its management and, where relevant, history of denture use. All these will influence subsequent treatment planning.

Medical history

This should include not only all those factors normally considered in any dental consultation, but also any of particular relevance to potential implant therapy. These principally relate to:

- Factors affecting the ability to cooperate;
- Unrealistic treatment aspirations;
- Factors prejudicing OI;
- Factors that contraindicate surgical procedures.

Examination

Extra-oral examination

This should take note of any facial asymmetries, restricted mouth opening, soft tissue abnormalities and the prominence of the teeth and alveolar mucosa when the patient smiles and talks.

Intra-oral examination

This must include all the factors normally covered in an examination of the partially dentate or edentulous patient. It must, however, also include those of particular relevance to implant treatment and, in particular, the following.

Access

It should be confirmed that there would be space to access potential implant sites and insert the implants.

Prosthetic space

There should be space to place a restoration, be it a single crown, fixed bridge or removable overdenture.

Size of spaces

The size of the edentulous spaces must be assessed from the viewpoint of implant placement.

Bone volume

Implants have certain minimum requirements with regard to placement and optimum requirements if the best outcome is to be achieved. It is therefore helpful to manually ascertain the dimensions of the bony contours of the potential implant sites, wherever possible. While this is not always feasible, and rarely accurate, it can indicate sites where there is clearly inadequate bone, or where further investigations are needed to confirm the appropriateness of implant placement. These usually involve radiography and possibly diagnostic casts and trial appliances.

Bone contour

The contours of the alveolar ridges, especially labially in the maxillae, are very important for they determine the emergence profile of the implant and can have a profound effect on its appearance.

Bone orientation

The bone of the jaws frequently has major and minor axes in the plane of implant insertion, which will determine the orientation of the implant body. If unfavourable, this may commit the surgeon to placing an implant where its angulation would make restoration difficult or impossible.

Dynamic and static space to restore the implant

It is important to confirm that the implant superstructure can be placed in the available space; where this is uncertain mounted diagnostic casts may be required, particularly to assess the effects of jaw movement on the superstructure space envelope.

Prognosis of remaining teeth

The prognosis of the remaining teeth will be of great importance, since dental implants have a high success rate and may potentially remain for the rest of the patient's life. Implant placement to manage one partially dentate scenario may be unsuited to another when more teeth are lost.

Status of existing prostheses

The status of these may help to indicate the likelihood of their performance being improved with new dentures, the significance of the patient's complaints and the probability of implant-based treatment being successful.

Special investigations

These typically include a range of radiographic techniques, study casts and diagnostic trial appliances.

Treatment alternatives

All treatment alternatives should be considered and a rational decision made as to the appropriateness of implant-based therapy. The absence or loss of a tooth does not indicate the absolute need for its replacement.

TREATMENT SEQUENCE

If it has been decided that implant treatment is to be preferred then a typical sequence of events would be as follows.

Patient information

The patient should be fully informed about the proposed treatment, including the treatment alternatives, their advantages and disadvantages, the probability of implant treatment failing and the alternatives if this occurs. Such essential information is the basis of informed consent. There are a number of aids to assist this process, such as published material, videos and CD-ROMs; however, the dentist remains responsible for the process.

Superstructure selection

At this stage the type of prosthesis to be potentially used should be identified since it is this which provides the desired outcome.

Implant placement sites

This stage involves deciding on the most suitable implant sites bearing in mind the following.

Bone volume

This has already been considered above.

Bone quality

Bone quality is widely recognized as a key factor in implant treatment, but has proved difficult to describe objectively. It is a combination of volume, radiographic density and structure. Two widely quoted scoring systems are those of Lekholm and Zarb and of Howell and Cawood.

Surgical factors

These have been outlined above.

Prosthetic considerations

These relate to the feasibility of placing a prosthesis, emergence profiles, ridge contour, the need to locate implant bodies in similar positions to the overlying crowns and possible requirements for prosthetic ridge recontouring by using a flange. Factors influencing the feasibility of placing a prosthesis and the appearance that it will produce include ridge contour, implant body location both mesiodistally and buccolingually, implant body orientation and the possible need for artificial gumwork.

Biomechanical considerations

Since mechanical overload is a key factor in implant failure, placement needs to take account of the resultant occlusal loads. Cantilevers, either lateral or distal, can result in forces in excess of those applied to the superstructure. The use of one or two implants presents a potential axis for rotation, the possible harmful effects of which are significantly reduced by using three widely distributed implants, in an effect referred to colloquially as tripoidization.

Resources

Implant treatment often requires a significant range of equipment, materials and components as well as considerable skill. It is therefore essential to ensure that adequate resources, both material and human, are available before embarking on treatment. Consideration must also be given to likely maintenance costs.

Implant placement

This may be carried out under local anaesthesia, with or without sedation, or under general anaesthesia. Antibiotic cover is widely recommended as it improves success rates. It is common to make use of a surgeon's guide to facilitate correct implant placement, and this is discussed in Chapter 5.

The bone is exposed surgically and a series of concentric holes drilled to accommodate the implant body. Details vary with the system; however, it is important in all cases to minimize thermal trauma to the bone. This is aided by the use of sharp instruments (often single use), slow drilling speeds and the external application of a coolant. Where the bone is hard it is commonly tapped to accept a threaded implant. Where less dense, a self-tapping design may be used.

Once the implants have been placed they are covered with a mucoperiosteal flap, unless a single-stage technique embodying immediate loading is being employed. Currently this is less common. To prevent ingress of bone into the internal connecting recess in the implant a cover screw is placed.

Where a two-stage implant procedure is employed it is important for the implant not to be externally loaded during the healing period, and patients are usually advised not to use their dentures for 2 weeks. After this they are adjusted to relieve the soft tissues, and often modified with a tissue conditioner.

Typically the implants remain buried for 3 months in the lower jaw and 6 months in the upper, after which they are exposed and connecting components placed. These may either be definitive or, more commonly, healing abutments. This marks the start of the prosthetic phase of treatment.

Prosthetic phase of treatment

This involves the fabrication of the prosthetic superstructure and its long-term maintenance. Treatment procedures vary in their details and complexity, and may involve more stages than indicated here; however, they involve the same basic sequence.

Primary impressions

Primary impressions are recorded to enable study casts to be produced. They usually indicate the positions of the implants by recording the location of the healing abutments; however, impression copings designed to fit directly on the implant bodies may be employed, and will provide more accurate information. The impressions are recorded in stock trays either using an elastomeric wash in a compound or elastomeric putty impression. An irreversible hydrocolloid (alginate) is often also used at this stage. Where there

are enough occluding pairs of teeth in a suitable and stable occlusal relationship, a jaw registration may be made.

Abutment selection

This may be done at the primary impression stage or alternatively following the recording of the working or secondary impressions. Abutments may either be manufactured or custom modified, depending on clinical circumstances.

Secondary impressions

These can be used either to record the positions of the abutments or the tops of the implant bodies, and the related dental arch and adjacent soft tissues. In both cases impression copings designed specifically for this purpose would be used. In the latter situation these are often referred to as fixture head impressions. Where this is done the cast is poured using a laboratory elastomer to represent the soft tissues adjacent to the implants and dental stone for the remainder. This cast can then be used to aid in abutment selection, following which a further working cast would normally be produced.

Registration

Where there are inadequate numbers of occluding pairs of teeth, or the patient is edentulous, a jaw registration using standard techniques will be required.

Trial prosthesis

This is frequently used to confirm the positions of the teeth on the prosthesis and the contours of any associated gumwork or flanges.

Trial casting

Once the tooth positions have been finalized, the metal framework on which the superstructure will be built is then fabricated and checked in the mouth. Usually this is made using a gold alloy casting; however, there are other techniques available using laser welding of titanium or spark erosion. These are capital intensive and thus only normally available via centralized facilities.

Trial with teeth

The casting would be finally confirmed with the teeth temporarily located.

Insertion

The superstructure is then finally checked and secured in place.

Inspection

A series of inspections will be carried out for the remainder of the working life of the prosthesis at increasing intervals. These will include routine radiographic assessment of adjacent bone levels.

Temporary bridges

It is possible and sometimes advantageous to make temporary polymeric bridges to assess potential treatment outcomes, and to facilitate construction of the final prosthesis, with particular regard to occlusal features and tooth positions and contours.

FURTHER READING

Albrektsson TO, Johansson CB, Sennerby L 1994. Biological aspects of implant dentistry: osseointegration. Periodontal 2000; 4: 58–73

Binon PP 2000. Implants and components: entering the new millennium. Int J Oral Maxillofac Implants 15(1): 76–94.

General treatment decisions

INTRODUCTION

Treatment alternatives to dental implants for the partially dentate case

It is important that treatment with dental implants is viewed in the context of overall patient care, and as one of a range of procedures that may be used to help the patient. Complex therapy is not inherently superior and simpler procedures may, in many situations, be more appropriate. When planning care it is important to understand the patient's perceived needs, which may differ markedly from those thought to be of importance by the dentist. Problems must be explained, options discussed and an agreed plan prepared. These options will often include a wide range of alternative approaches to the management of tooth loss, which must be considered if the patient's best interests are to be served.

NO REPLACEMENT

It should not be assumed that the absence of teeth is an absolute indication for their replacement, which should confer clear benefits (Fig. 3.1). The replacement of anterior teeth is almost always sought by the patient for aesthetic reasons (Figs 3.2, 3.3); however, missing posterior teeth may have much less impact. Where these are towards the front of the mouth then they can

influence appearance, although the replacement of more posterior teeth is usually only sought to improve masticatory efficiency. This can apply to a single molar for some patients, but tends only to affect chewing efficiency in the majority when several occluding pairs of teeth are absent.

There is little robust evidence that replacement of posterior teeth will prevent or resolve temporo-mandibular joint (TMJ) dysfunction, but it can sometimes prevent tipping or over-eruption of teeth.

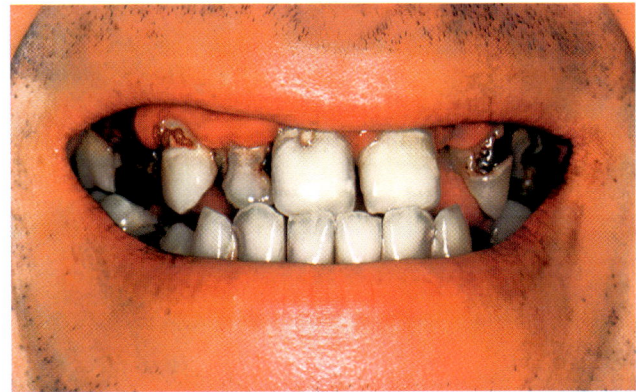

Fig. 3.2 This patient requested implant treatment to replace 22. It is evident that he has a range of oral problems requiring attention, in addition to a missing anterior tooth, and it would be important to consider all these, as well as his approach to advanced oral care, when preparing a treatment plan.

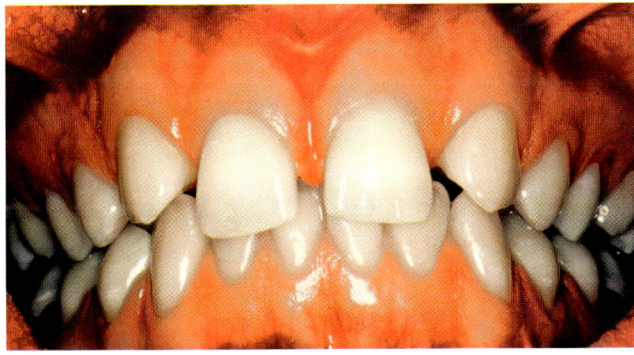

Fig. 3.1 Replacement of the congenitally absent maxillary lateral incisors would probably require orthodontic realignment of the teeth to create adequate spaces in the 12 and 22 regions. If the patient considered the appearance to be satisfactory then active treatment of the condition may be inappropriate.

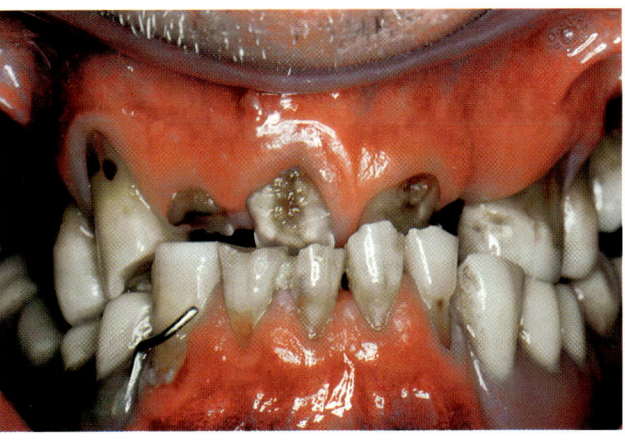

Fig. 3.3 The restoration of this patient's mouth is complicated by collapse of the occlusion, tooth surface loss, caries and over-eruption of posterior teeth.

Systemic factors

Residual life expectancy

A patient who has a very poor residual life expectancy may have little wish to receive extensive dental treatment, and prefer to have problems managed as they arise. In these situations implant procedures would be inappropriate. Nevertheless there are some situations in such cases where implant treatment is justified by the dramatic improvements it can bring in the patient's quality of life.

Patients' wishes

While a complete dentition is increasingly seen as very important by many individuals and societies, there are some for whom this is a low priority – a wish that should be respected provided that it is based on an informed decision.

Patients' availability

Where a patient is unable to attend for care for reasons of ill health or family or work commitments then little treatment may be feasible.

Ability to cooperate

Some patients suffer from systemic problems that severely limit their ability to cooperate with treatment, such as severe spasticity or reduced manual dexterity (Fig. 3.4). In these circumstances the patient is often best helped by placing the majority of effort on improving oral health to maintain the remaining dentition.

Local factors

These relate to oral status and the requirement to prepare a long-term plan for oral health commensurate with the patient's needs and wishes. This will involve an assessment of their oral status, the function of the dentition and the expected benefits of any possible treatment. Maintenance of oral health should take precedence over slavish restoration of the dentition. It is all too easy for both the patient and dentist to focus on the management of a small number of missing teeth, to the long-term detriment of oral health (Fig. 3.5).

Where it has been decided that spaces in the arch are to be restored then there are a number of options.

ORTHODONTIC MANAGEMENT

This is not often available as an option owing to technical problems or lack of suitable teeth to move into a defect. However, in appropriate circumstances it can be a valuable method of eliminating a space in the arch. It also has a role in facilitating implant treatment by realigning teeth adjacent to potential implant sites, so as to make the space a more suitable size for placing the implant(s) supporting a suitable crown(s). This is relevant not only for the edentulous span but also for the alignment of the roots of adjacent teeth.

Systemic factors

It is important to be sure of patients' ability to cooperate, and their willingness to undergo lengthy treatment, often with fixed appliances. Adults are less inclined to accept this for social reasons and added costs may also inhibit them from making this choice.

Local factors

Local factors to be taken into consideration include:

- **Technical feasibility.** There are the usual limitations on orthodontic treatment, including the skeletal pattern, musculature, bone volume and potential locations of anchorage.

- **Oral hygiene.** Orthodontic treatment is contraindicated in patients with poor oral hygiene and poor dental health.

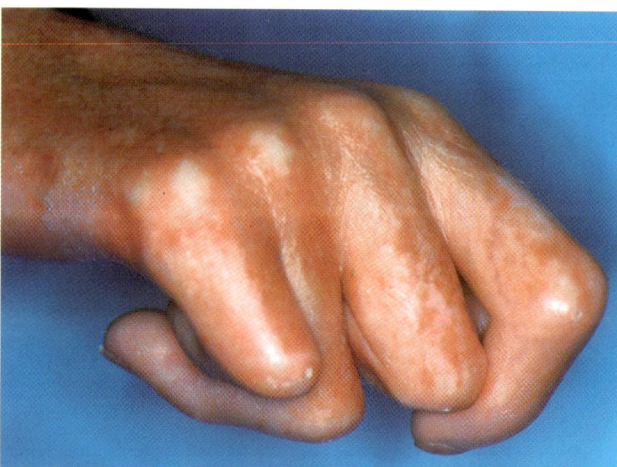

Fig. 3.4 Patients with very limited manual dexterity may be unable to maintain adequate levels of oral hygiene, or handle implant-stabilized removable appliances, making them less suited to implant treatment.

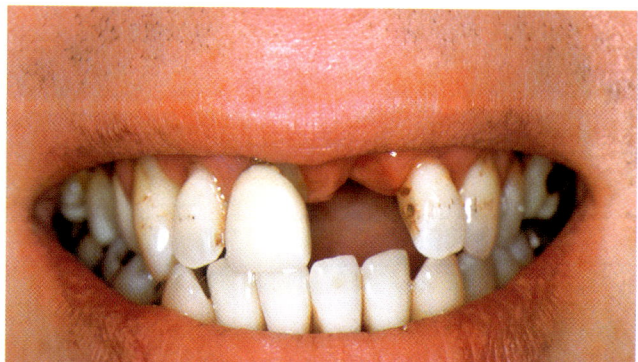

Fig. 3.5 This patient wanted to replace a loose partial denture restoring the 21 space with a single tooth implant. Local management problems include untreated carries, uncontrolled periodontal disease, an edentulous span wider than 11, alveolar resorption in the edentulous region and a high lip line when smiling.

- **Stable outcome.** Where orthodontic treatment results in teeth being placed in unstable positions then they will require stabilization to prevent relapse. This should be avoided where possible, as long-term stabilization can be difficult to achieve.

Advantages

The advantages of orthodontic treatment are as follows:

- No tooth preparation is normally required.
- The procedure does not normally involve surgical procedures.
- The resultant outcome has a projected lifespan similar to that of the remaining dentition, and has a natural appearance.
- The treatment, once completed, requires no further maintenance.

Disadvantages

The disadvantages of orthodontic treatment are as follows:

- The procedure is technically complex and requires special training.
- Orthodontic treatment can be labour intensive and hence expensive.
- The technique is not always applicable, particularly where there are significant numbers of teeth absent.
- If injudiciously used, then orthodontic treatment can occasionally result in tooth loss due to root resorption.
- The procedure can last over a long period and the commitment of the patient is therefore very important.

REMOVABLE PARTIAL DENTURES

Treatment with removable partial dentures (RPDs) is an extremely versatile procedure, which is widely used in the management of partial tooth loss, both as an interim measure and as the definitive treatment. Correctly utilized and supported by thorough oral hygiene and maintenance, it has minimal harmful effects on the oral cavity.

Systemic factors

Ability to cooperate

There are a small number of patients whose ability to cooperate with oral care is so limited that they cannot benefit from RPD treatment. Those patients who suffer from poorly controlled epilepsy and are liable to major fits may be at risk of inhaling or ingesting a denture or its fragments if it is broken or displaced during an episode. This problem can be minimized with a suitably designed RPD having a metal framework. It is not necessarily avoided by using fixed appliances, which can be more severely damaged in a fit.

Patients' wishes

While RPDs can effectively restore almost all partially dentate situations, they are by definition removable, which some patients consider to be totally unacceptable in principle. Particular objection is often made to the display of clasps. Where clinical circumstances and resources permit then such individuals may be better helped with alternative procedures using implant- or tooth-supported prostheses.

Resources

Treatment with RPDs can be very versatile and acceptable prostheses can be made in less challenging situations without specialist clinical skills, given sound technical resources. Metal-based appliances are usually to be preferred in terms of comfort, security, strength, longevity, tissue health and the ability to use more complex designs. These can include sectional dentures, precision attachments and overlays. The correct design and construction of these require specialist clinical skills and expert technical support, and are inevitably more expensive.

Local factors

There are few situations where an RPD cannot be used, provided that access to the mouth can be obtained to obtain the required clinical records. Partial dentures are sometimes used on a temporary basis where the long-term prognosis of the remaining teeth is poor. When made of acrylic resin they can provide valuable interim treatment, which is readily modified as dictated by changes in the mouth.

Advantages

The principal advantages of RPD therapy are:

- **Versatility.** There are few situations where an RPD cannot be used to provide tooth replacement, sometimes on an interim basis.
- **Speed.** An RPD can be made very quickly and thus is often suitable for the emergency management of tooth loss.
- **Diagnostic potential.** A simple RPD may be used to assess a patient's response to treatment without a major commitment of resources or irreversible oral modifications. Where the response is positive then more complex procedures may be planned, or similarly avoided where that is not the case. Partial dentures can also be used to assess the effects of changes in tooth positions, ridge contour and occlusal vertical dimension.
- **Wide applicability.** As has been indicated above, RPDs can encompass a wide range of complexities, and in their more straightforward designs can be suitable for use where specialist skills and more complex techniques are not available.

- **Flexibility of use.** Appropriately designed RPDs can be easily modified to allow for bone resorption and further tooth loss, which makes them highly suited to interim phases of treatment, or where the prognosis of the remaining teeth is uncertain.

Disadvantages

- **Potential increase in oral disease.** The use of RPDs has been demonstrated to be associated with increased oral plaque levels, caries, and periodontal and mucosal disease. Higher caries levels in abutment teeth, periodontal inflammation and breakdown, increased periodontal pocket depths and denture-related stomatitis have all been reported. These effects can be minimized by appropriate design and construction, avoidance of continuous wearing of the prosthesis, the maintenance of high standards of oral hygiene, and regular professional inspection and maintenance as necessary. There is sound long-term evidence that where these conditions are met, then RPDs can be used for many years with little resultant increase in oral disease levels.

- **Lack of security.** RPDs are by definition patient removable, and as a result may move in function, giving rise to problems. Where large numbers of teeth have been lost or there are extensive unbounded saddles, then it may not be possible to provide a high degree of stability under occlusal loads, or resistance to displacement when chewing adhesive food. The extent to which this will cause the patient problems is dependent on the degree of movement, their ability to control the prosthesis, and their subjective assessment of the degree of movement. Displacement, which can be profoundly disconcerting to one patient, may be of little concern to another.

- **Perceived quality.** Lack of security can also cause problems where patients equate a patient-removable prosthesis with inferior treatment, and consider a restoration which is permanently secured to abutment teeth or dental implants to be inherently superior. While there are situations where the use of such a prosthesis is the treatment of choice, this is not always the case.

- **Bulk.** A removable partial denture consists both of components that replace the missing teeth and their supporting structures, and components designed to maximize its stability. These inevitably increase the bulk of the prosthesis, although the extent to which they do so will be dependent on the material of construction and the particular design. Quite apart from the potential for increased levels of caries, periodontal and mucosal disease the greater bulk of the appliance can give rise to functional difficulties, particularly with regard to speech and mastication, as well as being poorly tolerated by some patients.

ADHESIVE BRIDGES

The development of adhesive techniques has made it possible to restore many edentulous spaces with resin-bonded bridges (RBBs), which can provide a very satisfactory replacement with minimal tooth preparation. This has the advantage of relative technical simplicity, and is less likely to place the abutment tooth at risk, particularly in the longer term. The procedure is not without its risks, particularly where the adhesive bond fails at one end of a fixed-fixed bridge, and the resultant failure is not corrected. It also has technical limitations with regard to its applications, particularly where the abutment teeth have short clinical crowns, there are occlusal difficulties, or the abutment teeth are unfavourably angulated. In addition the technique is not suited to replacing single teeth where it is desirable to have interdental spacing in the region of the pontic.

Despite these problems adhesive bridges are increasingly used to restore shorter edentulous spans, where they have proved to be clinically effective.

Systemic factors

There are few systemic contraindications to treatment with adhesive bridges and these largely relate to the patient's ability to cooperate. Where patients are subject to epilepsy, then in some cases treatment with such restorations is contraindicated as they may be dislodged. Treatment with adhesive bridges is a relatively straightforward procedure; however, it does require the availability of suitable technical facilities to produce the prosthesis.

Local factors

Treatment with adhesive bridges is much more likely to be influenced by local than systemic factors.

Feasibility

Technical limitations on treatment with RBBs relate to both access and the nature of the edentulous span and the abutment teeth. Where the edentulous span is very long or requires the use of a multi-unit cantilever, excessive loads may be placed on the adhesive bond to the abutment tooth or teeth, which are more likely to fail. Similar difficulties can arise where the edentulous span requires a bridge that is curved in the horizontal plane to follow the contours of the arch, as can occur when replacing teeth in the canine region. As a result the bridge will tend to rotate around the abutments, and the resultant torque can cause failure of the cement bond. A further problem relating to the length of the edentulous span occurs where it is necessary to place spaces on one or both sides of the pontic for aesthetic reasons. In these circumstances restoration with an adhesive bridge can be difficult or impossible since the connector linking the pontic to the abutment tooth or teeth cannot be disguised. This problem can sometimes be overcome by orthodontic realignment of the abutments, or modification of the adjacent teeth with a composite restoration so as to make the edentulous span slightly narrower.

Mechanical problems also arise where, as a result of the occlusion, heavy loads are placed on the pontic due to the close approximation of the natural teeth, either in ICP or in excursions of the mandible.

Difficulties can also arise if the edentulous ridge is markedly resorbed, since this will place restrictions on the alignment of the pontic. While the incisal edge or occlusal surface will have its position determined by the arrangement of the opposing dentition, the neck of the tooth is required to lie against the edentulous ridge, which can give rise to an unfortunate appearance. Suitable contouring can mask this, particularly if the patient has a low lip line when smiling so that the appearance of the pontic is not very evident. In other situations the problem may need to be corrected by transplanting bone or inserting a synthetic material. If bone grafting is contemplated, then there may well be a sound case for placing an implant, since long-term stability of the ridge contour following this procedure rarely occurs.

Further problems are associated with the abutment teeth, since these have to have adequate size to provide an appropriate area of enamel to provide a suitably strong bond. This relates not only to the area but also to the shape of the surface. Where this is severely tapered then in general the bond is more likely to fail. Difficulties can also arise if the abutment tooth is rotated around its long axis, so that the palatal metal coverage is more likely to be visible. This can be a problem with maxillary canine teeth used to retain adhesive bridges replacing missing lateral incisors. A further difficulty can arise where the abutment teeth are relatively thin labiopalatally, as a result of which the metallic wing lying on the palatal aspect of the tooth tends to cause some apparent discoloration when viewed from the labial aspect.

Oral hygiene

As with most restorative treatment, where the patient has poor oral hygiene then complex procedures are contraindicated, as they are likely to be associated with an increased risk of tooth loss if the plaque control cannot be improved.

Stable outcome

Where it is considered that the abutment teeth are unlikely to maintain their position as a result of periodontal disease or lack of occlusal stability, then treatment with an adhesive bridge is usually inappropriate.

Advantages and disadvantages

Since these have many similarities to treatment procedures, which have already been discussed, they are summarized in Box 3.1.

> **Box 3.1** Treatment alternatives for the partially dentate
>
> **OBSERVATION**
> - Missing teeth do not always need to be replaced.
> - Their replacement may not be in the patient's best interests, for example in the terminally ill.
>
> **ORTHODONTIC MANAGEMENT**
> - While of restricted applicability, this technique is very effective in suitable cases and has no long-term maintenance requirements.
>
> **REMOVABLE PARTIAL DENTURES**
> - Treatment with removable partial dentures is an extremely versatile procedure, which is widely used in the management of partial tooth loss.
>
> **ADHESIVE BRIDGES**
> - The development of adhesive techniques has made it possible to restore many shorter edentulous spaces with resin-bonded bridges.
>
> **CONVENTIONAL BRIDGES**
> - Prior to the development of reliable adhesive techniques in dentistry, conventional bridges were often considered the ideal treatment for restoration of the partially dentate arch. Extensive tooth preparation is a major disadvantage.
>
> **IMPLANT-STABILIZED PROSTHESES**
> - This is a complex technique, which can be used to stabilize both fixed and removable prostheses, and one which reduces the rate of resorption of alveolar bone. It is technically demanding and unsuited to many clinical situations.

CONVENTIONAL BRIDGES

Prior to the development of reliable adhesive techniques in dentistry, conventional bridges were often considered the ideal treatment for restoration of the partially dentate arch. The technique involves the reduction of natural teeth to provide space for the restorative material, and modification of their shape to maximize the retentive potential of the bridge abutments. With the rising numbers of partially dentate individuals in most age groups, more conservative attitudes to restorative dentistry and the emergence of newer techniques, treatment with conventional bridges is increasingly used only in those situations less suited to more modern methods.

Systemic factors

Systemic factors that may influence the choice as to whether to use a conventional bridge are essentially the same as those that apply for treatment with resin-retained bridges, although the work, particularly where it involves extensive restorations and occlusal modifications, is technically very demanding. In addition, the procedures are relatively expensive, which may place a limit on the amount of treatment that can be undertaken.

Local factors

Local factors of importance when deciding whether to treat a patient with a conventional bridge include the following.

Feasibility

Treatment with conventional bridges may not be possible where access is limited or the angulations of the teeth so extreme as to make it impossible to construct a suitable bridge, without the risk of pulpal exposure in order to obtain a single path of insertion.

Abutment teeth

The use of a conventional bridge is totally dependent upon the availability of suitable abutment teeth. This relates to their location, periodontal status and root length, crown height and condition, tooth angulation, endodontic status and the availability of space to place a suitable restoration, typically a full crown.

The status of the remaining teeth

This is also of great importance, since if any of these are lost subsequent to placement of the bridge the restoration of the resultant space may be technically challenging or impossible, and is often expensive.

Occlusion

A conventional bridge places additional loads on the abutment teeth, and care must therefore be taken not to use them where these are excessive. Long spans, bruxism, evidence of high masticatory forces and evidence of occlusal tooth surface loss all suggest that the restoration may have to resist heavy occlusal loads, with the risk of decementation.

Oral hygiene

Poor oral hygiene will predispose to caries and periodontal disease, putting the abutment teeth and indeed the remaining dentition at increased risk. Similarly, a history of indifference towards oral health, recurrent caries around restorations and periodontal disease all argue against treatment with a conventional dental bridge.

Alveolar resorption

Where there has been significant alveolar resorption, then the problems of placing a bridge with a satisfactory appearance will be similar to those described for adhesive retained bridges.

Advantages

Appearance

Conventional dental bridges, particularly where they are fabricated from porcelain, or porcelain fused to gold alloy, can provide a very natural appearance which is extremely hard wearing and durable.

Minimal bulk

Conventional bridges can often be made to be little larger than the tissues that they replace, and thus suffer from few functional problems as compared, for example, with a removable partial denture.

Security

Conventional bridges can usually be made so as to be extremely secure.

Disadvantages

Among the principal disadvantages of conventional bridges are the following.

Technical complexity

Conventional dental bridges range in complexity from those with a single tooth pontic to large constructions restoring the entire dental arch and modifying the occlusion, often in an extensive manner. Such devices are expensive to make and require high levels of skill from the dentist and technician. While their fixed attributes offer a number of advantages, the difficulty of modifying them once completed and in place, as compared with RPDs, is significant and on occasions may prove troublesome.

Expensive

Conventional bridges are expensive to make.

Lifespan

The projected life of a conventional dental bridge varies markedly depending upon its location, size and design; however, studies on survival times report failures of 5%, 10% and 40% after 5, 10 and 15 years respectively.

Restricted applicability

Conventional dental bridges can only be used in a limited range of cases. While they are suited for the definitive restoration of missing teeth in some situations, their irreversible nature and the difficulty of modifying them make them ill suited to more temporary situations.

Difficulty of repair

Conventional dental bridges may be difficult or impossible to repair should they fail, and in these circumstances may need to be replaced.

Poor retrievability

Unlike screw-retained implant-stabilized bridges, conventional dental bridges can rarely be removed for servicing since they are almost invariably cemented in place. Occasionally, they can be removed; however, this is difficult and can lead to fracture of the bridge or the abutment tooth.

SELECTING AN APPROPRIATE TREATMENT

While different conditions have a range of approaches to formulating a treatment plan, a typical sequence would include the following:

Systemic factors

1. What are the patient's wishes and aspirations in relation to their oral health?

2. What are the patient's views in relation to treatment procedures? Would they prefer a more straightforward approach or a technically complex procedure?

3. What are their views on the costs of oral care?

4. Does the patient have any systemic contraindications to any of the potential forms of treatment?

Local factors

1. Is it possible to gain adequate access to the mouth for treatment procedures? If this is limited then some types of treatment may be impossible or very difficult (Figs 3.8, 3.15).

2. Does the patient have missing teeth that require replacement?

3. Is the situation in the mouth stable so that restoration of the space will provide a functioning dentition for a significant period? If that is not the case, then what is the likely prognosis of the remaining teeth?

4. What is the status of the teeth adjacent to the edentulous spaces? Would these form suitable abutments for a resin-retained bridge or a conventional bridge? Do they require the placement of restorations, which may suggest the appropriateness of a conventional bridge, or are they sound, in which case a resin-retained bridge may be the more appropriate?

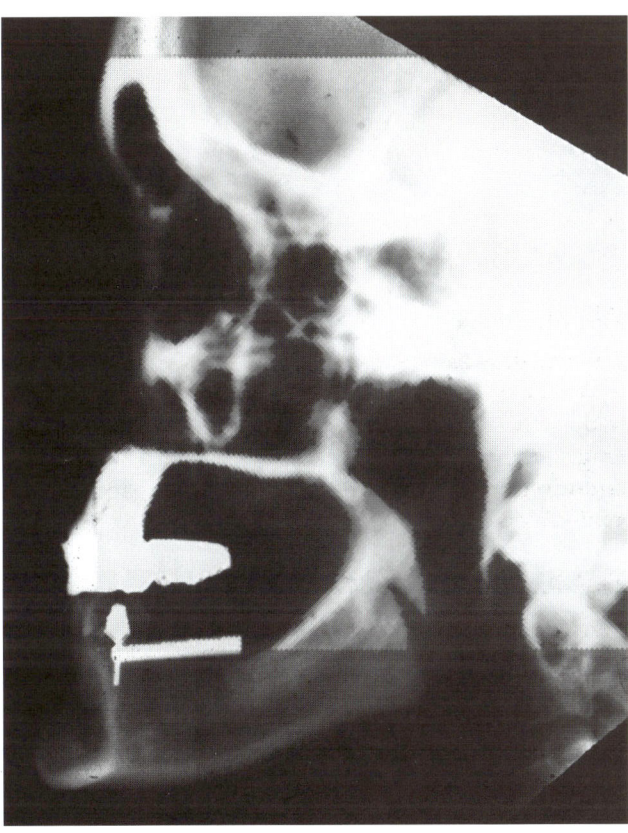

Fig. 3.7 Bone resorption in the maxilla has resulted in the need to cantilever the fixed prosthesis labially to provide an acceptable appearance.

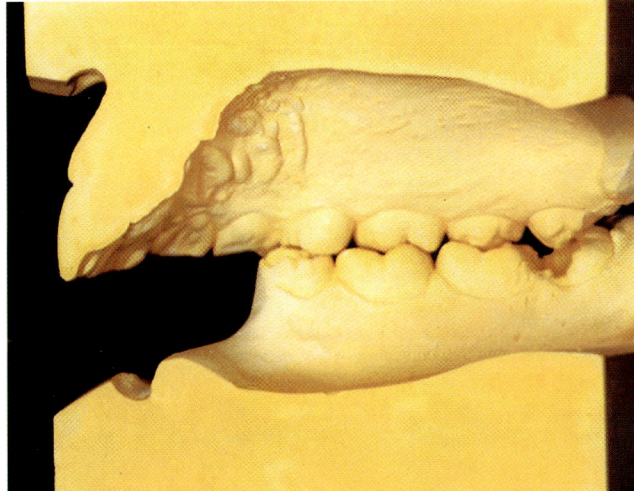

Fig. 3.6 This patient had a Class I incisor relationship in the natural dentition. If dental implants were placed in the residual ridge, then the teeth on the prosthesis would require considerable cantilevering to provide a similar relationship.

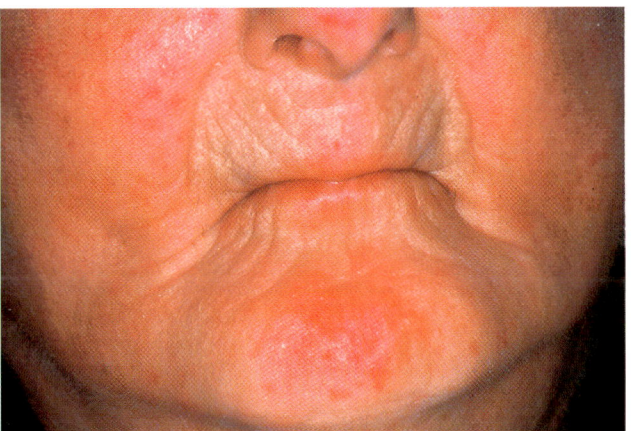

Fig. 3.8 Conditions such as scleroderma can result in a limited gape, creating access problems that often preclude implant treatment.

5. Is there a high lip line when smiling or talking, which makes the front of the mouth evident, thus placing great potential demands on the appearance of any restoration that involves the front of the mouth?

6. Does the patient have good oral hygiene, or is the situation one in which increased caries and periodontal disease are likely to occur if a prosthesis were placed?

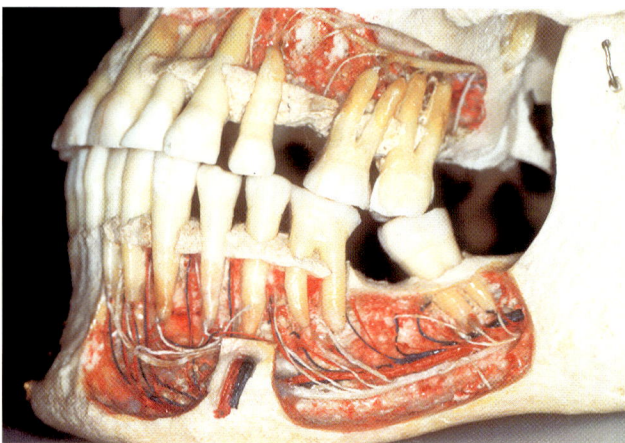

Fig. 3.9 Bone loss following removal of the natural teeth can be extensive. In the edentulous mandible the mental foramen may come to lie level with the crest of the alveolar ridge, while the mandibular canal may be relatively superficial. Both create potential hazards for implant insertion. Bone resorption in the maxilla will often result in inadequate bone volume for implant insertion.

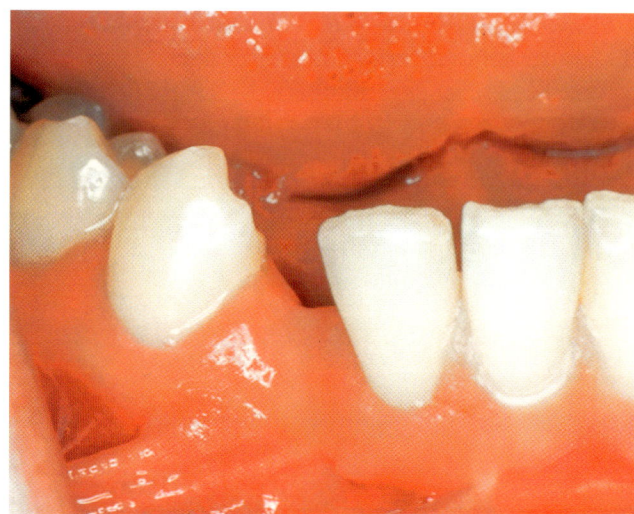

Fig. 3.12 Implant placement in the 43 region is contraindicated by the narrow alveolar ridge, high fraenal attachment and reduced space that is available between 42 and 44.

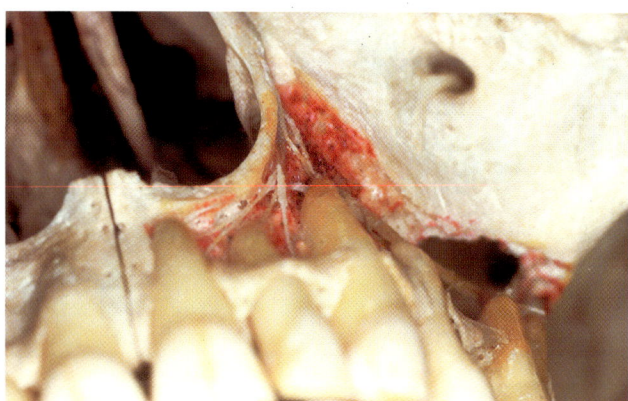

Fig. 3.10 The maxillary sinus and the floor of the nose lie close to the apices of the natural teeth. When these are removed the resultant resorption will often result in close approximation of the crest of the alveolar ridge to these structures.

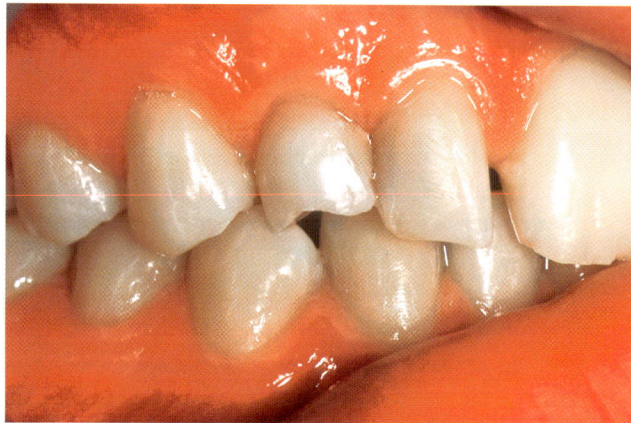

Fig. 3.13 Replacement of 53 with an implant is complicated by the dynamic relationship of this tooth to 43 in lateral excursions of the mandible, as seen in Figure 3.14.

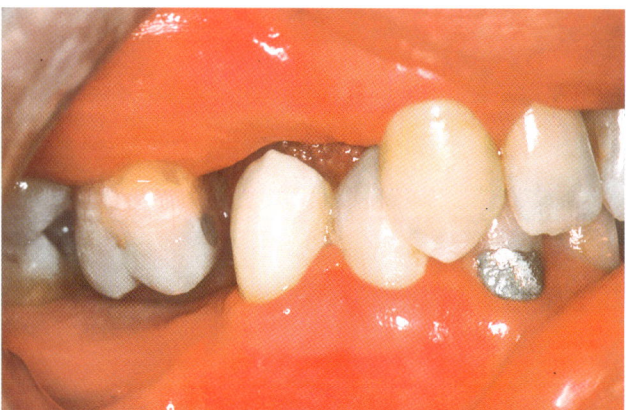

Fig. 3.11 There is a lack of vertical space for restoring any implants that might be placed in the edentulous regions of this maxilla and mandible.

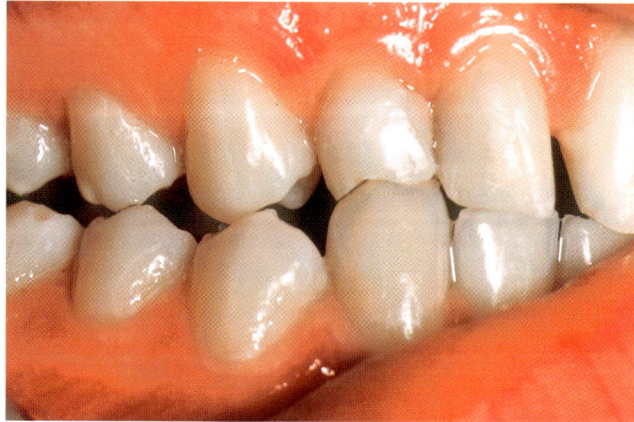

Fig. 3.14 The patient shown in Figure 3.13 during a right lateral mandibular excursion.

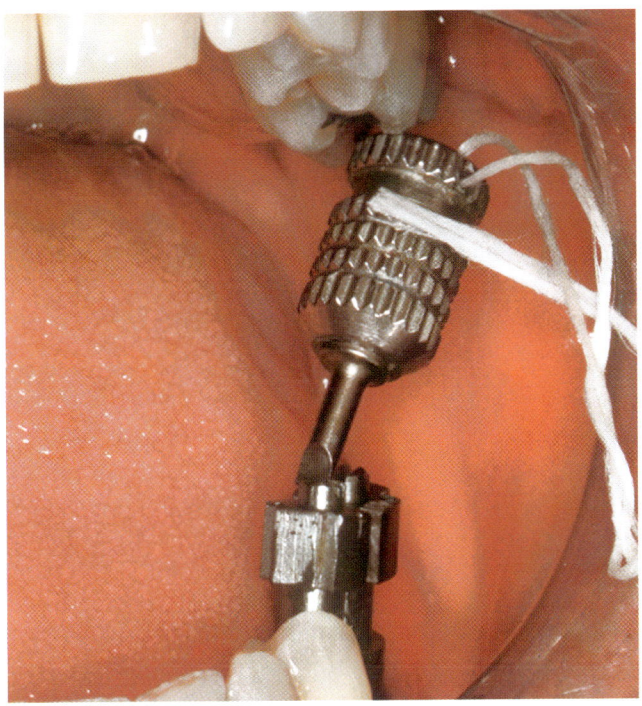

Fig. 3.15 Where the gape is restricted then access can be problematical.

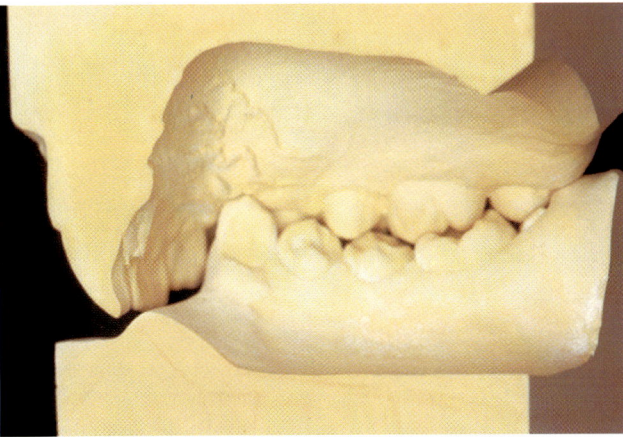

Fig. 3.16 Replacement of this patient's mandibular incisors with an implant-stabilized prosthesis would present major challenges owing to the restricted prosthetic envelope and the potential for occlusal overload.

7. Are there potential problems related to the prosthodontic envelope (Figs 3.9–3.14)?

8. Are there potential problems related to possible sites for implant insertion (Figs 3.15, 3.16)?

FURTHER READING

Awad M A, Locker D, Korner-Bitensky N, Feine J S 2000 Measuring the effect of intra-oral implant rehabilitation on health-related quality of life in a randomised controlled clinical trial. J Dent Res 79:1659–63

Esposito M, Coulthard P, Worthington H V, Jokstad A 2001 Quality assessment of randomized controlled trials of oral implants. Int J Oral Maxillofac Implants 16(6): 783–92

Feine J S, Carlsson G E, Awad M A, et al 2002 The McGill consensus statement on overdentures. Mandibular two-implant overdentures as first choice standard of care for edentulous patients. Montreal, Quebec. Int J Oral Maxillofac Implants 17(4): 601–2

Hobkirk J A, Brouziottou-Davas E 1996 The influence of occlusal scheme on masticatory forces using implant stabilized bridges. J Oral Rehabil 23(6):386–91

Hobkirk J A, Havthoulos T K 1998 The influence of mandibular deformation, implant numbers, and loading position on detected forces in abutments supporting fixed implant superstructures. J Prosthet Dent 80(2):169–74

Zarb G A, Schmitt A 1996 The edentulous predicament. I: A prospective study of the effectiveness of implant-supported fixed prostheses. J Am Dent Assoc 127(1):59–65

Zarb G A, Schmitt A 1996 The edentulous predicament. II: The longitudinal effectiveness of implant-supported overdentures. J Am Dent Assoc 127(1): 66–72

Gathering information and treatment planning

WHAT ARE THE OBJECTIVES OF GATHERING INFORMATION AND PLANNING IMPLANT TREATMENT?

The objectives of gathering information and planning treatment are to assemble all appropriate information about the patient's dental and medical history and conduct a clinical examination including evidence from radiographs and articulated study casts (Box 4.1). This will enable the patient to make a decision regarding the treatment options. The proposed treatments(s) should be sufficiently detailed for the dentist/ specialist to identify the surgical procedure(s), the positions for selected implants, the probable design of the prosthesis(es) including the supporting implant abutments, and the intended cosmetic and functional outcome of the restorations.

As a result, the dentist should be certain that restoration with dental implants is likely to confer a long-term benefit that will be superior to alternative treatments for replacing a deficient dentition with a dental bridge or removable conventional denture.

The consequences of ignoring a logical process are several. The most obvious are as follows:

- The intended design of the prosthesis does not match the position of the implants.
- After subsequent unplanned extraction of other teeth from the arch the dentist cannot guarantee the use of further implants to recover the function or appearance of these extracted teeth.

It is of course important for the patient and dentist to be aware that failure of osseointegration may arise from a number of causes, not all of which can be excluded by careful treatment planning (Box 4.2).

In which circumstances are dental implants most needed?

As a result of providing an initial consultation it is probable that the dentist will identify those patients who would possibly benefit because their needs are less likely to be met by more routine dental treatments.

The situations can be related to degrees of tooth loss.

The edentulous patient

Of those who are edentulous in one or both jaws, the following groups can often benefit particularly from implant treatment:

- those who report either severe denture intolerance or can be seen, because of a relatively young age, to be likely to be at risk from severe alveolar bone loss;
- patients with severe alveolar resorption;
- patients who find denture treatment emotionally disturbing.

Severe intolerance can be physical, where particularly palpation or coverage of the palatal vault evokes a strong retching reflex. It also often has a psychological overlay, where a patient may feel nauseous at the thought of an oral examination or use of a removable appliance. An implant-stabilized fixed appliance may be effective where the cause is physical, provided that it is feasible to carry out the treatment. In some patients the retching reflex is so extreme as to make this impossible.

Marked ridge resorption may be such that a well-constructed denture has unacceptable stability or

---

Box 4.1 Patient assessment leading to planned treatment

- Medical, dental and social histories
- Clinical oral examination
- Radiographic examination
- Possible psychiatric opinion
- Articulated study casts
- Evaluation of trial dentures/diagnostic wax-up
- Agreed surgical plan/template for surgery
- Discussion of options/agreed treatment plan
- Signed consent form

Box 4.2 Essential information

- What is the patient's complaint?
- Why has the patient requested implant treatment?
- Has the patient experienced successful routine prosthetic/restorative treatment?
- Is the patient aware of the requirements for implant treatment and long-term success?

causes chronic pain. This is typically seen in the edentulous patient with an atrophic mandible, or where a complete denture supported by a poor foundation opposes a well-maintained partially dentate arch.

A very few patients find extensive natural tooth loss emotionally disturbing and do not accept replacement dentures, however well constructed. While dental implants can help some of this group, many have unrealizable expectations of dental treatment. Such patients require very careful assessment, often by a psychologist or psychiatrist, since those who suffer from conditions such as dysmorphophobia are unlikely to be treated successfully, even with dental implants.

The partially dentate patient

The partially dentate patients for whom implant treatment may be especially beneficial generally fall into three categories of tooth loss/absence:

- developmental anomalies/trauma;
- extensive loss of teeth in one arch;
- accompanied by extensive loss of oral tissue.

The first group will be identified as suffering from developmental anomalies or trauma where the preservation of the remaining healthy intact teeth is of paramount importance. Examination of those with hypodontia indicates a range of young patients, from those with one or two developmentally missing anterior teeth, including those with misplaced canines (where corrective treatment has failed), to those with few permanent teeth and poorly developed alveoli. In this group permanent teeth are often small and conical, and sometimes poorly related to those in the opposing arch. Those with repaired clefts of the palate, including patients who have completed orthodontic treatment and bone grafting, are also suitable for dental implant restoration. This should, however, be planned prior to surgical and orthodontic procedures to ensure the optimum outcome.

Trauma may affect younger patients who lose one or two anterior teeth in their early teens, sometimes after failure of endodontic treatment or post crowns. Loss of significant numbers of teeth and alveolus may be associated with facial fractures sustained in road traffic accidents. The resulting span in a partially dentate arch of well-conserved, minimally restored natural teeth may ultimately be best managed with an implant-supported fixed prosthesis.

The second group comprises patients with stable occlusions with extensive loss of teeth in one arch where alternative restorations are unsuitable. These cases include those with long bounded spans, where conventional bridges cannot be satisfactorily retained and supported. Implant treatment should also be considered in long free-end spans where short cantilevered bridges or removable partial dentures are inadequate, and shortened dental arches fail to meet the functional and aesthetic needs of the patient.

The third group of patients exhibit considerable deficiencies of intra-oral tissue arising from developmental disorders, treatment of tumours and extensive injury. Restoration of function and appearance may be achieved either by fixed prostheses or removable ones where both the edentulous saddles and implants combine to stabilize the prosthesis.

What specific information should be sought in the medical, dental and social history of the patient?

The general health status of the individual must be properly considered. As previously mentioned, there are a few specific medical situations where implant treatment may risk the health of the patient or be associated with high failure rates of osseointegration. It is therefore wise to confirm the suitability of the patient for this treatment by asking specific questions in addition to using a general medical questionnaire.

Implants are not recommended for elderly infirm persons who are unable to undergo prolonged surgical treatment, or numerous visits for the complex prosthetic rehabilitation, especially if their ability to sustain high levels of plaque control is compromised physically or mentally. Those whose cooperation and general well-being fluctuate should be advised against implant treatment. These patients include those with drug or alcohol dependence, uncontrolled depression and those with some specific psychiatric disorders (Figs 4.1, 4.2). Likewise, patients who would be compromised by elective surgery and infection should be counselled to avoid this treatment. These conditions include those having mitral stenosis, heart failure, uncontrolled diabetes (Type 2) and blood dyscrasias, and individuals who are immunocompromised (Box 4.3).

Lower success rates for osseointegration are expected in heavy smokers and those having received irradiation of the face and jaws. Assessment of the

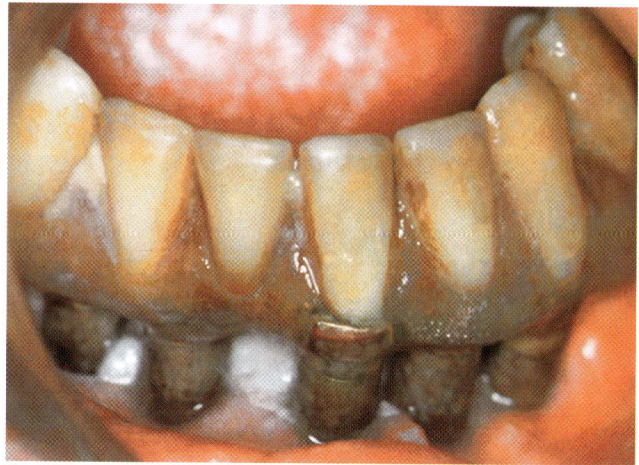

Fig. 4.1 Poor standards of oral hygiene indicate neglect of dental care by a patient suffering a relapse in general health associated with depression and alcoholism.

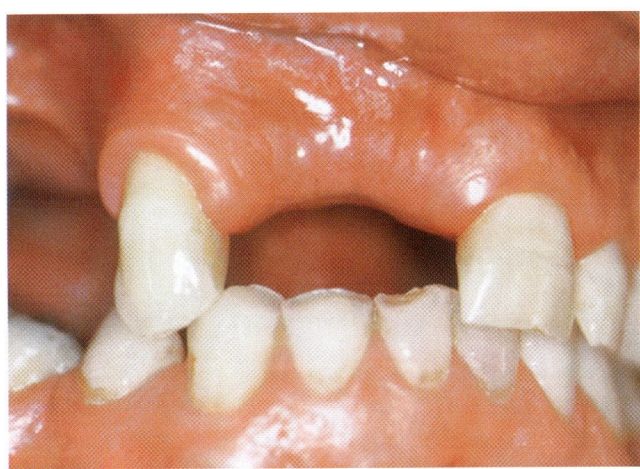

Fig. 4.2 Evidence of attrition and inadequate alveolar volume have excluded this patient with high expectations from receiving treatment with dental implants.

Box 4.3 Medical history contraindicating treatment

- Infirm elderly
- Medical/surgical risk, e.g.:
  - Uncontrolled diabetic
  - Immunocompromised
  - Blood dyscrasia
  - Impaired cardiovascular function
- Drug/alcohol dependence
- Psychiatric disorder, e.g.:
  - Paranoia
  - Dysmorphophobia
- Recent irradiation of orofacial tissues
- Smoking (?heavy use)

---

risks and benefits as well as the management of these patients are best undertaken in specialist centres.

Careful thought should be given to possible stabilization of dentures or their replacement by a fixed-implant prosthesis in patients exhibiting adverse neuromuscular control (e.g. cerebral palsy). Operative techniques should, however, be manageable and high standards of home care are necessary to produce effective levels of oral hygiene.

When establishing the dental history of the patient four aspects should be considered – the four 'A's' (Attitude, Awareness, Attendance and Appliance experience). Two extremes of patient attitude should be guarded against. Those who eagerly anticipate that replacement will restore completely all oral functions, and create a youthful appearance of natural teeth, are unlikely to be easily satisfied with any limitation of implant treatment. Similarly, those who have little appreciation or understanding of dental diseases and their own role in their prevention will usually have insufficient interest to maintain the health of their dentition and the desirable condition of the implant prosthesis. Previous patterns of irregular attendance

are usually indicative of those who participate poorly in follow-up monitoring and maintenance until a crisis arises. Careful consideration must be given to those who claim to have received unsatisfactory prosthetic treatment resulting in loose or painful dentures, or early failure of crowns or bridges. An examination may confirm if the complaint is justified, and indicate whether or not an alternative satisfactory solution may be reached by simple routine denture treatment carried out to a high standard.

Some occupations and activities contraindicate the use of dental implants. Young adolescents and those engaged in contact sports, e.g. hockey, rugby, football, water polo, squash, are liable to sustain further injury to the dentition. It is wise to delay complex care to later, when they cease playing competitively. Conversely, those facing the public in demanding situations, e.g. musicians, teachers, may gain considerable psychological advantage from implant treatment where the security of the prosthesis and lack of display of metal components are important issues.

What features should be considered in the extra-oral examination?

Three important features should be assessed in the extra-oral examination: the gape, the functional 'aesthetic zone' and the jaw relationship. Evidence of limitation in the gape is a clear warning that passage of instruments or insertion of the prosthesis through the lips or between opposing teeth will inhibit treatment (see Figs 3.8 and 3.15).

The morphology and function of the lips have a profound effect on the display of the dental arch and alveolus. Assessment is required when the patient is relaxed and while the history is being recorded, so that the extent of display of the oral tissues is evident during speaking, smiling and laughing.

In the edentulous patient, or those with one edentulous jaw, it will be apparent if the extent of resorption requires a flange to maintain the correct position of the arch and the facial profile. A short upper lip is likely to create a high smile line that reveals both the artificial teeth and flange (Fig. 4.3). Standard transmucosal abutments would be an inappropriate choice. This evidence may support the choice of a removable overdenture rather than a fixed prosthesis.

Assessment of the partially dentate patient is even more crucial since the length of the artificial tooth crowns, and the lack of gingival tissue either in the edentulous span or around the adjacent teeth, are likely to affect the design and display of the prosthesis.

Abnormal length, angulation and position of the artificial teeth, and the presence of dark spaces between the prosthesis and the natural teeth and gingivae, should be anticipated. Such an evident defect of tissue requires consideration to be given to ridge augmentation.

Abnormalities of the lips arising from previous surgical intervention and trauma may make access to

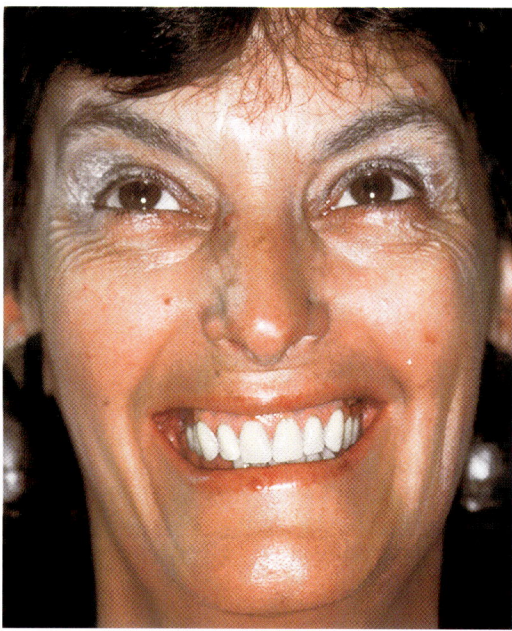

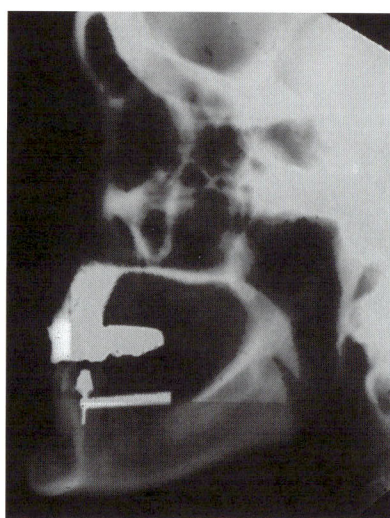

Fig. 4.4 One problem posed by restoring a Class II division ii malocclusion is that the crowns are angulated on the implant bodies, seen in the lateral skull radiograph.

Fig. 4.3 A difficulty foreseen at examination is that the patient has a 'high smile line'. A flange is necessary to provide artificial teeth of acceptable length of crown and to mask the abutments.

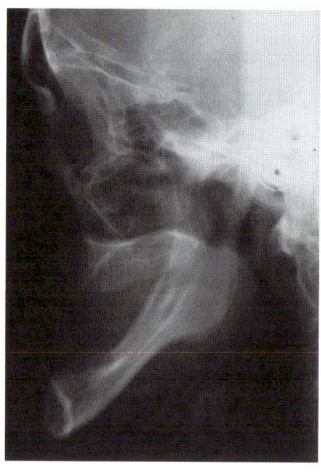

Fig. 4.5 An obviously unfavourable jaw relation makes implant treatment very difficult for this edentulous patient.

the jaw difficult, and result in distortion of the space available for the prosthesis. Patients who have undergone treatment for cleft lip and palate, or who have had resection of the mandible with reconstruction using nasolabial flaps for example, require detailed evaluation.

Obvious disproportion and malalignment of the jaws, present in skeletal Class II and III situations, and patients presenting with 'long or short face' patterns may create problems in the design of the prosthesis. There is the potential risk of unfavourable cantilevering and loading or inadequate space for components (Figs 4.4, 4.5).

What intra-oral aspects of the overall examination of partially dentate jaws are peculiar to implant treatment?

The clinical examination should be directed to gaining specific evidence. In the previous chapter general aspects have been considered and emphasis has been placed on selecting those patients with a well-restored stable occlusion and a high standard of plaque control associated with non-progressive periodontal disease.

The anticipated relationship between the arch restored by the prosthesis and the ridge will indicate potential key features in the design of the prosthesis. These are the likely extent of cantilevering between the occlusal surfaces and the implants, and any divergence between the angulations of the artificial crowns and the implants. The extent of the loss of alveolar bone will influence the potential length of these crowns. The width of the bounded span, which

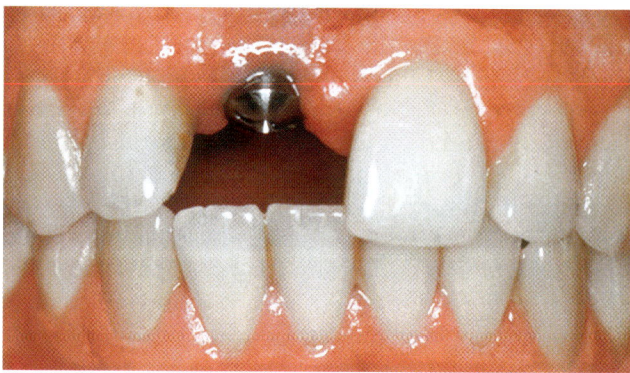

Fig. 4.6 One feature of the single-tooth span is unfavourable: the replacement crown will be potentially wider than the adjacent central incisor tooth.

will accommodate artificial teeth of an appropriately matched shape, must be noted (Fig. 4.6).

The initial inspection may give an early indication of the number of implants that may be suitably accommodated in the span, and whether or not there

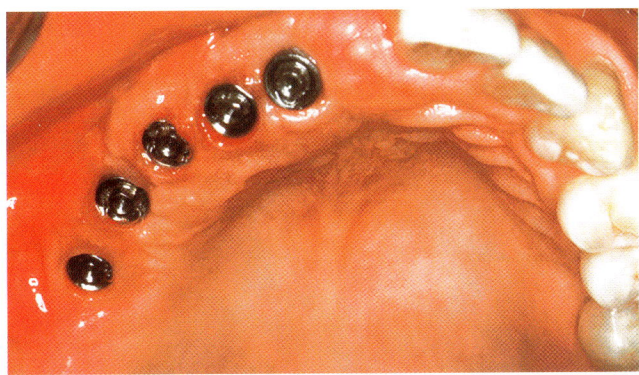

Fig. 4.7 The long free-end span of the edentulous area of the maxilla is appropriate for restoration with dental implants.

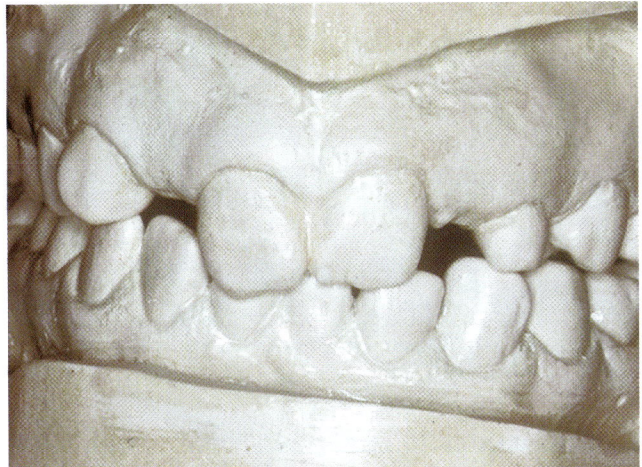

Fig. 4.8 Natural teeth adjacent to the spaces in the lateral incisor areas are unfavourably inclined.

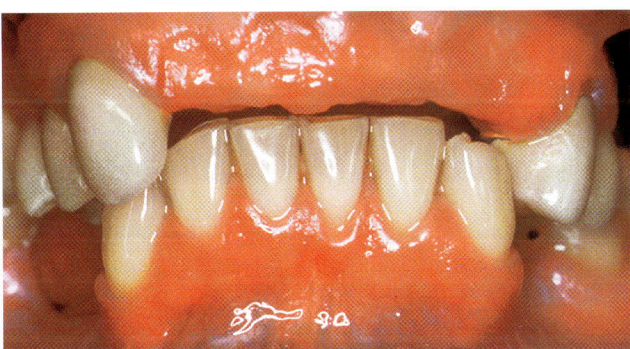

Fig. 4.9 Clinical examination shows the anterior ridge is narrow and the vertical incisor relation is unfavourable, inhibiting the choice of implants.

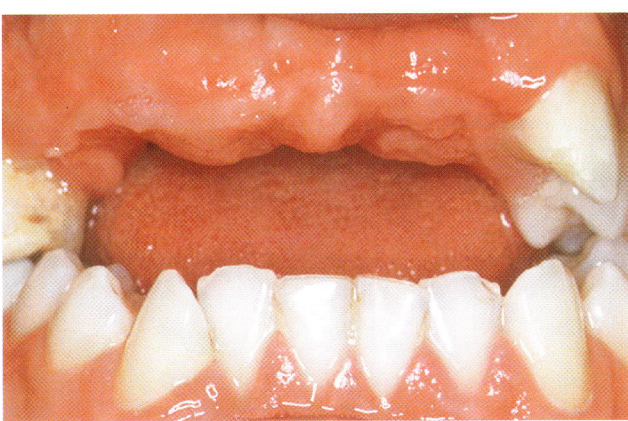

Fig. 4.10 Traumatic tooth loss in a patient with a Class III malocclusion has resulted in an unfavourable relation between the residual anterior maxilla and the natural mandibular incisor teeth.

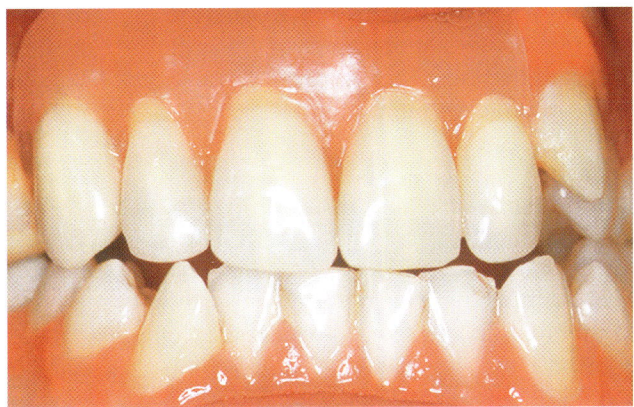

Fig. 4.11 A possible solution with the arch supported by a flange can be judged with a trial insertion.

is tilting of the adjacent natural teeth which may influence their positions (Figs 4.7, 4.8).

Examination of the opposing arches in the inter-cuspal contact position will indicate the extent of the vertical space between the opposing arch and ridge. A deep vertical overlap of the natural anterior teeth, typically associated with a Class II division ii malocclusion, will suggest that a potential problem may exist in accommodating implant abutments (Fig. 4.9).

Conversely, excessive vertical separation may identify problems of restoration of the occlusion, typically associated with a Class III jaw relation (Figs 4.10, 4.11).

What intra-oral aspects of the examination of the edentulous jaw(s) of the patient are significant to implant treatment?

Careful oral examination and assessment of the patient's existing complete dentures will indicate if shortcomings in the design of the prostheses have created problems affecting their performance. In such circumstances routine dental treatment may be a possible solution.

In the edentulous situation one denture, usually the upper, may be considered satisfactory by the patient who seeks a solution to problems with the other. Inspection may suggest some obvious changes that could overcome these problems. However, if a fixed prosthesis in one jaw offers a possible solution, the effect upon a hitherto satisfactory removable opposing prosthesis should be considered. Where there is jaw atrophy, will changes in the base and occlusion of the conventional denture be sufficient to create the desired

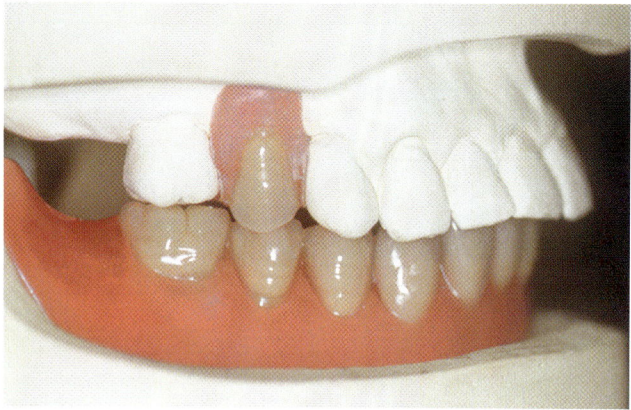

Fig. 4.12 The occlusal table is appropriately restored with an overdenture opposing a natural arch.

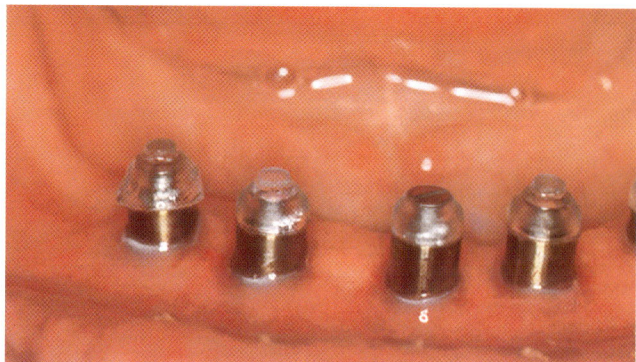

Fig. 4.13 A flat anterior edentulous ridge has been successfully restored with implants stabilizing a fixed prosthesis.

solution? If both dentures are poorly designed, have worn teeth or a poor fit then the examination may indicate that new conventional dentures are desirable before implant treatment is considered.

Where one jaw is partially dentate, or the arch is intact, very careful consideration must be given to the presence of irregularities in the natural arch and occlusal table created by tilting or overeruption of the teeth. Lack of balance with the opposing prosthesis produced by eccentric interferences may readily destabilize it. Further investigation using articulated study casts will reveal any lack of space for the prosthesis or implant components. The anticipated length of the occlusal table will influence the choice of a fixed cantilever or removable overdenture (Fig. 4.12).

Inspection and palpation of the jaw and ridge produce an immediate impression of the volume of available bone potentially available for implant insertion. The mandible may have a flat or inverted oral contour, but palpation may indicate an adequate volume of bone in the anterior part sufficient to accept implants as short as 7 mm or as long as 20 mm (Figs 4.13, 4.14). However, palpation may indicate a narrow ridge crest, and in the posterior area significant lack of height above the mental foramen, indicative of an unsuitable volume of bone for implantation.

Evidence of a well-formed maxillary ridge should include assessment of possible labial concavities, which may dictate the angulation of the future implants. In the presence of advanced resorption doubt concerning the appropriate treatment plan can only be resolved with supporting radiographic evidence. Palpation will obviously indicate where substantial fibrous replacement of the bone has already occurred (Box 4.4).

What evidence should be gathered about the soft tissues enveloping the dental arch or covering the edentulous ridges?

Both the thickness and position of the mucoperiosteum must be assessed. Part of this examination will

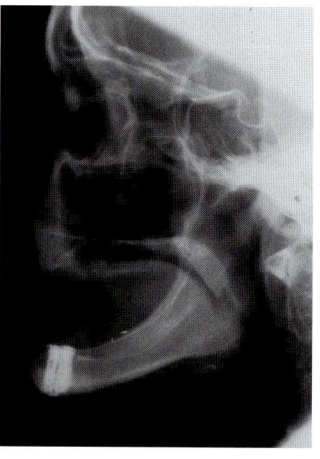

Fig. 4.14 A lateral skull radiograph showing a flat mandibular surface with a good depth of bone for implantation.

Box 4.4 Important local features

- Is the residual dentition healthy?
- Is there adequate gape for instrumentation?
- Does sufficient inter-tooth space allow positioning of fixture(s), abutment(s) and prosthesis?
- Does inter-arch space permit restoration?
- Is the occlusion stable, without evidence of excessive tooth surface loss?
- Is there overeruption of opponent teeth?
- How many sites require restoration?
- Are the gingivae evident ('e.g. high lip line')?
- Will the prosthesis replace coronal or coronal/alveolar tissue?

include appraisal of the extent to which the restored arch will be displayed on speaking and smiling. The so-called 'aesthetic zone', which is assessed during oral examination, therefore involves the dental and alveolar tissues including those to be restored by the implant prosthesis. Those patients who only display the occlusal third of the arch below the 'smile line' (high lip line) are sometimes more willing to accept a compromise in the resulting appearance, but this should not be a forgone conclusion, and possible

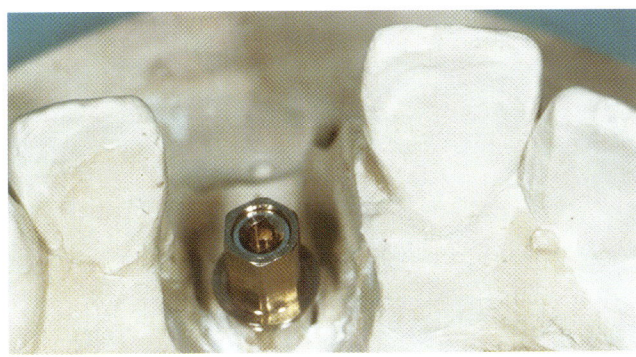

Fig. 4.15 A reduction in the alveolar width following healing of the socket has resulted in palatal positioning of the implant. The cast shows that the crown secured on the abutment is likely to be extensively ridge lapped.

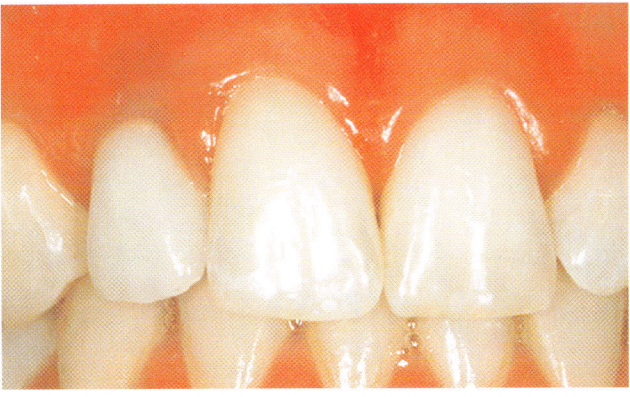

Fig. 4.17 The resulting 'gingival line' is associated with a good profile for the single-tooth crown emerging from the mucosal cuff.

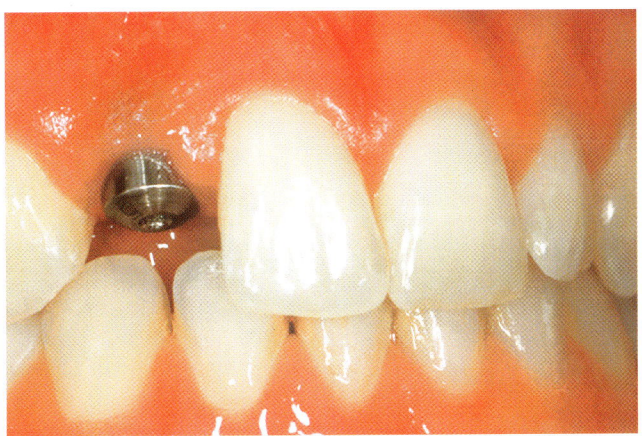

Fig. 4.16 Favourable soft-tissue contours exist adjacent to and around the natural teeth that abut a single-tooth span.

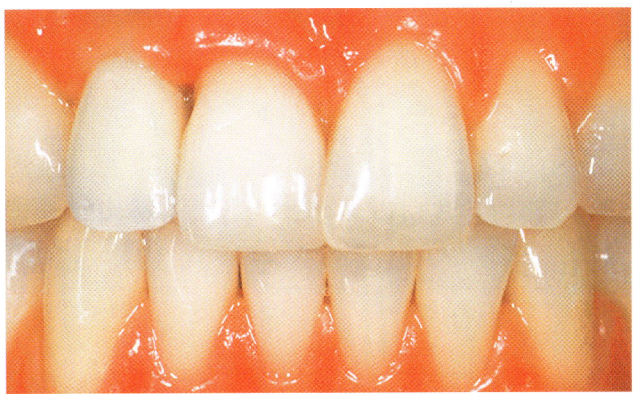

Fig. 4.18 A 'black triangle' is evident between the single-tooth crown on 12 and the adjacent central incisor tooth due to a deficient papilla.

shortcomings should be explained with the aid of a 'diagnostic wax-up/trial denture' before a treatment plan is finally agreed. For example, the design of a crown for a single tooth restoration will be influenced by the position of the head of the implant body. Hence, previous resorption of the alveolus may result in a longer clinical crown than those of the adjacent natural teeth, unless grafting of the alveolus and soft-tissue surgery can recapture the original form of the tissues. Evidence of labial resorption will suggest that an implant is likely to be positioned more palatally, with the prospect of the crown being ridge lapped and formed with a more bulky emergence profile (Fig. 4.15).

Visual inspection and periodontal probing of natural teeth adjacent to an edentulous span will confirm if the crevices are healthy and of normal depth. Also it will be evident if the gingivae have a normal architecture or exhibit recession. Surgical planning will aim to maintain the position of the gingival margins and not alter the form of the papillae around the tooth (Figs 4.16–4.18). Prosthetic planning will consider the likely height of the artificial crown, access for cleaning and the required position of the implant in any fixed design.

When examining the mandible it is important to consider the position of the ridge crest and determine whether well-keratinized masticatory mucosa is likely to surround the future position of a transmucosal abutment (Fig. 4.13). When resorption is advanced, the prosthetic space is often narrow, with mobile mucosa lying close to the centre of the anterior aspect of the body of the jaw. A partly mobile or completely mobile cuff around the abutment may be accommodated, although allowance must be made for the varying sulcus depth when constructing the prosthesis. However, misalignment of the implant with the prosthetic space can have important consequences. These can include complaints of impairment of tongue movement, difficulties with speech, abutment hygiene and recurring soreness as a result of inflammation of the cuff. It is therefore crucial to record an accurate impression of the prosthetic space, especially when removable overdentures are planned.

'Ridge mapping' may be employed to determine the thickness of the mucoperiosteum overlying the jaw (Fig. 4.19). This would subsequently form a cuff around the abutment, and will influence the choice of transmucosal abutment. The technique is described in Chapter 5. Similar information can be obtained from a

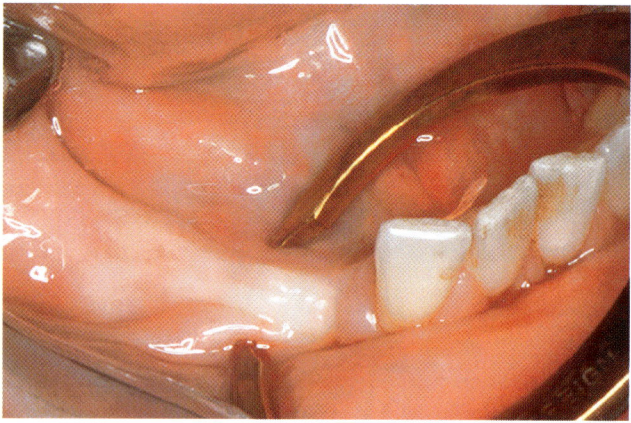

Fig. 4.19 Ridge mapping also assesses the available width in the alveolar process.

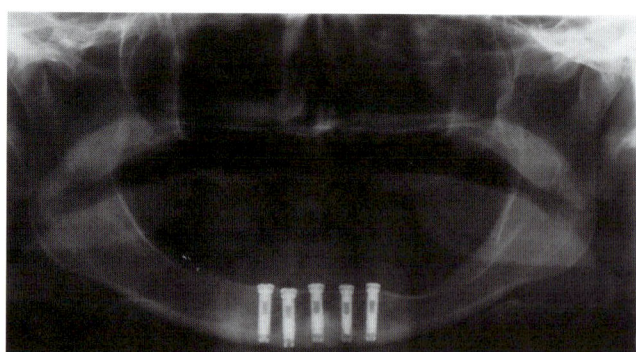

Fig. 4.20 The anterior body of the mandible is suitable for accepting five dental implants supporting a cantilevered fixed prosthesis.

CT scan where a radio-opaque marker has been placed on the mucosal surface.

What diagnostic radiographic images are required for planning purposes?

Both routine dental radiographic views and more complex imaging procedures are useful in case planning. The volume, and to a certain extent the quality, of bone available for implant insertion can be anticipated from such investigations.

Evidence exists from prospective studies that the outcome of implant treatment is significantly altered by the volume and quality of the bone into which implants are placed. Hence short implants placed in poor-quality bone are more likely to fail when loaded. Manufacturers have attempted to overcome these problems with implant designs with micro- and macro-surface modifications and greater diameters to enhance the surface area potentially available for contact with bone.

In an attempt to prejudge bone quality and quantity radiographic examination has been used to assist the findings at surgical operation, which influences the choice of implant. Lekholm and Zarb have classified the form of the edentulous jawbone, the extent of resorption being depicted in one of five categories ranging from minimal resorption of the alveolus to extensive reduction involving the base of the jaw. Cawood and Howell further divided the classification according to patterns of resorption seen in the anterior and posterior mandible, with the intention of identifying patients in need of augmentation by autogenous bone grafting. Assessment is usually made from images recorded in orthopantomographic (OPT) and lateral skull films. Lekholm and Zarb identified four qualities where the radiographic images depicted the extent of cortical bone and that of trabecular bone within it. Bone with thin cortices and a sparse trabecular structure, generally thought least able to withstand loading and provide good initial stability, is most commonly seen in the posterior maxilla.

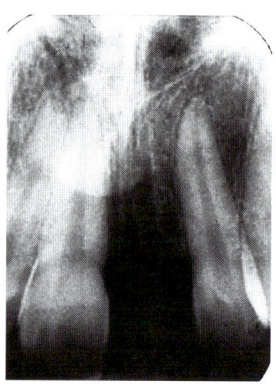

Fig. 4.21 'Open weave immature bone' in the lateral incisor site of tooth loss in a younger patient is unsuitable for implantation.

However, extremely dense, poorly vascularized bone may also be associated with poor integration.

Dental pantographic films (OPTs) provide useful initial evidence of the general status of the dentition and the relationship between alveolar bone or basal bone and key anatomical features that may preclude routine implantation, e.g. the inferior dental canal in the mandible and the maxillary antra. Also, although the image is magnified, an estimate can be made of the length of implants and the number that may be placed in an edentulous span to support a prosthesis (Fig. 4.20).

Intra-oral 'periapical' radiographs are especially useful for:

- examining the bony density (Fig. 4.21);
- assessing the available space in spans between adjacent tooth roots, especially in the anterior aspects of the jaws (Figs 4.22–4.24);
- determining the position of the surface of the alveolar ridge in comparison with that housing the natural teeth. Orthoradial projections are required for effective assessment.

Transverse images using tomographic or computerized techniques can show the cross-sectional form of the jaws and thus identify varying widths. This can confirm the adequacy of the bone to encompass dental implants, which may be selected from a typical range of diameters of 3–6 mm. Also, the outline form will

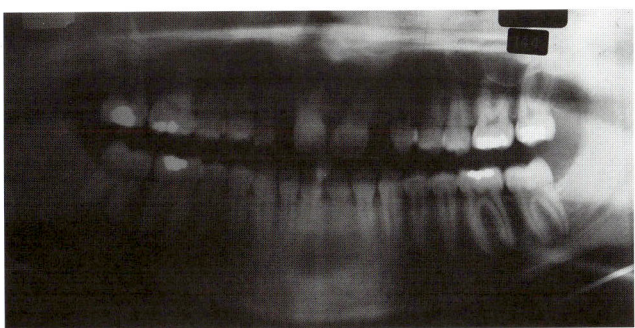

Fig. 4.22 The radiograph confirms a lack of interradicular space for the dental implants.

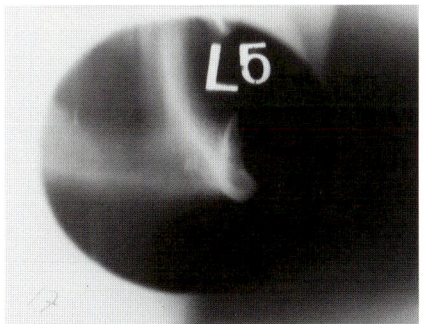

Fig. 4.25 A tomographic slice in the edentulous canine region shows an unfavourable narrowing of the mandible.

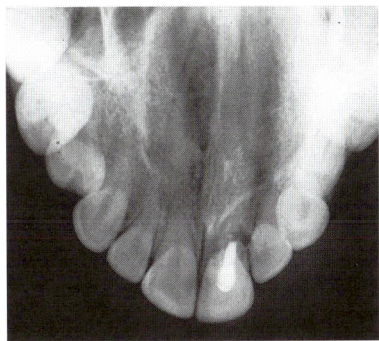

Fig. 4.23 An intra-oral anterior occlusal X-ray identifies potential space for an implant to replace a failing incisor tooth.

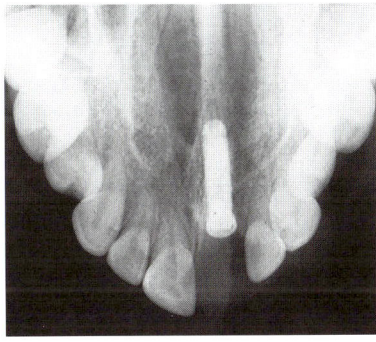

Fig. 4.24 The implant body in relation to the incisive canal.

indicate the direction of the surgical bony canal so as to avoid a dehiscence in placing an implant. If the film is recorded with a radio-opaque diagnostic prosthesis in situ, then the potential to achieve axial loading of the implant can also be judged. This will indicate the likelihood of significant cantilevering, where resorption has created a disparity between the alignment of the dental arch and the jaw.

The Scanora® unit, for example, first records a 'scout image', which confirms the correct positioning of the patient and the appropriate exposure values. The dental 'panorama', which focuses on the teeth and alveolus, has a magnification of 1.7. Dental images are usually recorded with an orthoradial projection. 'Maxillodental' programs create cross-sectional and lateral tomography with wide-angle spiral tomography. Layers of 2 mm or 4 mm are often selected. Cross-sectional images of the jaws will identify narrowing and concavities in the alveolus or body of the jaw and, for example, provide an opportunity for measuring the depth of bone that exists between the surface cortical layer and the inferior dental canal (Fig. 4.25).

Recent developments in data processing have increased the benefits from CT scanning of the jaws, where it is planned to undertake autogenous bone grafting in association with implant treatment. The increased levels of radiation are especially justified where successful implant restoration is dependent on the effective outcome of onlay and sinus infill procedures, segmental osteotomy or jaw resection and the prospective use of zygomatic implants.

A radio-opaque scanning template incorporating barium sulphate in the teeth, which will restore the arch, is prepared by a conventional 'denture duplication' technique of the 'diagnostic wax-up'. The patient wears this with the teeth in occlusion during scanning of the jaw that is to be treated. The resultant digital CT images may then be analysed on a PC using suitable software. A panoramic curve is drawn in the axial images and cross-sections perpendicular to the panoramic images are automatically constructed. Each image is cross-referenced to the others. Overall, the reformatted image of the jaw is related to the proposed reconstructed arch and the appropriate segments can be selected in relation to each intended tooth crown. Available size and patterns of implants are selected from a database, and each one is drawn and positioned appropriately in three dimensions within the jaw. Likewise, a suitable abutment can be chosen and the size of the prosthetic space identified. When 'virtual' planning is completed the data can be downloaded to a rapid process model machine.

A stereolithographic model of the jaw and/or a stereolithographic surgical guide can be prepared. The former represents an exact dimensional copy of the jaw to be operated upon (Fig. 4.26). The surgical template is designed to have a precise fit upon the jaw or residual teeth in the arch, and is constructed with cylindrical guides that correctly localize the drill used for preparing the bony canals which receive implants of matched size. The benefits of this technique may therefore extend beyond case planning, to assistance with surgical implantation (Fig. 4.27).

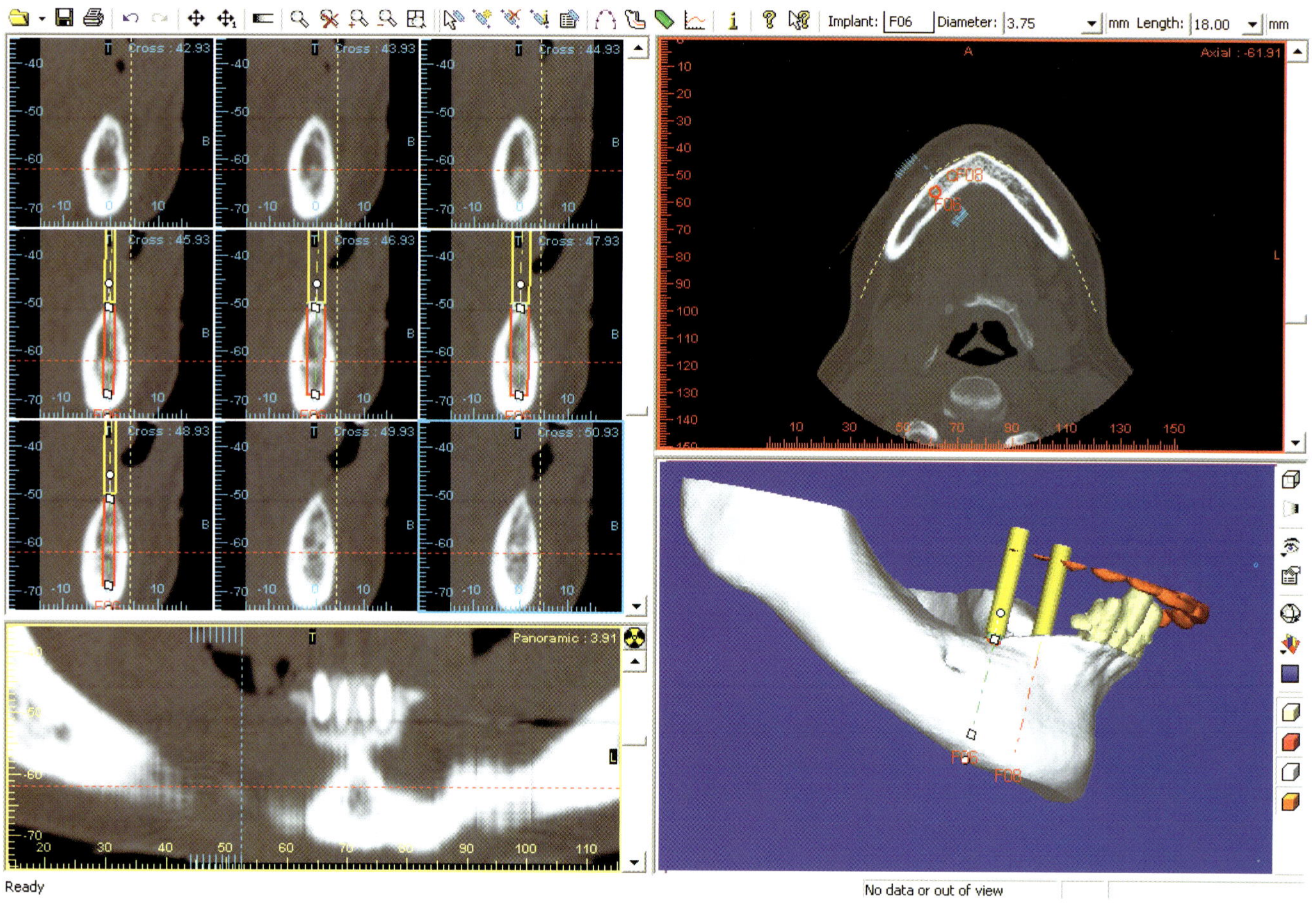

Fig. 4.26 Data from CT scan can provide information on the available volume of the jaw at sites selected for possible implantation. The intended position of the dental arch will assist in assessing the suitability of these sites. (Courtesy Image Diagnostic Technology)

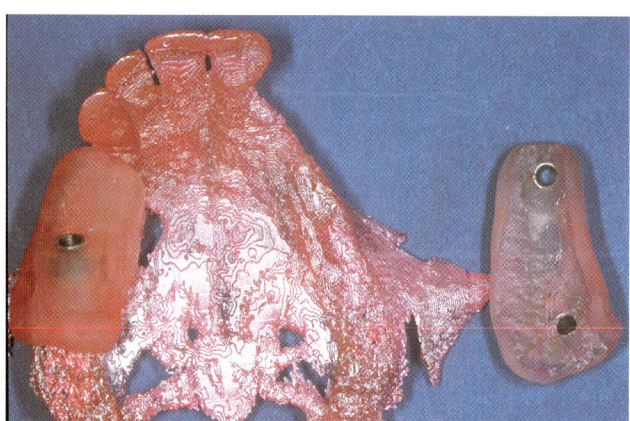

Fig. 4.27 A rapid process model produced from the data derived from a CT scan of the maxilla.

Such programs also allow prediction of bone densities at various sites in the jaws, and allow for the selection of implants with various surface characteristics, e.g. for 'soft bone' in advance of the operation.

In what ways may study casts contribute to decision making and treatment planning?

Well-made study casts, which represent the exact contours of the oral surfaces of the edentulous jaw(s) and residual dentition, should be prepared. It is normally necessary to articulate the casts to identify important details that affect the design of the proposed prostheses. These help in assessing potential space for positioning implants and components, as well as recognizing any problems associated with the relationship of the jaws and the existing or future occlusion of the dental arches.

Articulated casts enable a diagnostic wax-up or trial denture insertion to be prepared, which contributes to surgical planning, especially where computerized radiographic scanning, rapid process modelling and surgical templates (surgeon's guides) have not been produced by advanced data processing.

The patient will also benefit from seeing planned evidence. Any shortcomings in the likely appearance of the prosthesis or need for augmentation of the jaws are apparent, and less liable to lead to misunderstandings of proposed treatments and their predicted outcomes.

Although data processing with software exists that can simulate the implant position in relation to the restored arch, study casts may be used to incorporate replica abutments (Figs 4.28, 4.29). The dental technician can then identify preferred options or possible problems before the implants are inserted.

Study casts incorporating replica implants may also be produced from impressions immediately the

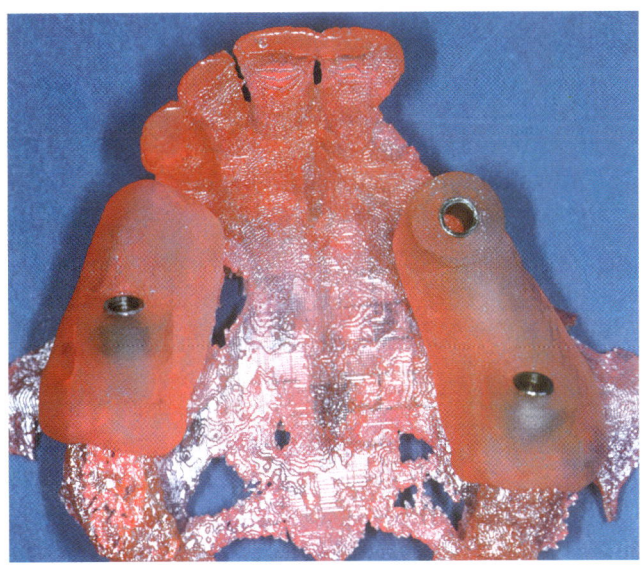

Fig. 4.28 Surgical guides for drilling the jawbone in the planned sites, including the pterygoid areas, fit exactly in position when the mucoperiosteal flaps are raised.

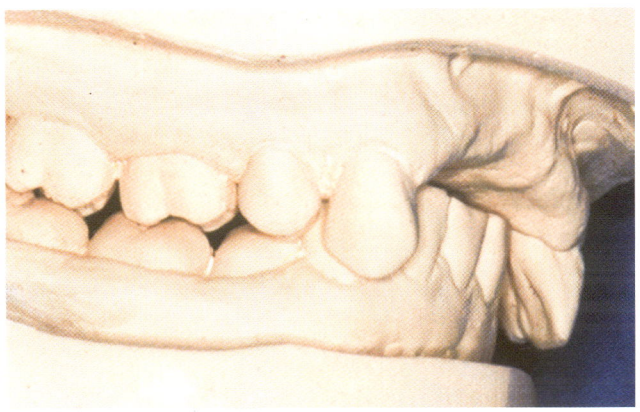

Fig. 4.29 Articulated study casts enable an assessment of potential positions for dental implants in the anterior maxilla.

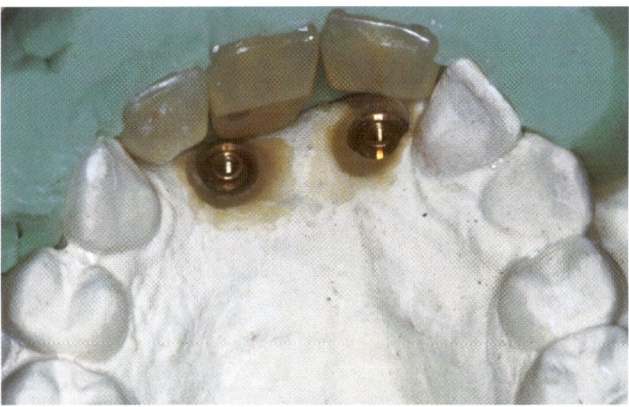

Fig. 4.30 Possible abutment sites in relation to the trial arch may be evaluated in the laboratory. The right implant would be better positioned under the central incisor, if the incisive canal does not conflict with it.

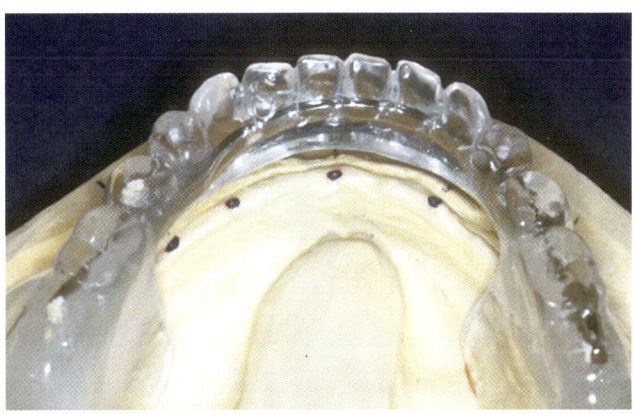

Fig. 4.31 A surgical template, positioned on the edentulous study casts, is produced by duplicating the trial denture. A wire reinforcement is necessary to prevent fracture. Greater stability is achieved in partially dentate arches when it is extended onto the adjacent teeth.

implant(s) is surgically positioned, or following exposure of the implant for abutment connection. Both diagnostic and transitional prostheses can then be prepared. The latter are usually constructed with a simple cast metal frame to which artificial acrylic teeth are attached. This may optimize the emergence profile of the prostheses and allow revision of the design before the final (definitive) restoration is made.

How may diagnostic wax-ups and trial dentures assist planning the treatment?

Diagnostic wax-ups and trial dentures are essential in preoperative planning. They are often of considerable benefit when prepared during the surgical phase, or immediately after the completion of surgery, in order to secure optimum functional and aesthetic outcomes from implant treatment.

These devices may be converted directly into surgical templates to assist the surgeon in correctly orienting the osteotomy in relation to the intended prosthesis. They may also be used to fabricate radio-opaque devices to provide suitable data from CT scanning, to enable the precise planning of both the surgical location of the implant and suitable abutments to support the intended prostheses. Such information will then be used in preparing rapid process models (e.g. stereolithographic) of the jaws and/or surgical templates that fit the jaw and adjacent teeth (Figs 4.30, 4.31).

Where partially dentate arches are to be restored, the diagnostic wax-up may be used to create a duplicate cast of the intended arch form, upon which a thermoformed template is moulded.

At the time of implant insertion an impression can be recorded with transfer impression copings so that a cast may be poured containing replica implants. Using appropriate components, a temporary acrylic resin single-tooth crown can be prepared and inserted immediately, or a short-span implant-supported bridge fitted within a few weeks, after soft-tissue healing. In either situation immediate loading would be avoided.

There is an essential difference between the wax-up for a fixed prostheses and a trial denture. The area to be covered by the base of a removable overdenture should be correctly produced in the dental cast and trial dentures. Hence the arch is supported by a flange. Conversely, in planning a fixed-implant prosthesis it may be more appropriate to have prepared the wax-up with anterior teeth gum fitted to the maxillary ridge, unless the crowns will obviously be excessively long (Fig. 4.11). In this case a decision must be made as to whether to change the level of the occlusal plane by reducing the incisor overbite (vertical overlap) or by recognizing the need for a short flange. This in turn will affect the choice of materials from which the prosthesis is to be constructed.

In what form should a surgical template be produced?

Surgical templates (guides) assist the operator in the appropriate placement of the dental implant to support the planned prosthesis. It is essential that the template should fit securely upon the residual arch or edentulous jaw and provide appropriate access to guide the drill in preparing the bony canals.

Traditionally templates have been manufactured in the dental laboratory. Recent changes now permit them to be commercially created by rapid process modelling using data from CT scanning. Where good clinical evidence and routine radiographs suggest that difficulties in positioning an implant are unlikely, a custom-made clear acrylic guide is appropriate. It is usually sufficient to represent the labial face of the restoration and for the surgeon to work within the long axis of both the tooth crown and below/above the template. (Fig. 5.9) Alternatively, direct vision and use of channels cut along the sagittal plane in the line of the arch will assist in precise location of the canal. However, difficulties arise if the study cast and radiograph are not correlated. The surgeon may find insufficient labial/buccal bone to encompass the implant, while if the directions of the adjacent natural roots have been insufficiently examined there may be a risk of damaging them. These difficulties may be minimized with suitable planning and an appropriate template as a guide.

What are the essential features of the treatment plan from the patient's and dentist's perspectives?

Formulation of a treatment plan usually takes place after a minimum of two assessments.

From the initial examination a basic understanding is gained of the patient's expectations in the context of their previous experience and need for dental treatment. This is evaluated against the principal features in the medical and social history and clinical examination.

The patient should understand whether it is appropriate to replace the missing teeth and, if so, the alternative means of doing so. Where implants are an option, the patient should understand the potential outcome of this treatment, e.g. whether there will be aesthetic or functional limitations, the prospects of failure and the likely maintenance requirements for the treatment.

The dentist must indicate whether it is technically possible to provide an implant prosthesis and whether it is desirable to do so. A simple discussion should make clear to the patient the risks, time, typical estimated costs and treatment required to achieve the result.

At this point it will often have become clear that alternatives to implants are more appropriate, such as:

- providing a conventional dental bridge;
- redesigning a removable prosthesis to achieve or assess the outcome more simply and at less cost.

Patients must also be made aware that many health schemes, such as the NHS in the UK, which provide treatment at no or limited cost to the patient at the point of delivery, do so only for specific priority categories that are not negotiable on behalf of the patient by the dentist.

Following a more detailed extra- and intra-oral examination, radiographic assessment and the production of study casts with or without a diagnostic trial prosthesis, the dentist may show the patient clinical photographs of results from similar cases and/or introduce a previous patient who is willing to share their experiences of this treatment. The patient will be aware whether a fixed or removable implant prosthesis has been proposed, with different expectations of function, aesthetic results, coverage of the oral tissues and maintenance. For example, initial adjustments and frequency of replacement of removable implant-stabilized complete overdenture may require more follow-up care in a given period than a fixed prosthesis.

The patient should agree to the proposed surgery for implantation being undertaken in one, two, or more phases where bone grafting etc. is proposed. The use of local anaesthesia with or without sedation or the use of general anaesthesia and admission to hospital where specialized care decrees it to be necessary must be explained.

Patients should understand that with few exceptions some periods of time are needed when an existing prosthesis cannot be worn immediately after implantation in order to allow healing and avoid immediate loading of an implant.

If further soft-tissue revision is needed to improve the emergence profile of the prosthesis or a transitional implant prosthesis is proposed in order to test or improve the outcome, then this must be explained.

Since all prostheses require monitoring and maintenance, the purpose and frequency should be discussed, together with cost implications. Routine dental radiography initially after fitting the prosthesis and at 1- or 2-year intervals will help to identify the response of the bone to loading, judged by the horizontal bone levels around each implant.

Clinical examination will judge the mechanical integrity of joints and the response of the peri-implant soft tissues and those acting in combination to support the prosthesis when a removable design is used. For example, the dentist may choose to place more implants in the posterior maxilla using patterns with an optimal surface area, since failure rates are known to be higher. Similarly, the dentist may advise the patient that the possible use of a removable prosthesis stabilized by fewer implants may become necessary, and that a subsequent surgical revision may not be feasible.

It is wise to provide the patient with a signed and agreed copy of the treatment plan and estimated costs of carrying out the work in order to minimize the risks of dispute and dissatisfaction with well-intentioned care.

FURTHER READING

Cawood J, Howell J 1998 A classification of edentulous jaws. Int J Oral and Maxillofac Surg 17: 232–236

Gröndahl K, Ekestubbe A, Gröndahl H-G, (eds) 1996 The Scanora multi-functional unit; spiral tomography with the Scanora unit. In: Radiography in oral endosseous prosthetics. Nobel Biocare A B, Göteborg Sweden pp11, 45

Lekholm U, Zarb G A 1985 Patient selection and preparation In: Tissue integrated prostheses, osseointegration in clinical dentistry. Brånemark P-I, Zarb G A, Albrektsson T (eds) Quintessence Publishing Company Inc. Chicago pp 199–209

Verstreken K, Van Cleynenbreugel J, Marchal G, Naert I, Suetens P, van Steenberghe D 1996 Computer-assisted planning of oral implant surgery: a three-dimensional approach. Int J Oral Maxillofac Implants 11 (6): 806–10

5 Basic implant surgery

INTRODUCTION

The main purpose of implant surgery is to establish anchorage for an implant so that a prosthesis may be most effectively secured in position. In some circumstances, surgical and restorative procedures will be carried out by the same operator, while in others a team of surgeon and prosthodontist will provide the overall clinical treatment. In either situation careful planning of the overall clinical treatment is essential if optimum results are to be obtained. Thorough preoperative planning is a key prerequisite for effective surgical placement. Good teamwork between the prosthodontist, surgeon and technician is essential to achievement of the desired results.

Previous chapters have dealt with the information gathering required for each patient; however those of particular significance to the surgical phase of treatment are considered here in more detail.

The traditional sequence of history, clinical examination, special tests, diagnosis, consideration of treatment options, preparation of a treatment plan, and delivery of care and review, has much to commend it.

INFORMATION REQUIRED AT THE SURGICAL STAGE

A detailed clinical examination should have been undertaken prior to surgery, any necessary special tests completed, a diagnosis made and a treatment plan prepared and agreed by the team, with the patient. This will also ensure that all involved understand the scheduling timetable. Speculative insertion of dental implants solely within a surgical context is to be condemned.

On the day of surgery all available information should be present at the operative area. This includes:

• Comprehensive documentation of past dental history.

• Special tests. These are almost invariably a prerequisite for the insertion of implants and the results should also be available on the day of surgery. These will include the appropriate radiographs for each individual case, which can range from periapical views to orthopantomographs and tomographic views.

• Mounted study casts. Study casts showing the diagnostic wax-up (Fig. 5.1), the intended final position of the teeth and a sterilized surgical stent or guide should be available for more complex cases. Where the situation is relatively straightforward, then only a surgeon's guide may be needed.

INFORMED CONSENT

Before any examination or treatment can begin it is essential that the patient has given informed consent. This requires the patient to have received an adequate explanation of the problems, the treatment alternatives and their advantages and disadvantages, and to have consented to the proposed plan. The patient should be fully aware of all possible complications, e.g. bleeding, infection and failure of integration. While written consent may not necessarily be informed consent, information provided in a written form may be more readily understood and can provide a more robust proof than purely verbal consent. For implant surgery all patients should give written consent, especially if general anaesthesia or sedation is to be administered. The medico-legal importance of accurate records cannot be overemphasized.

MANAGEMENT

The stages of surgical treatment in this chapter will be divided into three sections:

• pre-operative management;

• operative placement;

• postoperative management.

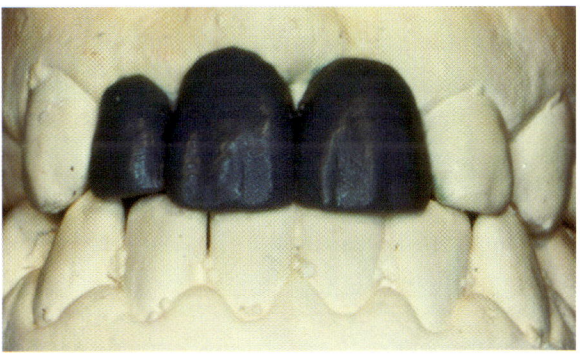

Fig. 5.1 Diagnostic wax-up of upper missing 12, 11 and 21 showing contours of final tooth positions.

Preoperative management

Patients receiving any surgical procedure must be medically, physically and psychologically able to undergo the demands of the procedure. The same rules apply to implant surgery as to other types of operation, where both absolute and relative contraindications to treatment may apply. Some medical and clinical situations, as well as chronic health problems, may present relative contraindications for implant surgery. However, as long as conventional precautions for these situations are fully considered during the surgical interventions, it may still be feasible to safely perform implant surgery.

Cardiovascular disorders

Hypertension

Pre- and postoperative monitoring is required, since increased blood pressure can result in a greater risk of postoperative bleeding. It should be noted that the patient taking antihypertensive drugs may be susceptible to hypertension when undergoing general anaesthesia.

Coronary artery disease

Patients suffering from recent infarctions, i.e. within the previous 6 months, should not have surgery. Patients with coronary artery disease and angina require careful monitoring of the amount of lignocaine and adrenaline administered. Glyceryl trinitrate tablets or sublingual spray should be readily available when undertaking the surgery in the case of patients with angina.

Infective endocarditis

As with all intra-oral surgical procedures, antibiotic cover will be necessary for patients who have:

- heart valve lesions;
- septal defects or a patent ductus arteriosus;
- prosthetic heart valves;
- a history of bacterial endocarditis.

No long-term studies have been reported on the relative risks of placing implants in patients with these conditions. A careful decision has to be made as to the risk–benefit ratio. There must be a very good reason why an implant is placed in these cases over any of the alternative treatment options for filling the space. Therefore, the patient should be fully aware of all the alternatives and the potential dangers of infective endocarditis in the placement of implants.

Anticoagulant therapy

Anticoagulant therapy may result in extended pre- and postoperative bleeding, as well as postoperative haematomas. For patients taking either heparin or warfarin following a thrombosis or cardiac surgery, the INR (international normal ratio) should be determined in the period immediately preceding surgery and be within a therapeutic range of 2.0–4.0. It should be less than 2.5 for safe surgery.

Psychological disorders

Patients with psychological disorders need to maintain their medication; however, this may interact with the anaesthesia required for the surgical procedure. Problems can also arise with patients with a drug abuse problem who may engage in non-therapeutic self-medication prior to surgery, which can give rise to pharmacological and handling problems. Full cooperation of the patient is essential, both at the time of surgery and subsequently if the outcome is to be optimum. While psychological problems are not in themselves an absolute contraindication to implant treatment, most clinicians experienced in this field have treated patients whose personality problems have subsequently given them cause to regret their original decision.

Smoking

It is well known in general surgery that smokers pose a higher risk of postoperative complications and poorer healing. This is also the case in dental implantology, where the patient who smokes tobacco is known to have a higher failure rate of individual implants of the order of 10%. In a smoker who has habitually smoked for a number of years it can be seen that the blood supply to the soft and bony tissues is much reduced, and that there are higher risks of postoperative infections. All health care workers have a role in helping patients to reduce or cease their smoking habit, and patients should be encouraged to stop smoking for at least 1 month prior to their implant surgery, and for at least 2 weeks postoperatively.

Diabetes

There is an increased risk of possible complications and reduced healing in the diabetic patient, and implant surgery should be avoided in the poorly controlled diabetic, although the condition is not in itself a contraindication to implant therapy.

Preoperative diets

As most implant treatment is carried out under local anaesthesia, patients should take normal meals before the procedure. If a meal has been missed then a glucose drink preoperatively may be necessary.

Local measures such as the use of a preoperative mouthwash of 0.2% chlorhexidine and peri-oral cleaning are also thought to be beneficial.

Antibiotic cover

The use of antibiotic cover for implant surgery has been proposed, as it is thought to reduce the incidence of

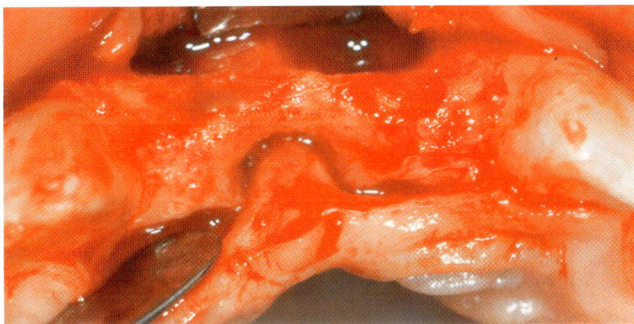

Fig. 5.2 Crestal incision showing local anatomy, including the large incisive canal.

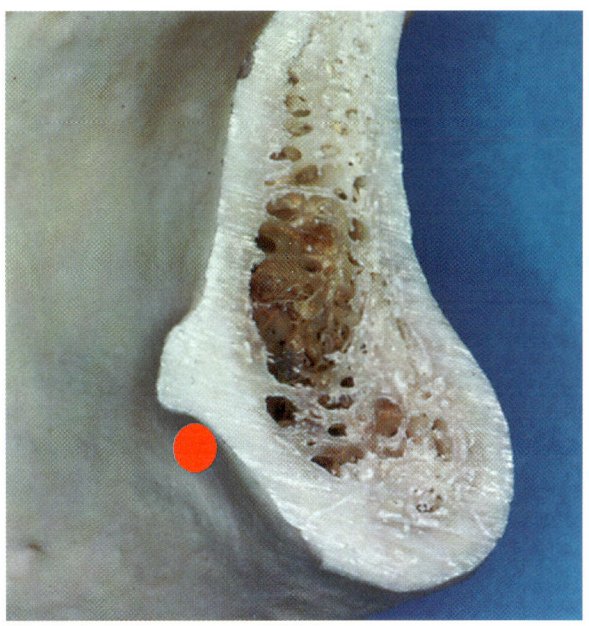

Fig. 5.3 Section through a cadaver mandible illustrating the position of the arteria submentalis.

postoperative problems. It is currently recommended that postoperative antibiotics, such as amoxicillin, be prescribed to decrease the risk of any infection.

Anatomical considerations

A detailed knowledge of the orofacial anatomy is necessary. This includes the following.

Maxilla

When planning the surgical procedure, a detailed knowledge of the region's anatomy, aided by appropriate radiographs, mounted study casts and diagnostic models, will enable the surgeon to form a view as to the lengths, diameters and orientations of implants suitable for insertion into the area. Following flap reflection, the goal in the posterior region of the jaw is to insert an implant so that it engages the cortical plate of the floor of the maxillary sinus, and anteriorly to engage the cortical plate of the nasal cavity. The object of this is to improve primary stability of the implant. This is not to say that implants must be inserted into the sinus or nasal floor, but to engage the walls of these structures. Anteriorly, careful reflection of the flap, together with radiographic evidence, will show the position of the nasopalatine canal and midline suture; it is important that the implants do not engage these (Fig. 5.2).

Mandible

Of particular concern in this region is avoidance of the mandibular canal and the need to ensure that implants do not penetrate the lateral or inferior aspects of the jaw, and thereby traumatize either the arteria submentalis (Fig. 5.3) and/or vena facialis. Concavities on the lingual aspect of the mandible may lead to perforations while drilling. Trauma to either of these significant sublingual vessels could result in postoperative bleeding, swelling and in some cases life-threatening situations.

Careful reflection of the flaps should reveal any concavities in the sublingual areas. In raising the flap care must be taken not to traumatize or damage the mental bundle. The use of sharp or metallic instruments around the nerve should be avoided so as to

minimize the risk of trauma. The incisal branch of the inferior alveolar nerve may extend from the mental foramen towards the incisal teeth and patients must be warned that if long implants are placed in this region trauma to the nerve may result in altered sensation associated with the lower incisor teeth. In the posterior region it is important to identify the position of the mylohyoid ridge. Careful palpation of the lingual aspect of the jaw may reveal a concavity below the mylohyoid ridge, as will tomographic views of this region. Implants placed in the posterior mandible are at risk of entering this region, which is highly vascularized, with resultant risks of haemorrhage.

Mandibular canal

It is imperative that the surgeon has a clear picture of the location of the inferior alveolar nerve, from either a long cone periapical radiograph or a tomographic view, typically a spiral tomograph or CT scan.

A clearance of at least 2 mm from the top of the inferior dental nerve should be allowed for to avoid the possibility of any surgical trauma.

Some authors have suggested that, in order to locate the nerve and select the appropriate implant length, the clinician should use a local anaesthetic infiltrated on the buccal and lingual aspects of the mandible. A pilot drill may then be slowly inserted inferiorly and medially drilling down towards the nerve until the patient feels a sensation. This will then indicate the appropriate length of the implant. This technique is definitely not supported by the authors owing to the high degree of risk of permanent damage to the mandibular bundle. The authors recommend that appropriate radiographs should be available, and a clear definition of the superior border of the nerve identified before any surgical procedure is undertaken

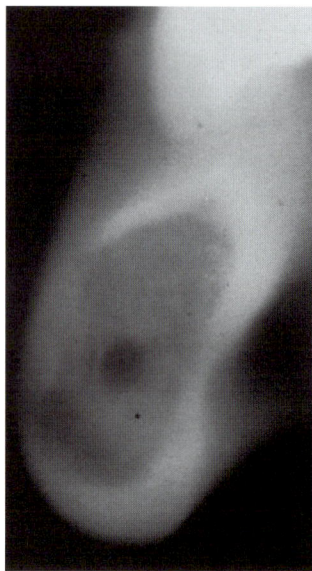

Fig. 5.4 Tomograph of the mandible, clearly showing the position of the mandibular canal and its relationship to the superior cortical bone.

(Fig. 5.4). Failure to identify the nerve and subsequent surgical trauma would leave the patient with anaesthesia or paraesthesia of the distribution of the mandibular nerve, a serious outcome for the patient which it would be difficult to defend.

Teeth

The positions, lengths and angulations of teeth adjacent to the implant site must be carefully evaluated. In any situation where teeth are involved near the proposed implant site, long cone periapical radiographs are the most appropriate choice. These will give the clinician guidance on both implant angulation and position. Failure to take appropriate radiographs may lead to the implant touching or penetrating the adjacent teeth, with possible damage to their root surfaces or apical tissues and loss of vitality, as well as an increased risk of implant failure.

Bone

Bone quality and volume are of key importance in implant success. This has been considered in previous chapters, and it is vital that this parameter is assessed both prior to and during implant placement.

At the time of surgical preparation the surgeon can gain some concept of the quality of the bone. For example, working in the anterior part of the mandible it may well be that the bone quality is of type 1 with very little cancellous bone, so that the surgeon may modify the surgical drilling technique so as to:

- avoid overheating the bone;
- ensure a less tight fit of the implant by using slightly larger drills before implant placement, or pre-tapping the site before insertion of the implant.

In areas where the bone quality is poor, e.g. the posterior part of the maxilla, the reverse may apply

and the surgeon in his drilling technique may use slightly smaller drills and avoid the necessity to tap the sites, relying on the implant engaging and compressing the bone to achieve primary stability.

In general, implants tend to be more successful when placed into better quality bone in terms of quantity and radiographic density.

When should implant surgery immediately follow tooth loss?

There has been some debate about the validity of placing implants in extraction sockets and a variety of approaches is adopted. It must be remembered that an important goal of implant placement is to achieve primary stability. This is achieved by close contact between the implant and the surrounding bone. It is therefore necessary that appropriate bone volume is available.

There are three options to the timing of placing implants following extraction of teeth:

- delayed implant placement to optimize bony healing;
- delayed implant placement for soft tissue healing;
- immediate implant placement.

Delayed placement to optimize bony healing

Historically, it was held that the most beneficial situation for the implant site was to allow a period of 3–4 months from tooth extraction to implant placement. Allowing full bone healing in this manner would, in theory, result in optimal bone volume and density.

Delay for soft tissue healing following extraction

Some authors believe it is not necessary to wait until there is complete bony healing and that a delay for soft tissue healing is sufficient. One month after tooth extraction is thought to be an appropriate interval. The two disadvantages of implant surgery at this early stage are the difficulty in reflecting a flap due to the thin, friable tissue and the difficulty in achieving primary stability of the implant body due to the lack of optimum bone volume and density.

Immediate placement at the time of extraction

Immediate implant placement has become more popular in the last few years and may be considered on the day of extraction. In order to ensure safe placement of implants the clinician should ensure that there is no evidence of peri-apical infection. Sufficient bone (5 mm is recommended) apical to the extraction site will permit primary implant stability and avoid endangering nearby structures such as the mandibular canal. Consideration should be given to the length of implants available for use, as longer devices may be required to gain primary stability in the apical bone while replacing the missing tooth. Immediate placement is much more appropriate for single-rooted teeth, and should be avoided when replacing multi-rooted teeth, due to the difficulty of obtaining adequate bone–implant contact and primary stability.

One- and two-stage surgery

There are two schools of thought as to whether implants should be inserted, covered and allowed to integrate for a period of 3–6 months (i.e., two-stage surgery) or left exposed at first-stage surgery (i.e., one-stage surgery). Most manufacturers now provide products that allow for either option.

While there are extensive data relating to the two-stage technique, which have shown very high success rates, the information relating to the single-stage technique is less extensive but suggests that in carefully controlled circumstances good results can be obtained, although possibly not as good as with the two-stage method. This is a rapidly evolving area; however, it is suggested that a cautious approach be adopted and that unless there are clear advantages to be gained from the one-stage technique the two-stage procedure should be used. This should also be the approach of choice where patient factors make the outcome less certain. In the case of immediate placement of the implant after extraction of a tooth, it may well be very difficult to achieve primary closure of the flap over the implant and a one-stage technique is preferred.

Surgical guide

Close collaboration with the prosthodontic members of the team will facilitate the preparation of a surgical stent/surgical guide using the diagnostic wax-up. This will help the surgeon to predict the position of the final prosthesis and facilitate correct placement of the implants. Most stents are made in self-curing acrylic resin and are based on the diagnostic wax-up or an existing prosthesis. Their function is to ensure that the implants are optimally placed. In some circumstances this is achieved by their rigidly defining the implant location, while in others they merely indicate the prosthetic envelope, which serves as a guide when placing the implant bodies. Recent developments in digital imaging offer the possibility of implant positions and superstructure design being determined using 3-D digital images, which can then be employed to fabricate proscriptive stents. There are numerous ways in which a stent can be constructed, the principles of which are that the device should be:

- rigid;
- capable of being sterilized;
- indicative of the final shape and form of the teeth to be replaced;
- well stabilized in the mouth.

Design of a surgical template/surgeon's guide

Surgical splints are used to assist in the optimum placement of the dental implants. They vary in the extent to which they are proscriptive; some can define the exact position of the implant, while others indicate the prosthetic envelope and by implication the range of acceptable implant positions from the restorative viewpoint. Their design will depend on both surgical and restorative criteria, since both must be satisfied if the treatment is to be successful.

From the outset it must be known whether the superstructure will be screw or cement retained. If it is a screw-retained prosthesis, especially in the anterior part of the mouth, then the access holes for the screws will need to emerge on the palatal aspects of the teeth. With a cement-retained prosthesis, the projection of the long axis of the implant may transfix the incisal tip of the crown or even its labial aspect without any risk of this affecting the appearance of the prosthesis.

Proscriptive design

A proscriptive splint design has an enclosed form with holes through the cingulum or occlusal surfaces of the tooth forms, which define the implant location by directing the drill into the bone. By incorporating a stop it can also control the drilling depth and hence extent of implant insertion. The disadvantage of this type of splint is that is allows no leeway for changing the direction of the drilling sequence if at surgical placement there appears to be some anatomical deviation from that suggested by preoperative clinical examination and radiographs. For example, an alteration in the direction of the drill to engage more palatal bone and still exit through the occlusal surface is more difficult. With all proscriptive designs the type of restoration will influence the degree of flexibility. There may be more freedom in an edentulous patient than one who has many teeth remaining. In situations where there are teeth present the splint may be more accurately located by being extended onto the adjacent teeth. Unfortunately, when using proscriptive stents in an edentulous patient, whether in the maxilla or mandible, it is extremely difficult to keep the reflected flap away from the surgical site if the splints are well extended. It can also be difficult to stabilize the splint within the surgical area. It is therefore probably better for edentulous cases to consider a less proscriptive design.

Freeform designs

This popular design embodies an arch form on a base in which the palatal aspect of the tooth forms has been cut away and thus only retains the outlines of the buccal faces of the final tooth positions. This will then permit surgical exposure of the bony site and allow for a change in direction of the drilling sequence, provided that the projection of the long axis of the implant does not penetrate the labial face of the final prosthesis. While such an eventuality can be managed

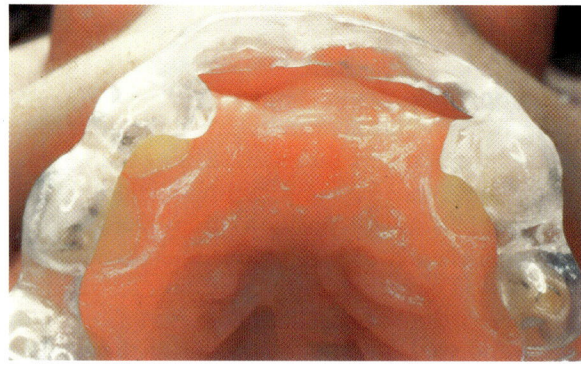

Fig. 5.5 This slide shows a performed surgical guide outlining the incisal edge and buccal contours of the missing upper three incisors.

Box 5.1 The prerequisites for surgery

- Preoperative study casts
- Diagnostic wax-up
- Surgical stent
- Appropriate radiographs
- Sterile surgical field
- Drilling unit with controlled speed and variable torque

---

with an angled abutment, this is not always possible and can create problems when designing the prosthesis. Some authors have suggested the use of a rigid splint with a palatal outline, but unfortunately this tends to impede the insertion of an implant on the more palatal aspect of the edentulous ridge.

OPERATIVE PLACEMENT
Operating conditions

Implant surgery should be performed under sterile conditions, and can be carried out in the general dental clinic, as long as the operating area is simple in design, uncluttered and easy to clean. There should be adequate illumination of the surgical field, with the use of a headlight when working in the maxilla and shadowed areas. High-volume suction should be available, and the radiographic viewer placed so as to be easily seen by the surgical team and without the surgeon having to move from the patient.

Local anaesthetic drugs

The gold standard for implant surgery is 2% lignocaine and (1:80 000) adrenaline (epinephrine). The maximum dose of this in a healthy patient is 4.4 mg per kg body weight. In patients with unstable coronary artery disease the use of prilocaine-phenylpressine may be required. The maximum dose of this drug should not exceed five cartridges. Bupivacaine, a long-acting local anaesthetic, may be used in a concentration of 0.5% with adrenaline (epinephrine) 1:200 000 to provide longer duration of anaesthesia for 6–8

hours when given as a nerve block. This is sometimes useful to decrease the amount of postoperative discomfort. The maximum dose is 1.3 mg per kg body weight.

Local anaesthesia with sedation

Sedation may be oral or intravenous. For the extremely nervous patient oral temazepam can be very effective, either in tablet form at a dosage of 10–20 mg preoperatively or as an elixir 10 mg/5 ml. This will decrease the anxiety of the nervous patient; however, for longer procedures it may be prudent to use intravenous sedation, although this would require the assistance of an anaesthetist, who would manage the patient's level of consciousness and respiratory and circulatory states, and a dental nurse with appropriate training. It is important to note that all patients will require an escort to accompany them home from the surgery.

The surgical team

The team should ideally consist of four people: the surgeon and their assistant, a second assistant and, where relevant, the anaesthetist. The fundamentals of an aseptic technique should be adhered to at all times, and both the surgeon and the surgical assistant should be correctly scrubbed and gowned throughout the procedure. They should remain in a sterile state at all times during surgery, while the second assistant, who does not scrub up, dispenses components and other items required during the operation.

Preparation of the patient

The final decision on suitable sedation and anaesthesia should be based on both the patient's individual requirements and the degree of surgical intervention.

Patient preparation prior to surgery

- Ensure that the patient fully understands the surgical treatment.
- Confirm that informed consent for the procedure has been given and is documented.
- Discuss postoperative care with the patient and carer, if present. This is especially important if sedation is to be used.
- Ask the patient to use an intra-oral mouthwash of 0.2% chlorhexidine, which should also be used to prepare the area around the mouth. This will decrease bacterial contamination.
- Administer local anaesthetic and sedation as required.
- Where a separate room is being used for surgery then this should already have been prepared and the patient may now be brought in.
- Provide the patient with a head cover and protective glasses.

Box 5.2 Reasons for failed integration

- Poor surgical site
- Inexperienced operator
- Failure to achieve primary stability
- Early loading
- Poor surgical technique
- Infection
- Heavy tobacco-smoking habit

- Apply sterile draping with a complete or upper body drape.
- The surgeon should now scrub- and gown-up.
- Ensure that there is good illumination of the operative site.

Instrumentation

As with all surgical procedures the surgeon should have the necessary surgical instrumentation which will allow for all eventualities during surgery, including a range of implant bodies. In most cases this may well be a personal decision on the part of the surgeon and assistant, who must be familiar with the instrumentation available and the appropriate requirements for each case.

Principles of incision design

The site, size and form of the incision should be planned to give the best possible access and ensure the least damage to important structures. This will also ensure good wound closure, minimize the risk of any possible nerve damage, and aid the visualization of defects, concavities and perforations.

Flap reflection is usually best done with a periosteal elevator or Mitchell's trimmer, avoiding tearing the flap.

An incision should:

- provide good access and visibility of the operative site;
- provide flexibility in positioning the surgical guide;
- allow identification of important anatomical landmarks, e.g. the mental foramina and incisal canal;
- facilitate the identification of the contours of the adjacent teeth, and concavities or protrusions on the surface of the bone;
- have clean edges, which will facilitate primary closure and optimize healing by primary intention;
- permit the raising of a full mucoperiosteal flap, ensuring that it has a good vascular supply;
- minimize scarring and avoid vestibular flattening.

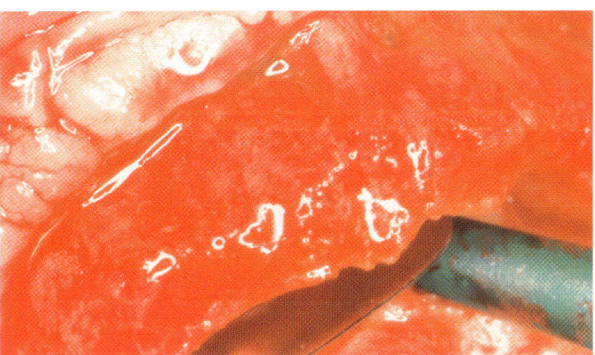

Fig. 5.6 A reflected flap, following crestal incision in the maxilla, showing the crestal ridge in the midline and buccal concavities.

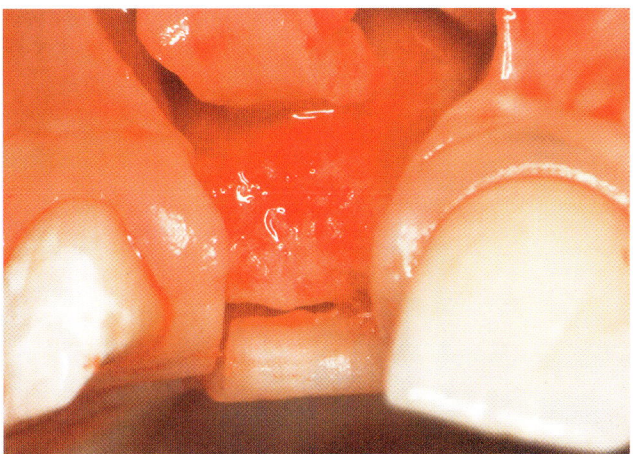

Fig. 5.7 A modified flap preserving the papillae of the teeth adjacent to the surgical site.

Maxilla

Crestal incision

This may be with or without a relieving incision. A relieving incision will:

- provide the surgeon with increased visibility. This is particularly important when concavities are present on the buccal aspect of the ridge (see Fig. 5.6);
- allow for good access for the surgical stent;
- result in less scarring;
- avoid vestibular reduction as a result of scar formation.

Vestibular incision

This incision was previously the standard procedure for two-stage implant placement, ensuring that the implant was completely covered and protected during the healing phase. It is also claimed to provide a superior vascular supply.

Originally, it was thought with all implant surgery that the incision line should be made away from the implant site itself. The advantage of this was supposedly that there would be no contamination of the implant from the oral environment and that the

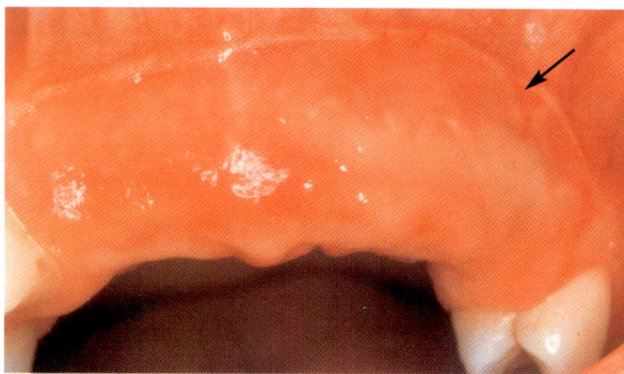

Fig. 5.8 Scarring from a buccal incision; a flap design previously recommended for implant surgery.

incision site was distant to the implant. Since then comparative studies between crestal and vestibular incisions have shown little difference in the outcome of both incisions.

Previously a horizontal mattress suture was the method of choice for replacing the flap; however, the disadvantages of this technique were that it caused vestibular flattening and increased scarring (Fig. 5.8). Vestibular flattening made it difficult to insert the denture after implant placement, unless extensive reduction of the buccal flanges of the denture was carried out. Failure to reduce these sufficiently resulted in the wound being opened.

Mandible

Crestal incision

This gives the same advantages as in the maxilla. A careful blunt dissection is required to identify the mental neurovascular bundle, and it is important to expose the mental foramina to identify any anterior loop. Tissue separation with a blunt instrument will show if the inferior alveolar nerve is approaching the mental foramen from a distal or a mesial direction, and should confirm what is already visible on the radiographs.

The use of metal instruments when reflecting the mucoperiosteal flap near the mental foramina should be avoided; reflection is better carried out with a damp piece of gauze.

Preparation of the implant site

General principles

The aim of the procedure is to provide close approximation of the bone to the implant surface, and to achieve primary stability to prevent micro-movement of the implant and minimize the risk of failure of integration.

The production of excessive heat, which can cause osteocyte death, may be minimized by the use of sharp burs, an intermittent drilling technique, and profuse use of saline irrigation. The drilling technique is extremely important, especially when working in

dense bone, for example the symphyseal region of the mandible.

Drilling equipment

Most implant systems provide a drilling unit with variable speed and torque settings, however, drilling units are available that are not device specific.

The osteotomy site is generally prepared at 2000 rpm to prevent overheating. Following preparation of the site, the insertion of the implant and/or tapping of the site are carried out at about 25 rpm and a torque limit of up to 40 N cm, depending on bone density.

Basic instrumentation

- surgical drapes;
- surgical hoses;
- dental explorer;
- dental mirror;
- scalpel;
- needle holders for suture material;
- various retractors;
- gauze.

A saline coolant must be delivered using an internal/external technique or both.

Drill sequence

The flap is next raised, and the surgical guide positioned (Fig. 5.9). A sterile surgical pencil can be used to mark the position and direction of the implants on the bone (Fig. 5.10).

The initial site is then prepared with a small rose-head bur (Fig. 5.11, and 5.12).

Irrigation: internal or external

The purposes of irrigation are to:

- prevent a rise in the temperature of the drill bits, which then overheats the bone;
- continually wash away bone chips and keep the drill bits clear of debris.

Manufacturers supply various drilling systems with the facility to provide either internal or external irrigation, or both, to the operative site. Both systems used appropriately will provide adequate cooling.

Generally, most implant systems will provide the surgeon with a range of drills, which allows for gradual enlargement of the osteotomy site, correct orientation of the implant and prevention of overheating and over-preparation of the site (Figs 5.13, 5.14). Drills vary in length and diameter, corresponding to the dimensions of the implants. The diameter of the last drill to be used is generally slightly smaller than that of the implant. This provides for good initial stability of the fixture. In very dense bone it may be necessary to tap the bone to ensure ease of implant insertion. Forcing an implant into a tight-fitting osteotomy can result in

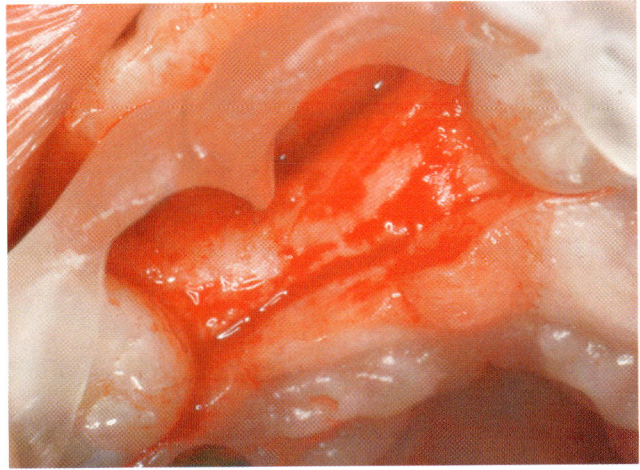

Fig. 5.9 Following raising of the flap the surgical guide is placed in position.

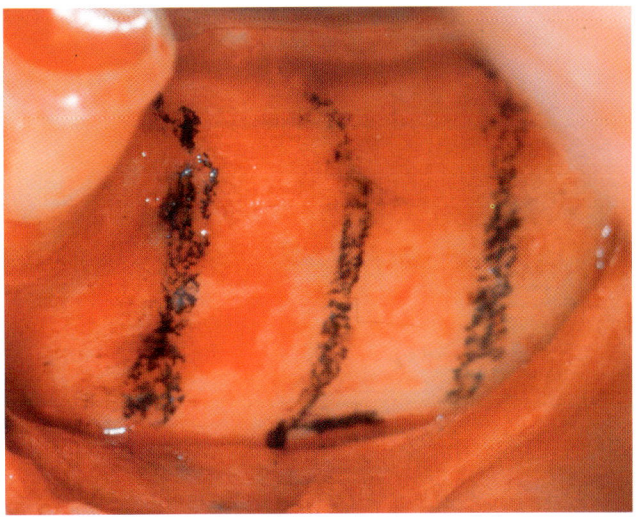

Fig. 5.10 A sterile pencil may be used to mark the position of the proposed implant site and direction. The horizontal outline marks the upper border of the mental foramen.

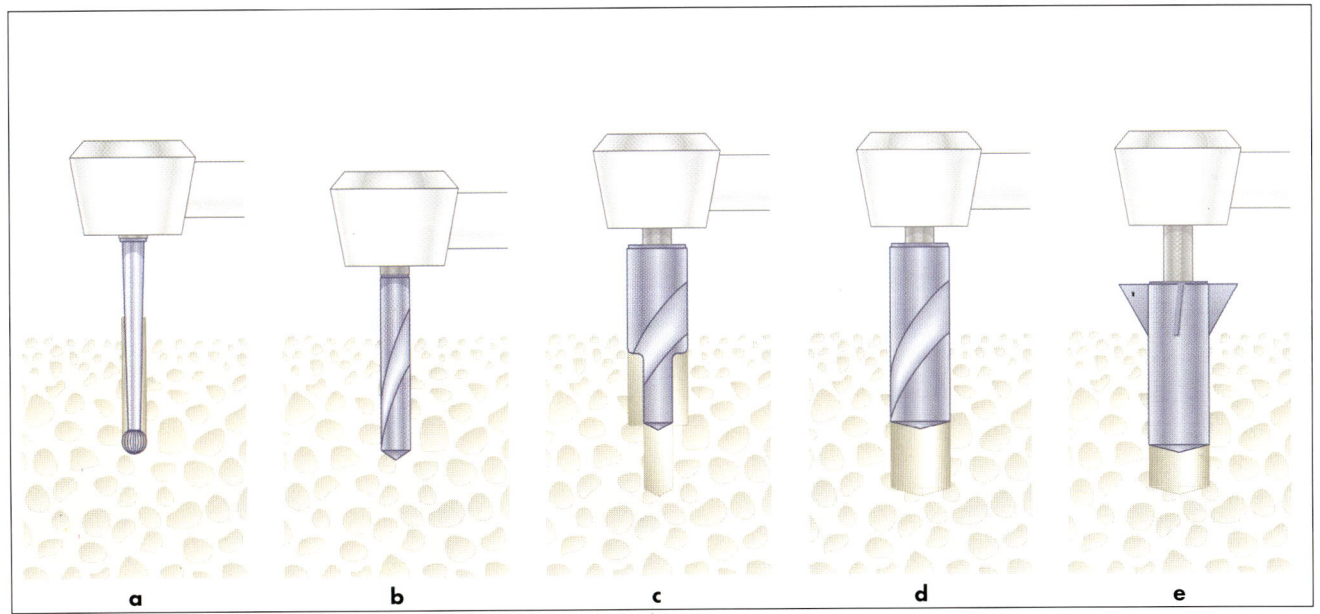

Fig. 5.11 Diagrams showing drilling sequence using initial drills at speeds of 2000 rpm. **a** Initial guide drill is used to start hole. **b** 2 mm drill is drilled to the full depth of the site. **c** Pilot drill is used to enlarge the site from 2 mm to 3 mm. **d** 3 mm drill is used to complete the preparation to the full depth. **e** Final drilling at 2000 rpm; a countersink drill is used.

excessive heat generation, failure to fully seat the implant and bone fracture.

As a general recommendation, whenever possible implants should be inserted in such a way that they engage two cortical plates to facilitate better primary anchorage of the implant. This is normally achieved by engaging the plates in the coronal and apical regions; however, buccal and lingual plates can also be used. This is particularly the case when working above the inferior dental nerve, where engagement of the inferior border of the mandible could be very hazardous.

In the maxilla it is often possible to establish bicortical stability using the sinus or nasal floor. Note that only the apical tip of the implant should engage the cortical plate.

Abutment selection

While abutments may be selected at the time of implant insertion, which can have logistic advantages, this is better done after second-stage surgery, either in the laboratory using a cast prepared from a fixture head impression or by direct measurement at the chairside.

Implant registration at surgery

The aim of implant registration at the time of implant placement is to record the position of the fixture so that, when using a two-stage technique, a temporary crown may be placed at second-stage surgery. The

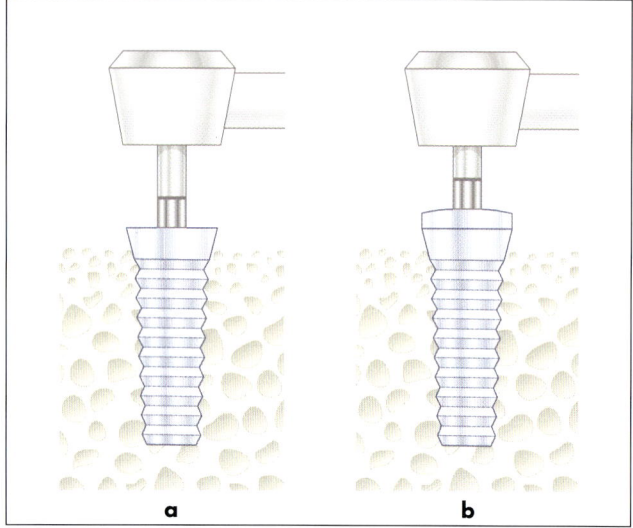

Fig. 5.12 a The implant is inserted at 25 rpm. **b** The final cover screw is placed in position.

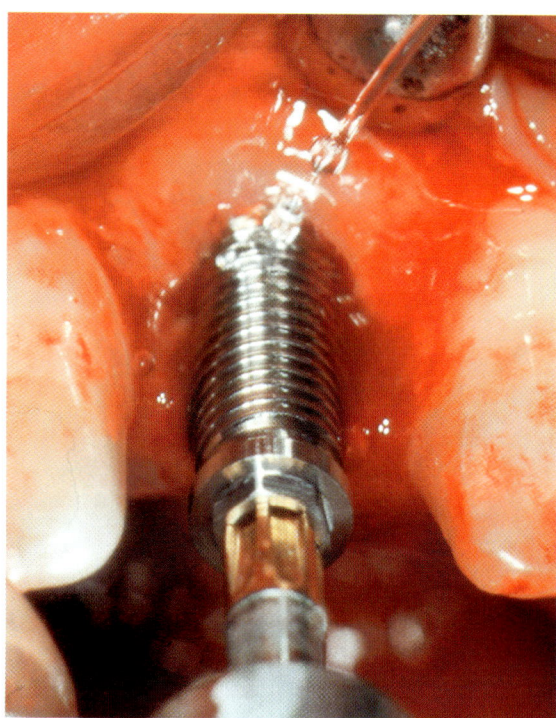

Fig. 5.14 An implant is placed in position with adequate external irrigation.

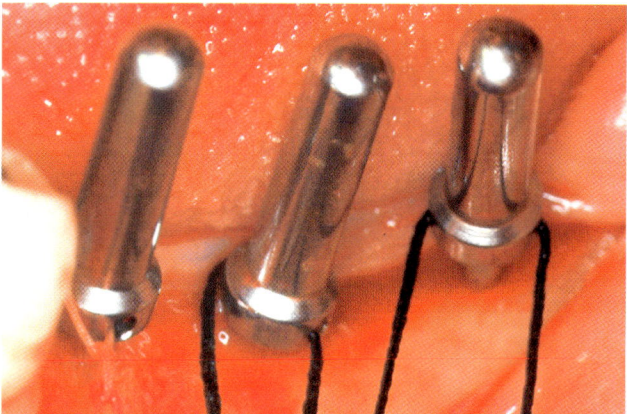

Fig. 5.13 Following initial drilling with the 2 mm twist drill, the direction indicators are placed in situ, with floss or suture material, to guide the surgeon through further site preparation.

Box 5.3 Surgical preparation

- Elevation of a full mucoperiosteal flap
- Placement of surgical stent
- Preparation of implant site
- Placement of implant
- Placement of cover screw or healing abutment
- Wound closure
- Adjustment and replacement of temporary prosthesis

Box 5.4 To minimize thermal injury to bone

- Intermittent drilling technique
- Copious irrigation
- Fresh, sharp drills
- Controlled cutting speeds

---

procedure may also sometimes be employed when making partial and complete fixed prostheses.

Advantages include decreasing the waiting time for the placing of temporary restorations (temporization) and greater potential for soft tissue contouring. The principal disadvantage is the commitment to laboratory work prior to knowing whether the implant has become integrated.

The procedure involves recording the relationship of the implant body to the adjacent dental arch. This is done once the implant is in place, but before cover screw placement, by placing an implant body impression coping on the implant, and then linking it to the surgical stent using either autopolymerizing or light-cured acrylic resin. A shade is also required and can be recorded at a prior stage of treatment. The laboratory will then use the record to cut a recess in the working cast. A replica implant is then mounted on the impression coping, the stent positioned on the cast, and the replica implant secured in position in the prepared recess using dental stone. This cast may then

be mounted on an articulator, using previous clinical records, so that a temporary crown may be made for insertion at second-stage surgery. This may be placed either directly on the implant or on a transmucosal abutment, which will, however, have to be selected at the time of implant placement. Should the result be unsuitable, then the crown would have to be remade.

Immediate loading

The aim of immediate loading is effectively to provide the patient with teeth on the day of surgery. The authors recommend caution when considering this technique, as some methods require surgical and

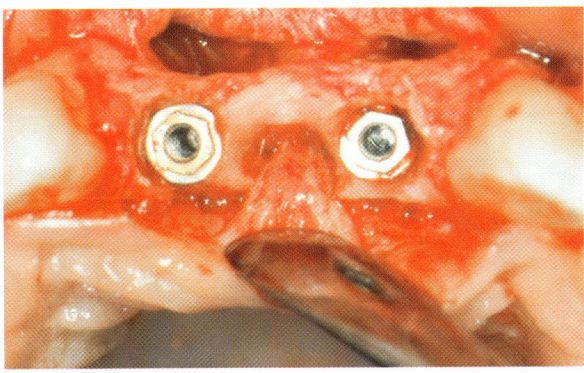

Fig. 5.15 Narrow implants placed in a thin ridge in the maxilla.

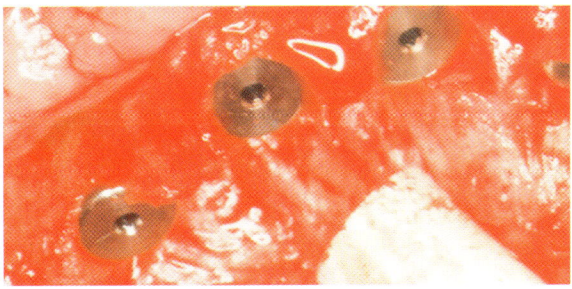

Fig. 5.17 Cover screws are placed on the implants to prevent ingrowth of soft tissue and bone while integration takes place.

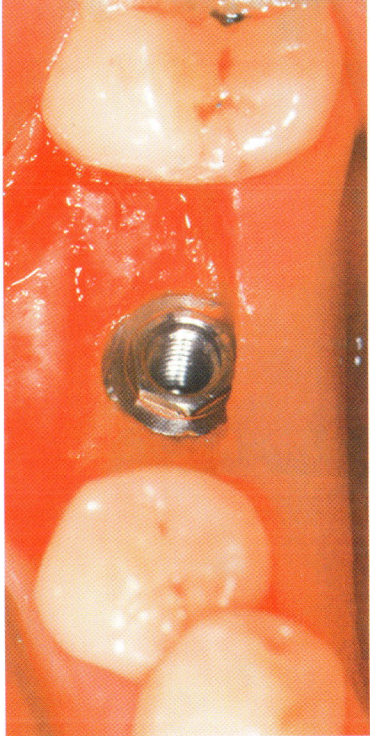

Fig. 5.16 A wide platform implant may be used for molar replacement.

restorative compromises, and may be associated with higher failure rates. This method may be considered in specific cases, such as the anterior mandible, which normally has a good quantity and quality of bone. Use in a single-tooth case may also be considered; however, it is extremely important to avoid any functional loading of the temporary crown in all mandibular movements. Patients demanding this technique should be made aware of the possibly of a higher than normal failure rate.

Augmentation of soft tissue and hard tissue at the time of surgical placement

While bone defects or exposed threads around the implant after insertion should be avoided, the bone anatomy and required implant location sometimes make these inevitable. In these circumstances the defect can be restored in a number of ways at the time of implant placement. These include the following:

- Autogenous bone grafting: this can be harvested at the time of drilling using a bone-collecting device on the suction line, or by removing bone from the drill bits manually. It can then be packed around the exposed implant threads and the flap replaced. Some clinicians recommend covering the graft with a resorbable or non-resorbable guided tissue membrane, to maintain the contour and reduce the ingrowth of fibrous connective tissue while healing occurs. These are available made from synthetic and natural materials such as expanded PTFE and collagen.

- Use of an allograft, such as freeze-dried demineralized bone: there are several products of this type available based on either human or bovine extracts. This material may be used to supplement an autograft; however, patients must be fully informed of the possibility of this procedure at the time they give consent to the treatment. Both auto- and allografts have been shown to be successful with or without membranes.

- Use of a block autograft, composed of cortical and cancellous bone: these are less easy to harvest due to the restricted number of donor sites; the anterior region of the mandible apical to the incisor teeth is sometimes used, and they are sometimes used to overlay a narrow alveolar ridge buccally and/or lingually.

Soft tissue augmentation may also be carried out if necessary at this stage, by using an interpositional connective tissue graft, which may be harvested from the palatal tissue.

Extensive bone grafting

Where there is a massive bone deficit then more extensive augmentation procedures may be necessary. These can involve the use of large bone grafts, and reconstruction using titanium mesh trays containing autograft or allograft material. The detailed use of these is beyond the scope of this book.

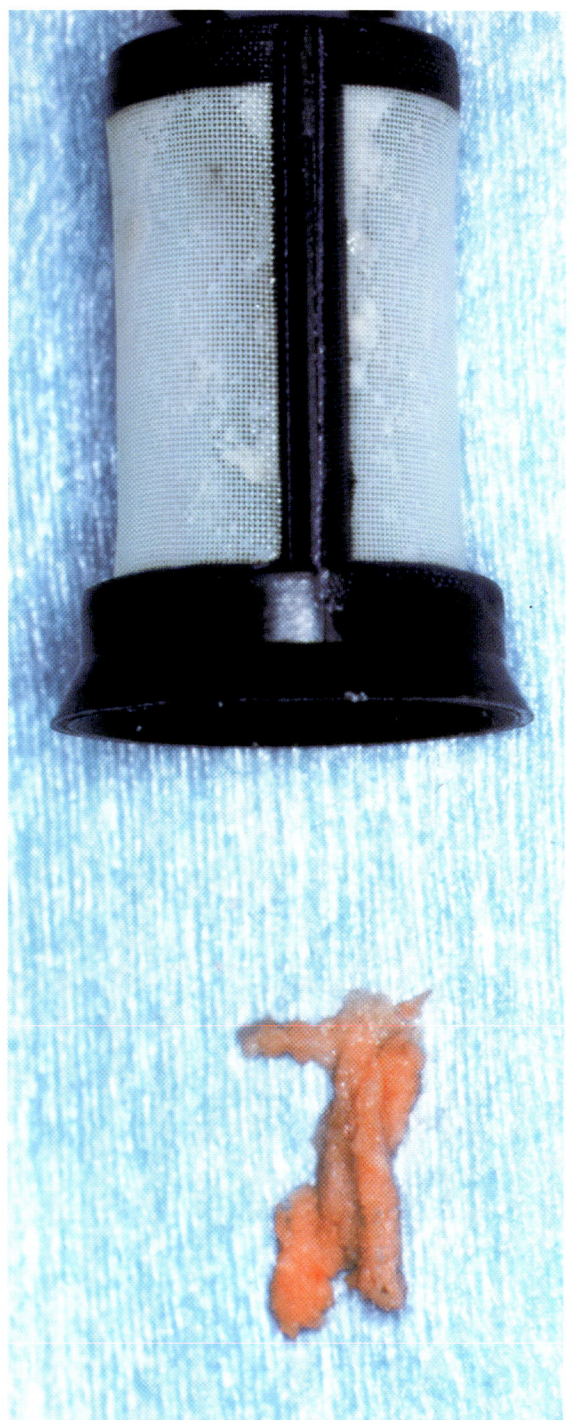

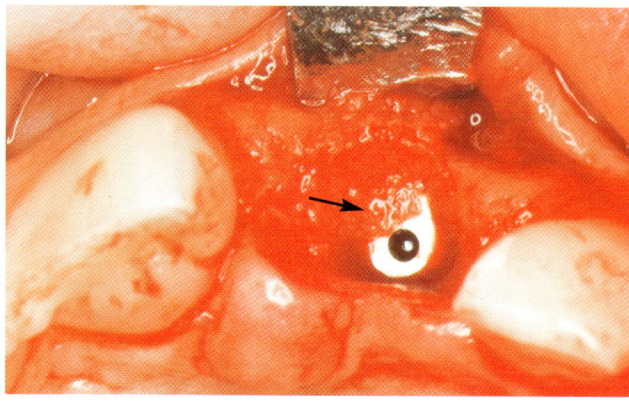

Fig. 5.19 Using bone collected from the bone trap the implant site is augmented to provide better soft tissue support and cover any exposed implant threads.

Box 5.5 Grafting material

What are the important properties?
- Sterile
- Non-toxic
- Non-antigenic
- Biocompatible
- Osseoconductive
- Osseoinductive
- Easy to use

What are the sources of autogenous bone grafts?

INTRA-ORAL
- From the drilling site
- Local to the implant sites
- From the mandible anterior to the premolars
- The retromolar region of the mandible

EXTRA-ORAL
- From the iliac crest
- From the cranium
- From the radius for maxillomandibular reconstruction

- Advise the patient of possible transient paraesthesia of the mental nerve where implants have been placed in the mandible.
- Insertion of the denture is recommended straight after surgery if the surgical technique has been planned using a crestal incision.
- Insertion of the denture is not recommended after surgery when using a vestibular incision and a vertical mattress suturing technique.
- Postoperative Corsodyl mouthwash is recommended to be used twice daily to assist in plaque control and reduce the risks of postoperative infection.
- A long-acting local anaesthetic should be considered, such as bupivacaine.
- Patients wearing dentures should be recommended to keep them in overnight to decrease post operative swelling.

Fig. 5.18 Using a bone trap during preparation of the implant site autogenous bone is collected and may be used for augmentation if necessary.

POST-OPERATIVE CARE
Wound management

This may include some or all of the following procedures:
- Warn the patient of swelling and bruising.
- Pressure or ice packs can be useful to control the above.
- Consider prescribing analgesics as necessary.

- It is recommended that the patient sleeps the first night after surgery slightly raised using an extra pillow, which decreases the possibility of more postoperative swelling.

Postoperative haemorrhage

This is best avoided by a careful history and examination and a thorough surgical technique. Petechial haemorrhages (purpurea) and bruising are typical of generalized vascular damage. If there is any suspicion of such disorders either as a finding in the medical history or as a result of a subsequent clinical observation then a haematological investigation should be considered. Similarly clotting disorders should be identified prior to surgery. Postoperative bleeding is usually controlled by pressure applied via a gauze pad. If not, then more extensive measures using standard surgical protocols may be needed.

Postoperative analgesia

This is best managed by the prescription of analgesic drugs with an anti-inflammatory action such as ibuprofen. If these are contraindicated then paracetamol may be used.

One-week review

At 1-week review the suture may be removed if not resorbable and the surgical site inspected; the denture, if present, may be adjusted.

SINUS LIFT/ELEVATION PROCEDURES

The maxillary posterior quadrant poses special challenges to the successful use of implant prostheses. Loss of alveolar ridge, particularly where there has been pneumatization of the edentulous posterior maxilla, means that there is frequently a lack of bone height for implant placement. This problem can often be managed by surgically augmenting the maxillary sinus floor. In the classic approach access to the sinus is gained via a bony window created in its buccal wall.

Contraindications

- There must be no sinus pathology.
- Patients with acute sinusitis.
- Tobacco smokers.
- Patients with an excessive inter-arch distance.

Careful radiographic analysis will indicate the proposed crown to implant ratio of the prosthesis, and the optimum length of implant that is to be supported in the implanted bone after the floor of the maxillary sinus has been elevated. The procedure can be carried out under local anaesthesia. Good access is obtained through a wide-based soft tissue flap; usually the sinus wall is thin and can be seen as a bluish-grey bony surface. Using a large rose-head burr and copious saline spray, a window can be gently removed in the bone, care being taken not to perforate the underlying sinus membrane. The inferior and lateral cuts are carried completely through the bone, while the superior cut should only partially perforate the bone to create a trapdoor effect, with the superior aspect acting as a hinge. Once the cuts are completed it is possible to move the window upward with gentle pressure. This effect will gradually elevate the sinus membrane, which should be gently lifted off the surrounding bone. It is important to keep the sinus membrane intact throughout the procedure; perforation is difficult to repair but may sometimes be accomplished with collagen strips. Elevation is continued until the desired size of void has been created.

GRAFT MATERIALS

At present there are four principal categories of material used to augment the bone which will form the floor of the maxillary sinus:

- intra-oral or extra-oral autographs;
- allografts;
- xenografts;
- alloplastic graft material;
- a combination of the above.

The intra-oral or extra-oral autogenous bone graft is readily available and is the first choice of bone grafting material for many clinicians. However, patient acceptance of autogenous bone grafting may be low, depending on the site of collection. The main advantages of autogenous bone graft are:

- biocompatibility;
- sterility;
- availability;
- osseoinductive and conductive potential.

The grafts act as a scaffold for the ingrowth of blood vessels and are a source of osteoprogenitor cells and bone-inducing molecules. The graft is eventually resorbed as part of the normal turnover of bone. The intra-oral donor sites are either the intraforaminal or retromolar regions of the mandible, depending on the volume of bone required. The latter site can provide good-size grafts of high-density bone. Careful radiographic assessment of the region is important in order to ascertain the amount of bone available. Once the mucoperiosteal flap has been raised by a sulcular incision, grafts may be taken as block specimens using a small trephine. Great care is needed in order to avoid compromising the blood and nerve supply to the anterior teeth when using this region of the jaw. Other materials can perform satisfactorily; however, the gold standard of bone grafting remains autogenous bone. There are, nevertheless, limitations on the amount

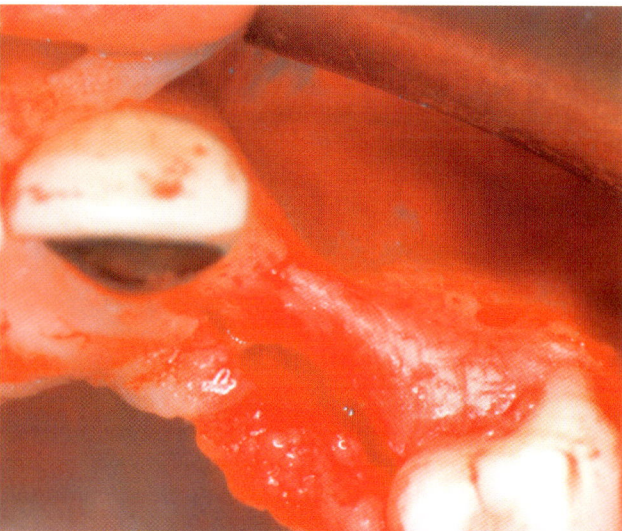

Fig. 5.20 Extensive bone loss from trauma is evident.

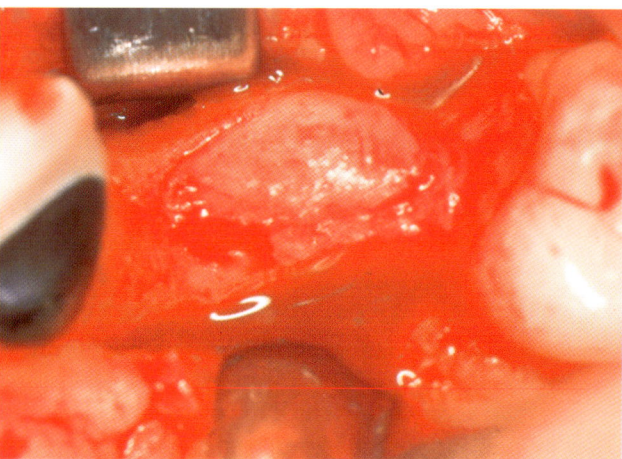

Fig. 5.21 Six months after placing an autogenous bone graft taken from the anterior mandible, a better foundation for implant placement has been created.

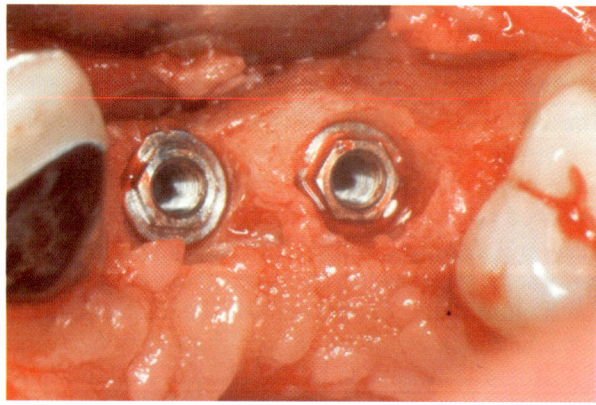

Fig. 5.22 Clearly the ridge augmentation has made implant placement easier and more predictable than would have been possible in the situation shown in Figure 5.20.

of bone available, and while these can be largely overcome by using extra-oral sites, such as the iliac crest, there is a potential morbidity associated with such techniques.

Allografts

These are graft materials available from the same species, i.e., bone derived from cadavers, and have been used widely in orthopaedic and periodontal surgery. The graft may be freeze-dried or decalcified freeze-dried material. It may be harvested from donors with well-documented medical histories and is tested for all common antigens during production. It is therefore considered a relatively safe source of grafting material.

Xenografts

Xenografts made from bovine bone from which the proteins have been removed are purely mineral grafts, but have been found to be effective when mixed with the patient's blood and packed into the sinus. As it is available in large quantities it is useful in sinus lift procedures as an alternative to an autogenous or allogenic graft.

Alloplastic grafts

Synthetic alloplastic grafting materials have a reduced risk of cross-contamination and may well act as a good framework for bone formation; however, caution should be used when considering using them for a sinus lift procedure.

SURGICAL PROCEDURES
Edentulous mandible: implant placement for two implants for retaining an overdenture

Suggested anaesthetic:
   Mental foramina infiltration.
   Lingual infiltration.

Suggested incision:
   Crestal. First premolar to first premolar, not necessary to dissect down to expose mental foramina.

Implant placement:
   Canine region approximately 2 cm apart. Where the form of the edentulous ridge is curved, then it may not be possible to link the implants rigidly without encroaching on the lingual space. In these circumstances it is usually necessary to use individual ball attachments.

Suggested abutments:
   Either ball- or bar-retained prosthesis.

Edentulous mandible implant placement for five implants for retaining fixed prosthesis

Suggested anaesthetic:
   Bilateral regional blocks.
   Lingual and buccal infiltration.

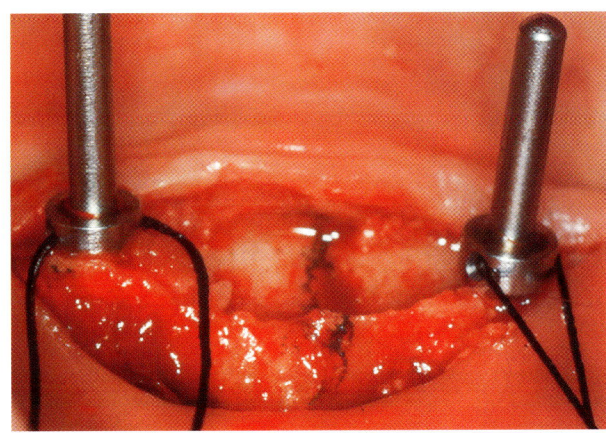

Fig. 5.23 Direction indicators placed in the lower edentulous mandible to assist in the placement of two implants to support a complete overdenture.

Suggested incision:
Crestal. First molar to first molar relieving incision anteriorly, if necessary blunt dissection to expose both mental foramina.

Implant placement:
Suggested locations 3 mm in front of mental foramina, minimum distance between implants 7 mm (centre to centre) following curve of anterior mandible, with access through, or slightly lingual to, the cingula of the lower teeth.

Suggested prosthesis:
Fixed with cantilever extension approximately twice the distance between the most anterior and distal implants, up to a maximum of 15 mm from the distal aspect of the abutment.

Edentulous maxilla: placement of four implants for retaining an overdenture

Suggested anaesthetic:
Buccal infiltration.
Regional blocks in the incisal canal and greater palatine foramen regions.

Suggested incision:
Crestal second premolar to second premolar. This is necessary to enable dissection to expose the incisive foramen. A buccal relieving incision is often needed to expose any buccal concavities.

Implant placement:
Canine and central incisor regions. Where there is lack of bone in the incisor region then implants may sometimes be placed in the premolar regions.

Suggested prosthesis:
Bar-retained complete overdenture.

Edentulous maxilla: implant placement for six implants to retain a fixed prosthesis

Suggested anaesthetic:
Buccal infiltration.
Regional blocks in the incisal canal and greater palatine foramen regions.

Suggested incision:
Crestal. First molar to first molar, necessary to dissect to expose incisal foramen. Buccal relieving incision to expose any buccal concavities.

Implant placement:
Depending on floor of maxillary sinus, and bone volume in second premolar, canine and incisor regions

Suggested prosthesis:
Fixed, with cantilever extension approximately one and half times the distance between the most anterior and distal implants, up to a maximum of 15 mm, depending on the lengths of the implants and bone quality.

Posterior mandible

Suggested anaesthetic:
Regional block, lingual and buccal infiltration.

Suggested incision:
Crestal, with relieving incision anteriorly to mental foramina and blunt dissection to expose these as necessary.

Implant placement:
Suggested spacing 3 mm distal to the natural abutment directly medial to the edentulous region. Optimum separation between implants 7 mm (centre to centre) using a surgical guide.

Posterior maxilla

Suggested anaesthetic:
Buccal and palatal infiltration.

Suggested incision:
Crestal with relieving incision anteriorly.

Implant placement:
Suggested 3 mm distal to the direct medial abutment. Optimum separation between implants 7 mm using surgical guide.

Single tooth

Suggested anaesthetic:
Buccal and palatal infiltration.

Suggested incision:
Crestal with relieving incision if necessary.

Immediate placement

Suggested anaesthetic:
Buccal and palatal infiltration. Osteotomes should be used to minimize the trauma associated with the extraction.

Following extraction of the tooth, careful debridement of the extraction socket should be carried out to remove any remnants of tissue. Using a surgical guide a small pilot hole is then made, usually on the palatal wall.

With immediate placement it is often difficult to follow the orientation of the tooth with a parallel-sided implant, and there is a significant risk of penetrating the buccal concavity. It is therefore preferable to engage bone on the palatal aspect of the socket. Following insertion of the implant, it is often preferable to follow a single-stage surgical protocol and place a healing abutment. In suturing the socket, primary closure of the soft-tissue wound should not be attempted (Figs 5.24–5.26).

KEYS TO SUCCESSFUL SURGERY

There are a number of ways in which the surgeon can reduce problems during or following surgery. These include the following:

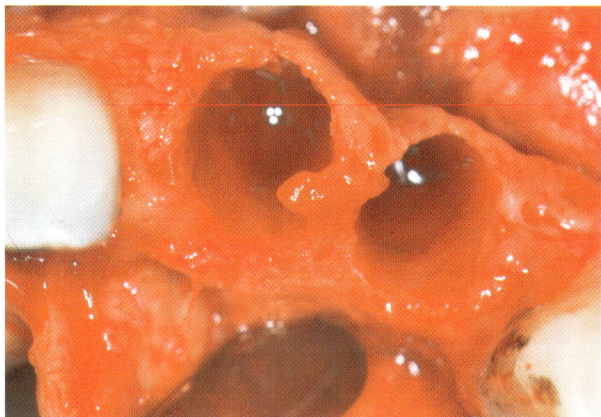

Fig. 5.24 The sites of two atraumatically extracted teeth in preparation for immediate placement of implants.

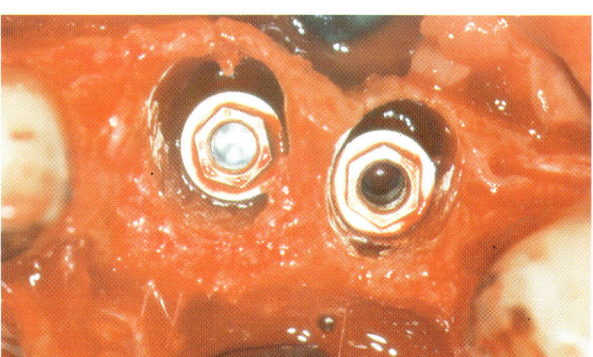

Fig. 5.25 Implants placed in the sockets of the extracted teeth. Primary stability is gained by securing the apical portion of the implants into bone.

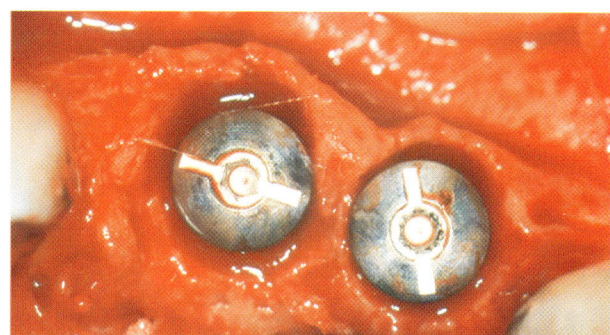

Fig. 5.26 Following immediate placement into extraction sockets healing abutments have been placed onto the implants. The flap is then sutured around the healing abutments.

- Minimize infection risk. One known cause of failure of implant surgery is infection of the surgical site. This can be minimized by careful preparation, draping the patient, using as sterile a technique as feasible, employing pre-sterilized packaged components wherever possible, and using appropriate antibiotic cover. Contamination of the implant surfaces should be avoided.

- Minimize tissue injury. A gentle surgical technique will minimize this, while sharp disposable drills employed in incremental sizes, and a light and intermittent drilling pressure with copious cooling irrigation, all help to minimize thermal trauma to the bone.

- Pain control. This can be achieved by adequate local anaesthesia, employing an experienced surgical team, adopting an aseptic technique and minimizing trauma.

POSTOPERATIVE RADIOGRAPHY

While it has been suggested that postoperative radiographs should be routinely taken, the validity of this is questionable as very little information will be gained. Previously it was thought that the radiation may cause localized bone necrosis but there is little evidence to support this view.

POSTOPERATIVE CARE

Initial pressure on the wound site by the patient using damp gauze for a minimum of 20–30 minutes will help to decrease postoperative swelling and bruising. The use of extra-oral ice-packs may also be valuable in this regard. Where the surgical placement of implants has been correct and has involved the use of a crestal incision and interrupted sutures, it is often possible to insert the denture immediately following the surgery. If one-stage surgery has been undertaken and the healing abutments are exposed, it will be necessary to prepare some relief of the internal aspect of the denture. It is not recommended at this stage that the denture be relined as the material may intrude into the suture line. The patient should be given postoperative instructions, including a warning of possible swelling and discomfort. It is recommended that the denture be left in place for the first 24 hours, after which the patient can rinse with warm saline. The denture must thereafter be thoroughly cleaned with a toothbrush and toothpaste.

POSTOPERATIVE ANALGESIA REVIEW

To help minimize any discomfort, analgesic drugs with an anti-inflammatory action, i.e., a non-steroidal anti-inflammatory such as ibuprofen, should be prescribed. If the patient's medical history contraindicates such drugs, then paracetamol is the next drug of choice. A nerve block using a long-acting local anaesthetic, such as bupivacaine 0.5% with adrenaline 1:200 000, will provide 6–8 hours effective anaesthesia and therefore decrease any postoperative discomfort.

The patient is usually reviewed 1 week following surgery, when the sutures are removed. Any adjustments to the denture can be made at this stage. At the 1-month postoperation review, if a denture is present and there have been evident changes in the contours of the denture-bearing tissues, a more permanent reline should be carried out.

SECOND-STAGE SURGERY

The aim of second-stage surgery is to uncover the implants and place healing abutments, which will:

- facilitate gingival healing;
- allow easy access to the implants following healing.

Second-stage surgery is by definition required if a two-stage technique is being employed. This involves exposure of the head of the implant body and the placement of a connecting component, either a healing or more permanent transmucosal abutment. This connects the head of the implant through the mucosal tissue. Where the implant is relatively superficial it can usually be located by palpation, and possibly probing, and then exposed with a local incision or surgical punch. Where the implant lies deeper, and is perhaps covered with bone, it is necessary to raise a full flap, depending on the position of the implant in the arch, while trying to keep the edges within keratinized tissue. Flap design at this stage is important as it gives the surgeon a chance to modify the soft-tissue profile. This procedure is almost invariably carried out under local anaesthesia, as it is relatively straightforward. In general, incisions are made directly over the implant head unless the surgeon wishes to relocate some of the available keratinized tissue. The use of relieving incisions should be avoided if possible and, if necessary, placed remote from the edges of the abutments, as wound breakdown may occur if the flap margins are not on sound tissue. Once the flap has been raised, the cover screw on top of the implant is removed. It may be necessary to remove excess bone from the head of the cover screw before this can be done, using purposed-designed mills or burs and chisels, and taking care not to damage the implant. An appropriate healing abutment is then removed from its sterile pack and secured on the implant. The healing abutment length should be chosen so that it just emerges through the soft tissue and does not require too much modification of the provisional prosthesis. There are two types of healing abutment:

- Conventional cylindrical design. These are usually supplied in varying diameters depending on the size of the implant, and of various lengths depending on the thickness of the soft tissue. The disadvantage of this type of healing abutment is that it does not follow the outline or emergence profile of the teeth to be replicated. Also, the width of the healing abutment can be extreme and compromise the soft-tissue profile. Narrower healing abutments are recommended, so that at final prosthetic placement the peri-implant tissue will be placed slightly in tension.

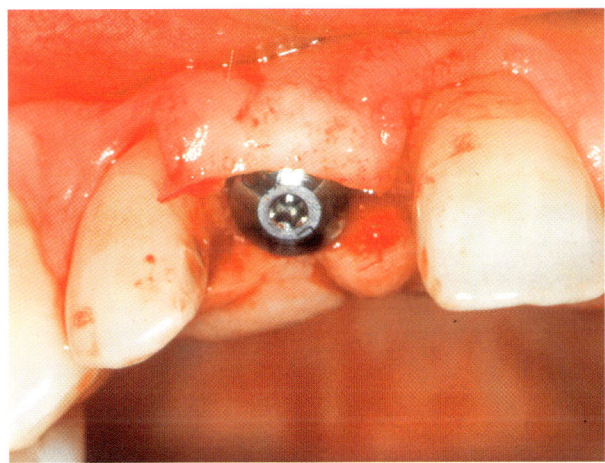

Fig. 5.27 A full-thickness flap is raised following integration of the implant and a healing abutment is placed in position.

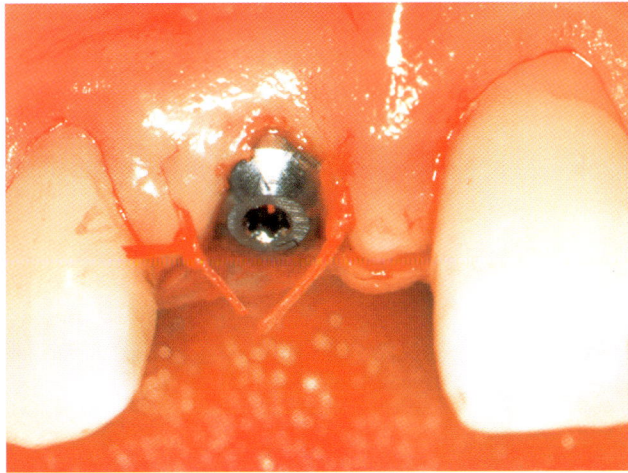

Fig. 5.28 The soft tissue is modified and contoured to the healing abutment, thereby maintaining the 'papillae'.

- **Custom-made anatomical abutments.** Customized healing abutments, which are in two parts, can follow the root outline of the teeth being replaced. This has the advantage of facilitating the reformation of the soft tissues to improve the form of the 'interdental' and the soft tissue contours.

The flap is then repositioned and sutured. Rotational flaps can be used to try to reconstruct some of the lost papillae. This technique may enhance the amount of interdental tissue, especially between implant and natural teeth. If at the time of stage one surgery a jaw registration had been taken, it may be possible to insert the temporary crown at this time.

COMPLICATIONS

Complications seen at the time of surgery

Careful surgical planning before the first incision may avoid or minimize many of the problems that may be seen at the time of surgery. A carefully positioned incision will ensure that the flap exposes the correct surgical site, while the use of a surgical guide will facilitate the correct positioning of the implant. Use of an appropriate sequence of drills will provide for optimum bone–implant contact, neither too tight nor too loose, and therefore optimize implant location and the achievement of good primary fixation.

Complications associated with unanticipated bone cavities and indentations

Despite careful radiographic assessment, it may be found at surgery that the bone contours are not as anticipated. It may then be necessary to reorient the direction of the implant, and hence that of the drills, bearing in mind the type of final restoration. If it is a retrievable system, or a screw-retained prosthesis, then the access hole needs to be located in the cingulum or occlusal surface of the prosthetic tooth. Careful knowledge of the selection of abutments available, e.g. angled abutments, is important for the

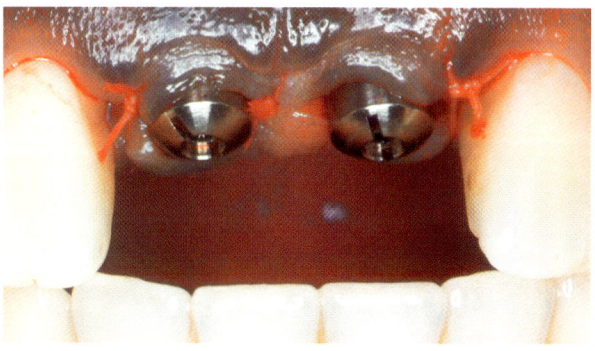

Fig. 5.29 The soft tissue is carefully contoured around two healing abutments in an attempt to recreate the patient's papillae to provide a more natural emergence profile.

surgeon, so that an unanticipated change in implant orientation does not compromise the restorative outcome.

Buccal perforations

Buccal concavities in the bone can result in some implant threads being exposed. Where these are very circumscribed and covered with a thick and well-vascularized soft-tissue flap, they may be left. Where not, then the situation can usually be managed either by placing bone chips, collected at the time of site preparation, so as to cover the exposed threads, or by guided tissue techniques.

In poor-quality bone the operator may find that the long axis of the site preparation may veer laterally and it is therefore necessary to use a secure finger rest to avoid this happening.

Problems seating the implant

This is usually caused by dense bone and is managed by removing the implant and either widening the hole with a slightly larger-diameter drill, typically about 0.15 mm wider, or pre-tapping the hole with a tapping device.

Excessive heat can be generated by attempting to fully seat an implant that is proving resistant to placement, and it has been suggested that compression necrosis of the bone may occur as a result.

Failure to achieve primary stability at the time of placement results in a high probability of failure, since initial stability is a virtual prerequisite for osseointegration. The situation may be retrieved by removing the implant and placing one of a slightly larger diameter.

Failure to place a cover screw or healing abutment over the implant

If the site has been incorrectly prepared and the implant is deep to the bone crest then excess bone may prevent the full seating of the abutment. Removing the abutment and trimming back any excess bone usually resolves the problem. Care should however be taken to ensure that this does not compromise primary fixation, or result in excessive loss of height of the alveolar ridge.

Failure to close the flap

It may be necessary to make periosteal relieving incisions to allow increased flexibility of the soft tissues to permit coverage of the implant.

Excess bleeding

Very occasionally there may be some aberrant vessels within the hard tissue of the osteotomy preparation site, and excessive bleeding may occur. This may also happen from either the sinus or nasal floor. After completion of placement of the implant the bleeding should cease; however, on these occasions the patient should be made aware that there might be excessive bruising following surgery.

Paraesthesia

Patients who have had mandibular implants inserted should be warned that they may have some transient paraesthesia of the lower lip, caused by localized surgical trauma around the nerve, or by compression from a haematoma. If the paraesthesia is still present after 2 days, appropriate radiographs may be necessary to check for evidence of potential damage to the

mandibular or mental nerves. If the radiographs do not suggest such a possibility, then the paraesthesia may be due to trauma associated with the injection of a local anaesthetic. This is usually transient, but may last for up to 6–9 months. Damage to the mandibular nerve due to the osteotomy preparation or implant placement may be permanent, and specialist advice should be sought.

Wound breakdown

With careful flap design and considerate tissue handling this is a rare complication. Provided that the breakdown is minimal then healing will be by secondary intention, and can be aided by the use of a chlorhexidine mouthwash.

Exposure of cover screws

This is not now considered a problem, and patients should be instructed to clean around the cover screws carefully.

Postoperative pain

Patients need to be warned that there will be some transient pain for about 24 hours after surgery. Persistent pain following implant placement is rare, and indicative of possible infection around the implant and failure of the integration process.

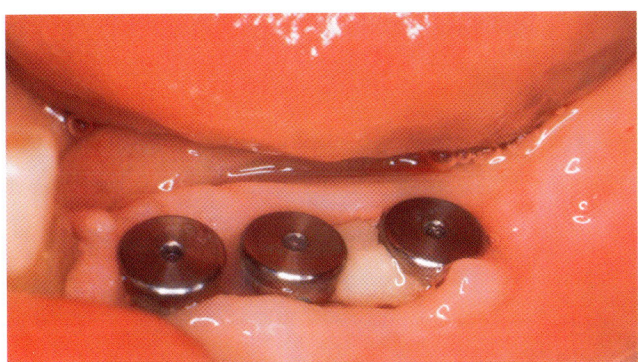

Fig. 5.30 Wound breakdown around these three recently inserted implants has led to their exposure. They are associated with necrotic bone, and all three have failed.

FURTHER READING

Esposito M, Hirsch J M, Lekholm U, Thomsen P 1998 Biological factors contributing to failures of osseointegrated oral implants. (I). Success criteria and epidemiology. Eur J Oral Sci 106(1):527–51

Esposito M, Hirsch J M, Lekholm U, Thomsen P 1998 Biological factors contributing to failures of osseointegrated oral implants. (II). Etiopathogenesis. Eur J Oral Sci 106(3): 721–64

Palacci P, Ericsson I, Engstrand P, Rangert B 1995 Optimal implant positioning and soft tissue management for the Brånemark system. Quintessence Publishing, Berlin, Chicago, London

Moy PK, Weinlaender M, Kenney EB 1989 Soft-tissue modifications of surgical techniques for placement and uncovering of osseointegrated implants. Dent Clin North Am 33(4): 665–81

6 The edentulous patient

INTRODUCTION: WHEN IS IMPLANT TREATMENT CONSIDERED APPROPRIATE?

Restoration of one or both edentulous jaws with a prosthesis stabilized by dental implants is appropriate in two distinctly different situations.

First, and most commonly, the procedure is proposed when a conventional complete denture is found to be unsuccessful. Various symptoms are complained of when attempts are made to wear one or both prostheses, such as retching, chronic pain and soreness, and looseness causing difficulty with oral functions, e.g. chewing. Coverage of the mucosa may also affect speech and taste and promote symptomless denture-induced stomatitis. Such problems may be compounded in some individuals by antagonism to wearing conventional dentures, which are emotionally associated with ageing and the embarrassment of tooth loss, and the sense of stigma associated with disease.

The second situation, less frequently appreciated, is the desirability of promoting the retention of alveolar bone and avoiding resorption and future atrophy of the edentulous jaw. Such situations are seen in younger patients with uncontrollable periodontal disease and those having poor-quality teeth with low resistance to caries as a result of inherited or developmental defects. Of course, among those with early tooth loss are many patients whose motivation and interest in dentistry are poor, such that extensive rampant caries can only be resolved by extraction and the provision of conventional complete dentures. For appropriately selected patients the early insertion of dental implants will considerably reduce the resorption and provide a less damaging solution with effective restoration of the dentition for several decades and probably life.

IN WHICH CIRCUMSTANCES IS THIS TREATMENT LIKELY TO BE PROVIDED?

Recent epidemiological surveys conducted in Great Britain, other European countries and North America show considerable changes in the experience of tooth loss, with fewer edentulous individuals and the persistence into old age of the partially dentate state.

However, in the past two decades the need to provide implant treatment has been commonly experienced by dentists caring for edentulous patients, particulary those exhibiting a 'flat mandibular ridge' that offers insufficient stability to a complete mandibular denture.

An equally difficult management problem is found in restoring the dentition of subjects with an edentulous jaw, either upper or lower opposed by an intact or nearly intact dental arch. Most often the problem of wearing a complete denture becomes apparent with significant resorption of the supporting tissues. The combination of a poorly supported complete denture opposed by an irregular occlusal table frequently requires the patient to have considerable experience in which the neuromuscular skill needed to control the denture has been acquired, together with tolerance of the compressive forces applied to the supporting oral mucosa. Many patients do not adequately meet such demands.

The third category for whom this treatment is appropriate is younger edentulous patients who are judged to have prospects of severe bone resorption of the jaws. This is most likely where the jaws are of small volume and where tooth loss is associated with periodontal disease.

HOW MAY THE EDENTULOUS OR POTENTIALLY EDENTULOUS JAW BE TREATED?

From the previous chapters it is clear that the provision of implant treatment is only one option in restoring the dentition. The choice rests between conventional complete dentures, removable complete implant-stabilized overdentures and fixed-implant prostheses (Boxes 6.1–6.3). The treatment may involve a prosthesis of one type or a combination of any two where the patient is edentulous. Hence an edentulous maxilla, for example, may be restored with a complete denture,

---

Box 6.1 Complete dentures – influencing factors

- Favourable previous experience of denture wearing
- Adequate stability from ridge form
- Simple reversible treatment
- Lower cost
- *Surgery precluded*

Box 6.2 Complete implant-stabilized overdentures(s) – influencing factors

- Adequate quality/volume of bone for a minimum of two implants
- Enhanced stability and retention by anchorage from implants in a resorbed jaw
- Improved resistance permitting improved tooth positions in the dental arch
- Facial support provided by denture flange
- Occlusal table may oppose an intact natural arch
- Complete denture occlusion favours stability of an opposing denture having limited support from the jaw
- Easy cleaning for oral hygiene
- *Higher maintenance requirements*

Box 6.4 Problems associated with conventional complete dentures

- Unpredictable ridge resorption
- Unpredictable fibrous replacement of ridge
- Occlusal instability of prosthesis
- Labiolingual displacement of prostheses
- Intolerance of mucosal coverage
- Unpredictable denture-induced stomatitis
- Variable levels of acquired muscular control
- Changes in facial support
- Variable retching responses
- Reduced masticatory efficiency
- Emotional distress from tooth loss

Box 6.3 Complete implant-stabilized fixed prosthesis(es) – influencing factors

- Adequate quality/volume of bone for a minimum of five implants in the maxilla, four in the mandible
- Total retention and stability of prosthesis
- Reduced volume/mucosal coverage improving tolerance
- Optimal masticatory function
- *Resorption may not be easily compensated*
  - *(i) increased leverage on implants*
  - *(ii) poorer alignment of implants with dental arch*
  - *(iii) appearance and phonetics may be compromised*
- *Cantilevering limits occlusal table*
- *Risks destabilizing an opposing complete denture*
- *More difficult to clean and achieve good oral hygiene*
- *Presence of periodontally compromised natural teeth may compromise implant support*
- *Initial costs greater than overdenture*

a complete implant-stabilized overdenture or a fixed prosthesis.

The provision of conventional, well-designed complete dentures has the advantage of being a reversible treatment where doubt exists about the patient's capacity to undergo dental care, e.g. the frail elderly and those with a history of intolerance. Such treatment is more likely to be successful where good ridges exist in a normal jaw relationship. Less than ideal situations may be best assessed by considering changes that have the potential to improve function or appearance of the patient (Box 6.4).

The retention of natural teeth (usually endodontically treated roots or those prepared for telescopic crowns) has been employed as overdenture abutments in order to resist resorption and retain a more favourable jaw form. Where excessive loading is anticipated because of clenching or grinding habits, preservation of the periodontal proprioception from carefully chosen natural teeth is an advantage.

However, high standards of patient motivation and maintenance are needed for long-term survival of these natural teeth due to either the progression of gingival recession or recurrent caries in the root face.

HOW MAY THE EDENTULOUS JAW BE TREATED WITH IMPLANTS?

Removable overdentures

Complete dentures may be successfully stabilized by a limited number of implants sited in the edentulous jaw (usually two in the mandible and four in the maxilla). Two implants usually provide sufficient stability, although the support is shared with the tissues covered by the denture base (Figs 6.1, 6.2). Four evenly distributed implants may contribute the majority of the support for the prosthesis and a maxillary overdenture may be reduced to a horseshoe, exposing the mucosa of the palatal vault, for example.

A sufficient volume of bone for implantation is usually present in the canine eminence and anterior to the antrum in the maxilla and in the canine/first premolar area of the mandible (although the central incisor site may also be available). Generally, standard

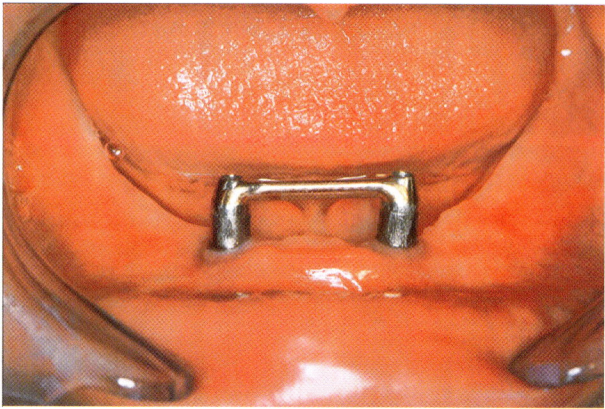

Fig. 6.1 Resorption of an edentulous mandible has been treated with two implants stabilizing a complete overdenture. Standard abutments support gold cylinders linked by a Dolder bar.

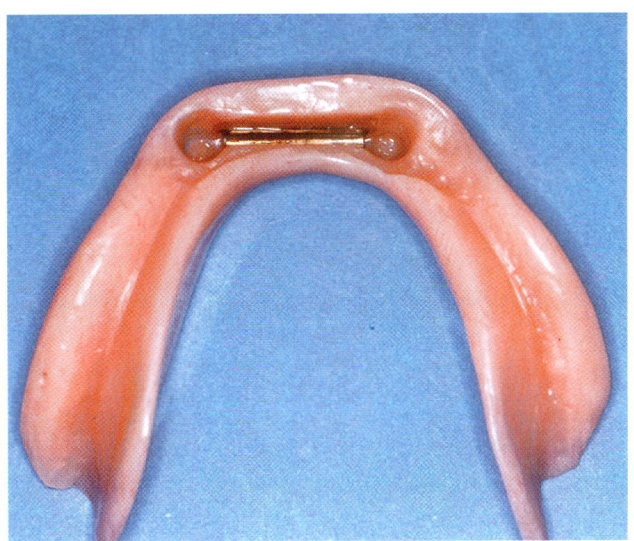

Fig. 6.2 Maximum coverage of the supporting tissues is achieved with the complete overdenture base, which encloses the retentive Dolder sleeve.

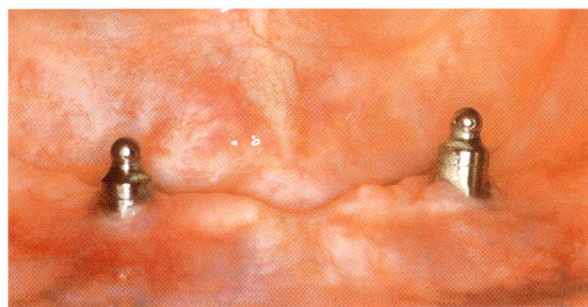

Fig. 6.3 Separate stud anchorages may be retained on implants.

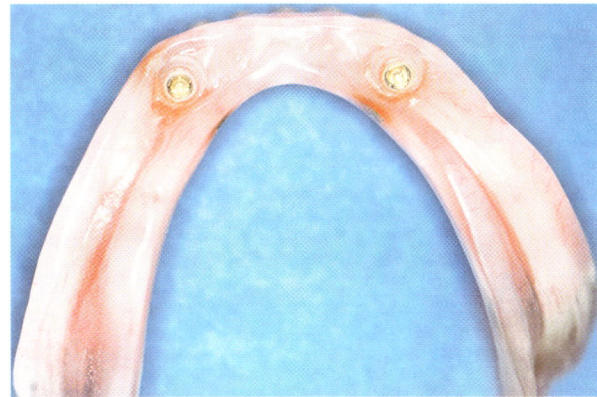

Fig. 6.4 Retentive caps are retained within a well-extended base.

implants of approximately 4 mm diameter and at least 10 mm length are considered adequate to sustain load in the maxilla, whereas even 7 mm is a sufficient length to engage the more dense basal bone of the anterior mandible. Obviously, the longer the implant the better are the prospects for osseointegration and the reaction to loading.

Standard transmucosal abutments that project approximately 1–2 mm above the mucosal cuff may secure an independent ball anchorage to the implant or provide a source of screw retention for a gold alloy cylinder to which a bar may be soldered. Hence retention for the overdenture may be gained from an individual cap, which fits over the ball, or small clip or longer sleeve that fits over the bar. These are secured within the fit surface of the denture (Figs 6.3, 6.4). The precision joints are manufactured either to allow a small element of rotational and/or vertical movement in the anchorage when dissipating occlusal forces applied to the overdenture, or none. Since there is inevitably some malalignment of each implant there must, of course, be sufficient allowance for undercuts present in the path of insertion to allow the prosthesis to be seated. This requires the abutments to be surveyed and 'blocking out' to be practised, including relief to the margins of caps or clips/sleeves so that opening and closing are also permitted in the retentive element. Clinical experience recommends that maxillary implants be linked by connecting bars to share the load since the supporting bone in the maxilla is less dense. There is as yet no prospective evidence to indicate that linked or isolated implants demonstrate better survival rates, or continuing bony support judged from radiographic evidence. The choice may therefore depend on the space available or clinical and technical expertise required. Obviously, isolated implants must be well aligned to permit insertion of the prosthesis on the retentive element. Similarly, implants require to be appropriately

spaced to allow sufficient length of bar to be accessible to the clip or sleeve. More recently manufacturers have produced 'low-profile attachments', which screw directly into the implant, that have a matched element to provide retention. Where one component is manufactured in 'plastic' the degree of alignment is less stringent for isolated implants. A particular advantage of complete overdentures is the provision of a labial flange to compensate for the reduction in volume of a resorbed ridge (Figs 6.5–6.8). This masks the abutments and produces a satisfactory arch with normally positioned artificial teeth of expected size that create support for the facial tissues and thus a pleasing appearance.

With vertical loss of the anterior maxillary alveolus problems exist in placing the artificial teeth, which can be resolved by recreating the appropriate alveolar contour with the overdenture. This avoids the escape of air and saliva that can arise with a fixed prosthesis supported by implants, where the abutments are inevitably placed palatally and superiorly to the arch.

Where one edentulous jaw is opposed by a dentate arch it is possible with an overdenture to create an occlusion fully interdigitated with the natural teeth. Care must be taken to avoid creating eccentric interferences that will readily destabilize the prosthesis. While it may be impossible to create the artificial arrangement expected from opposing arches in edentulous jaws, it is important to avoid creating immediate canine or incisal guidance associated with a deep overbite and inadequate horizontal overjet (Fig. 6.9).

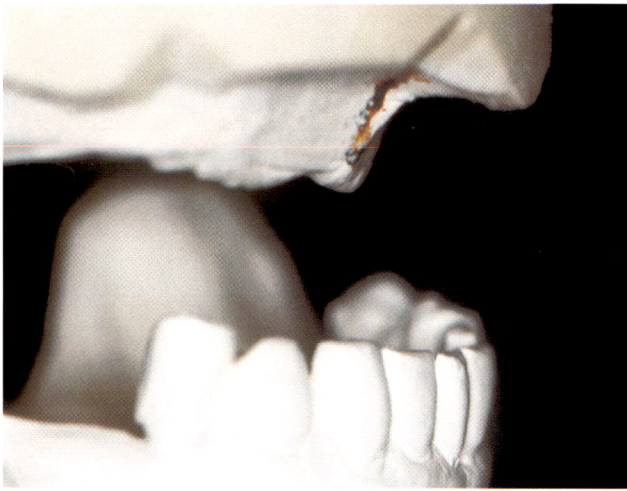

Fig. 6.5 Study casts identify a skeletal III relation between an edentulous maxilla and partially dentate lower arch.

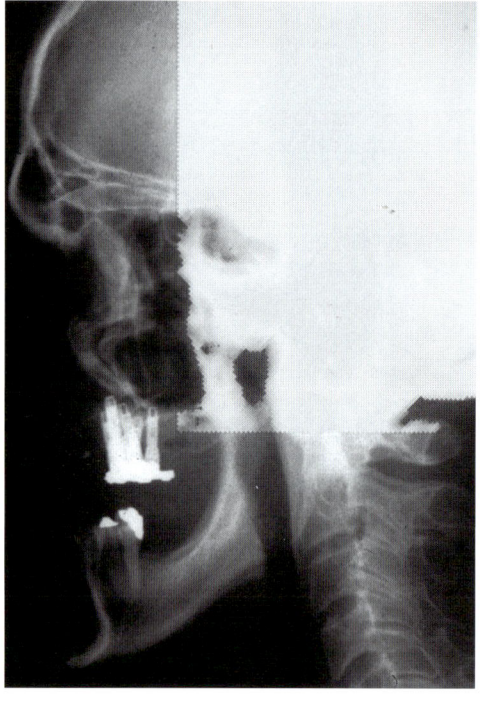

Fig. 6.6 A lateral skull radiograph of the patient shown in Figure 6.5 depicts the maxillary dental implants in situ.

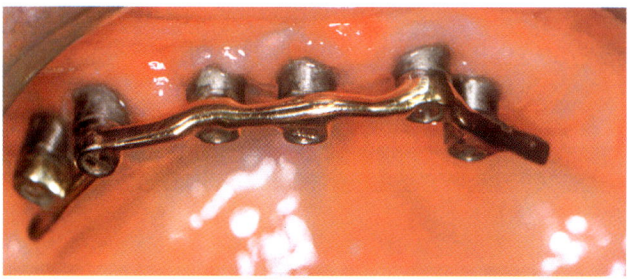

Fig. 6.7 A bar anchorage is used with clips for retention.

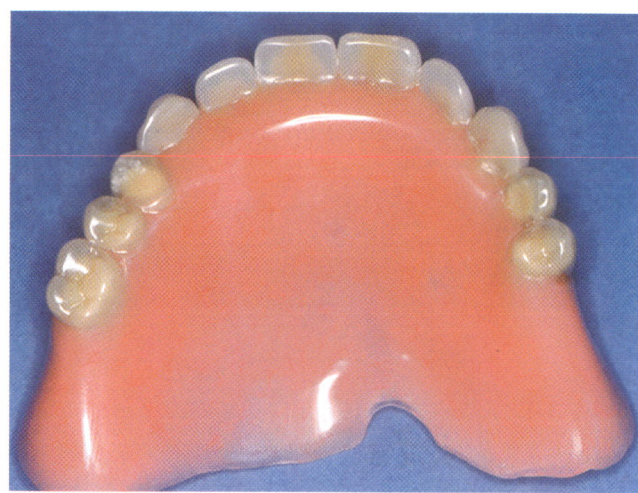

Fig. 6.8 The overdenture restoring the maxilla has a favourable palatal contour. Sufficient bulk exists over the anchorages to avoid fracture of the resin base.

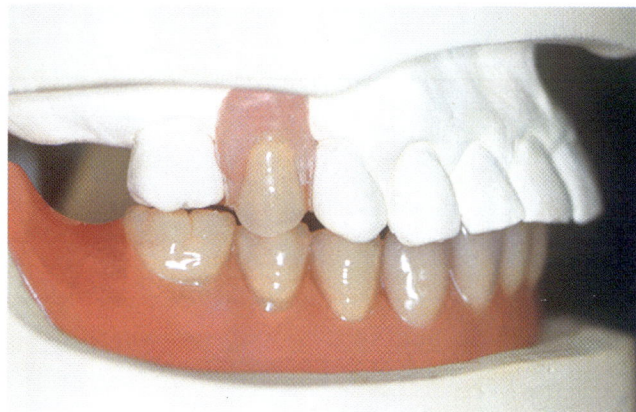

Fig. 6.9 A trial implant-stabilized complete overdenture restores the occlusion made with a partially dentate maxilla.

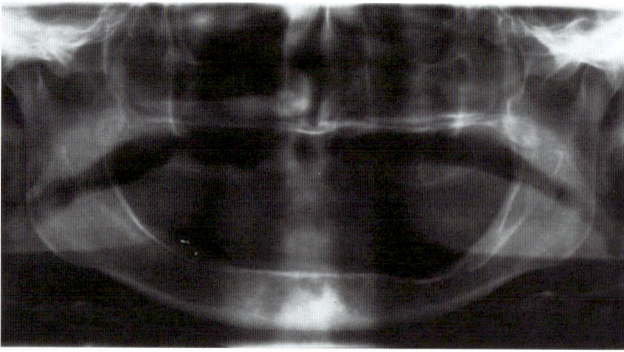

Fig. 6.10 An OPT demonstrating the edentulous atrophic mandible.

It is appropriate to select an implant-stabilized complete denture when the opposing removable denture is supported by a poor foundation that offers limited stability. A well-balanced occlusion established between the opposing dentures is least likely to create problems. For example, patients frequently exert good muscular control over a maxillary denture, while finding the conventional lower denture difficult or impossible to manage without experiencing trauma and limited ability to chew. Once stabilized by implants both prostheses can function satisfactorily (Figs 6.10, 6.11, 6.12). However, the choice of a fixed mandibular prosthesis in such a situation may create unexpected problems in the opposing jaw.

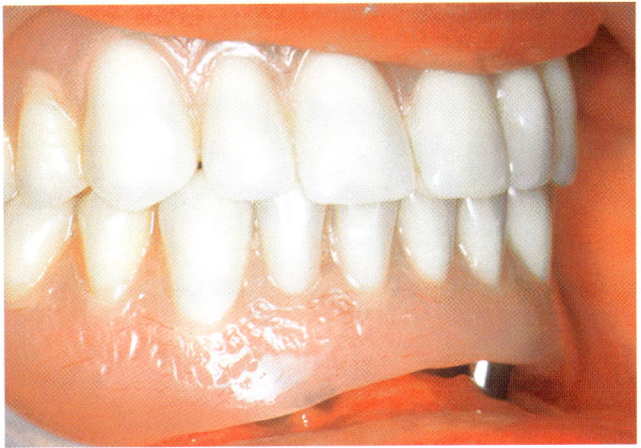

Fig. 6.11 The restored occlusion is made between a complete upper denture and a mandibular overdenture. Notice that the abutments are placed within the denture space.

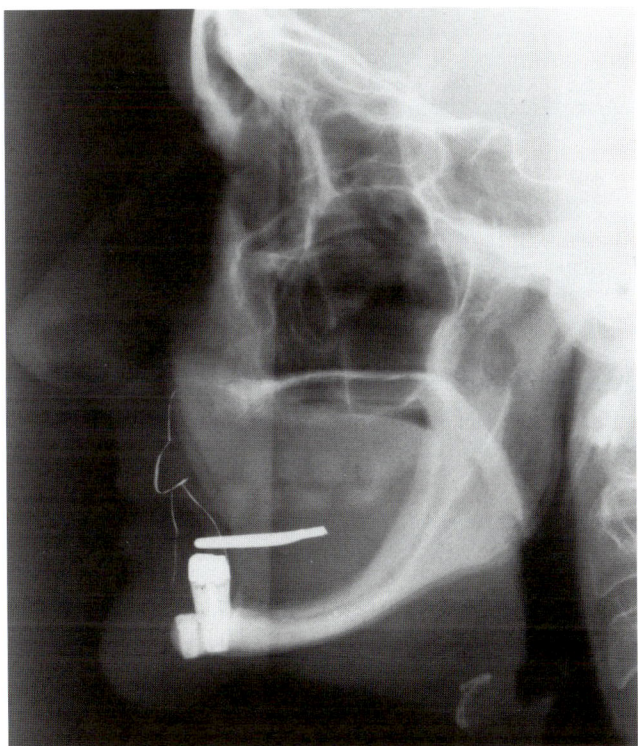

Fig. 6.12 A lateral skull radiograph identifies atrophic jaws. The mandible has been restored with an implant-stabilized overdenture.

Overdenture treatment is less costly to provide, being less demanding technically and using fewer implants than a fixed prosthesis. However, it is likely that there will initially be an increased number of attendances by the patient to perfect the tolerance and comfort expected. Regular monitoring and maintenance are needed since it is likely that replacement or rebasing will be required at regular intervals of between 5 and 10 years, as a result of loss of fit and abrasion of the artificial teeth.

It is possible that the overall cost of the treatment and maintenance of prostheses involving overdenture construction may, in the lifetime of the patient, be no less that the initial cost and maintenance of a fixed

Box 6.5 Comparison of a complete implant-stabilized overdenture with a complete fixed prosthesis

- *Load bearing.* Fewer implants imply load sharing between the edentulous jaw and implants supporting an overdenture
- *Retention/stability.* Total security is provided by a fixed prosthesis. Small amounts of movement exist with a removable overdenture
- *Occlusion.* Limitations of the length of occlusal table arise with a cantilevered fixed prosthesis. An artificial balanced occlusion is obtained with an overdenture versus a complete denture
- *Prosthetic space.* Less space is required for a fixed prosthesis; tolerance may be enhanced
- *Appearance.* Atrophic loss of alveolus is more easily replaced with an overdenture using a flange
- *Hygiene.* Good standards are more easily achieved with a removable overdenture
- *Cost.* Initial cost is higher for a fixed prosthesis. Maintenance costs may be higher for an overdenture

implant prosthesis if the latter is designed as a metal–ceramic or metal–composite structure (Box 6.5).

COMPLETE FIXED PROSTHESIS, RETAINED BY IMPLANTS

Restoration of the dentition with a fixed prosthesis may usually be achieved with six implants in the edentulous maxilla and five in the edentulous mandible. Prostheses are secured to the abutments supporting a cantilevered shortened arch extending approximately 10–13 mm beyond the distal implant. The volume and quality of the bone supporting the implants are influential upon the outcome; the better the quantity and quality the longer the available implant length and survival of osseointegration. Hence it is advised not to place implants of less than 10 mm in the softer bone of the anterior maxilla. Where resorption has created inadequate height and width to the jaw, autogenous grafting may be used in the form of an inlay or onlay.

The design of the prosthesis and the type of abutments secured to the dental implants usually differ in the upper and lower jaws. A well-formed maxillary alveolus with an optimal thickness of covering mucous membrane offers the prospect of a good aesthetic result. Shouldered tapered abutments will allow the artificial crowns to be produced with a good emergence profile, provided the implants have been positioned apically and slightly palatally to each artificial tooth. The crown is usually formed in composite resin bonded to the metal frame of the prosthesis since this material is much easier to repair or replace than damaged porcelain (Figs 6.13–6.16). In the mandible, standard abutments projecting through the mucosa support a cast gold alloy or welded/milled beam of titanium alloy con-

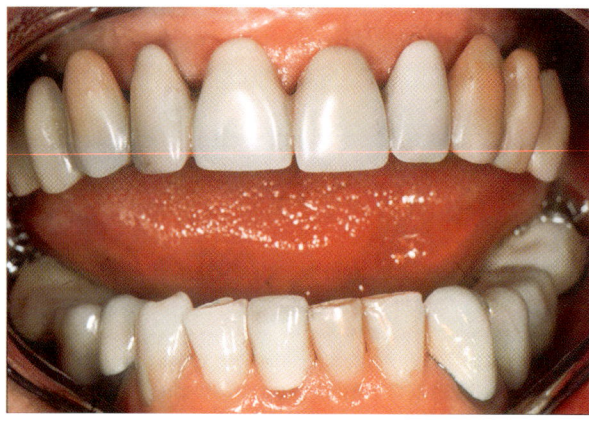

Fig. 6.13 The maxillary fixed prosthesis is satisfactory at a review appointment 4 years after placement.

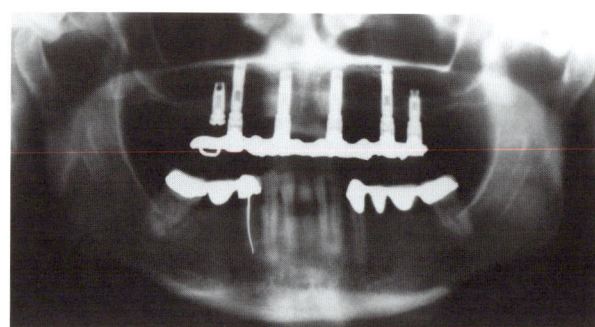

Fig. 6.16 Radiograph of the completed fixed restoration. The implant in the 15 region has not been exposed and may be used if the adjacent implant fails.

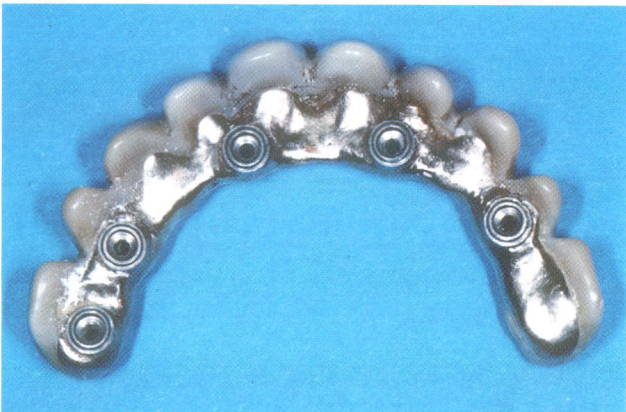

Fig. 6.14 The superstructure has been removed and demonstrates the high level of oral hygiene that the patient has been able to maintain.

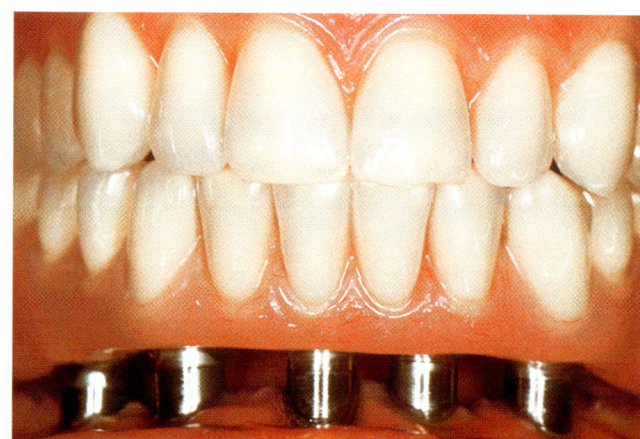

Fig. 6.17 The complete fixed prosthesis occludes with a complete overdenture.

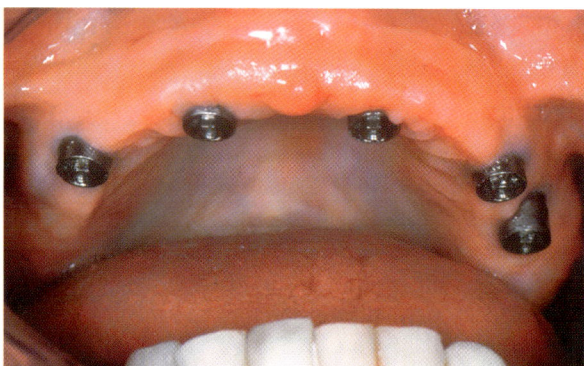

Fig. 6.15 The mucosal cuffs around the abutments remain healthy.

structed with clearance between the prosthesis and the mucosa, (so-called 'Zarb' or 'oil rig' design). In the mandible the titanium abutments are not visible during extremes of lower lip movement in laughter and speech and access for cleaning below the prosthesis is easier. Either artificial teeth embedded in acrylic resin or composite resin bonded to the frame may be used to form the mandibular dental arch (Figs 6.17, 6.18).

Where alveolar resorption necessitates replacement of a significant volume of bone a combination of metal

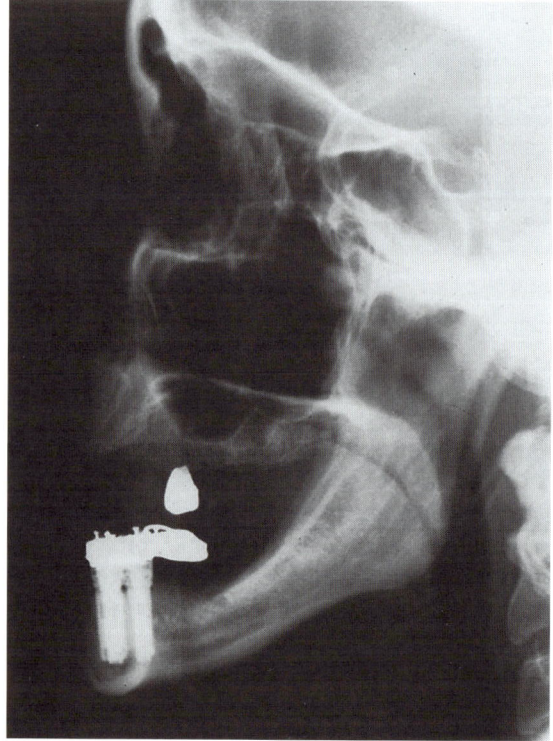

Fig. 6.18 A radiograph shows the completed restoration of the occlusion.

alloy and acrylic resin is used to recreate the arch and its supporting tissue.

A fixed prosthesis may be chosen to oppose an intact or partially dentate arch of natural teeth. However, if the entire length of the occlusion is to be restored either sufficient bone must exist above the maxillary antrum or inferior dental canal to accommodate implants of at least 6–7 mm length and 5–6 mm diameter. If not, then an auxiliary surgical procedure must be considered, e.g. a maxillary sinus lift, in order to create an increased volume of bone. A fixed mandibular prosthesis occupying a reduced prosthetic space may be provided to oppose a complete maxillary denture, if the upper foundation offers good support and retention. Monitoring is essential to evaluate changes in the opposing edentulous ridge as loads tend to be concentrated about the anterior aspect of the jaws.

The reduced coverage of the edentulous jaw provided by a fixed prostheses is appreciated by the patient. However, there may be unforeseen disadvantages especially associated with designing the maxillary prostheses. These are alteration in speech articulation, escape of saliva leading to the complaint of spitting while speaking, and difficulties in cleaning, with adverse effects of plaque stagnation. Most of these problems are not encountered when the jaw has a well-formed alveolus and the dental arch can be appropriately sited close to the ridge with artificial teeth of the expected crown form.

When resorption is greater the arch may be cantilevered labially and either longer crowns or a flange may be required. It is then that problems arise. Usually anterior dental fricative sounds, e.g. *s*, *sh*, *t*, *th*, are affected. If the fixed prosthesis has been designed for easy access for cleaning, a solution may only be found by providing the patient with a removable silicone veneer that can be introduced into the space between the inferior surface of the prostheses and the ridge.

The design of a short flange for a fixed prosthesis is inappropriate for a patient with a high smile line and may cause irritation to the lip, resulting in a hyperplastic fold if it is spaced from the residual alveolus.

HOW IS THE CHOICE MADE BETWEEN THE OPTIONS?

Although it may appear logical to meet the patient's request for a fixed replacement of missing teeth, this may not be straightforward. Enthusiasm for the option may soon disappear if it is immediately apparent that only a bone-grafting procedure can provide sufficient volume to accommodate the implants and create a suitable appearance.

When the patient's previous experience has been heavily biased by the lack of success with a poorly made conventional denture, it may be more appropriate to construct a new prosthesis(es). The patient's responses can then be closely monitored. For example, well-made complete dentures may completely resolve the problems, at lower cost. Alternatively, they may play a key part

in success when implants provide the required stability necessary for function.

On the other hand, where it is clear that other options for tooth replacement in the terminal dentition will result in unsatisfactory function or damage to the residual tissues this risk should be explained to patients suffering early tooth loss. It is little consolation for a patient to have all their natural teeth extracted early in life as a result of intractable periodontal disease, only to have to face severe problems with malfunctioning complete dentures at a later age.

PLANNING TREATMENT

What are the key issues in obtaining the history and carrying out an examination?

The general principles of recording the history and examination have already been explained in Chapter 4. Specific answers should be sought to the following questions:

- Has the patient worn successfully a complete denture?
- Is the patient able to undergo the necessary extensive treatment and be motivated to achieve a high standard of oral hygiene?
- Has the patient undergone a dramatic change in dental status/health that can be resolved by implantation?
- Are there obvious physical, functional defects that could be resolved, especially by implantation of the edentulous jaw(s)?
- Are there obvious physical, functional or emotional defects that are unlikely to be resolved by implant treatment with or without allied surgical procedures?

What are the procedures?

Preoperative planning:summary

The clinical examination

Examination of the jaws should identify whether the bone is of sufficient width and height to accommodate suitable implants, the likely thickness of the mucous membrane and the relationship of one jaw to another (or to the opposing dentate arch). Evidence of fibrous ridge replacement, atrophy in height or width likely to preclude implant placement, or mucosal pathology must be identified. Extra-oral changes associated with limited jaw movement or ageing and the effects of tooth loss affecting the profile should be recorded.

The radiographic examination

Where favourable features are identified clinically it is often appropriate to rely on assessments based on simple examinations such as intra-oral radiographs, an orthopantomogran (OPT or DPT) panoramic view and a lateral skull radiograph at the established jaw

Table 6.1 Critical local features in the clinical examination of the edentulous patient

Favourable	Unfavourable
Ridge well rounded, minimally resorbed	Severely atrophied/narrow or flat
Class I jaw relation	Gross Class III, Class II relation
Keratinized masticatory mucosa	Encroaching mobile mucosa or fibrous ridge replacement
Adequate inter-ridge/ interocclusal space	Restricted inter-ridge/ interocclusal space
Opposing arch with level occlusal plane	Opposing arch with irregular occlusal table
Well-formed opposing ridge	Atrophied opposing ridge
Normal gape	Restricted gape
Low lip line on smiling	Short upper lip or high lip line on smiling
Well-formed lips with good profile	Thin, creased lips typical of ageing
'Gentle' lip behaviour	Dynamic activity in speech/ smiling
Minimal retching tendency	Highly active gag reflex
Clearly articulated speech	Tendency to lisp/tongue-tie
Normal saliva	Dry mouth

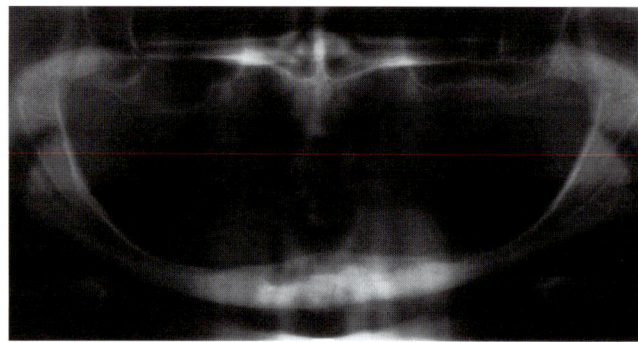

Fig. 6.19 An OPT is valuable for routine examination of edentulous jaws.

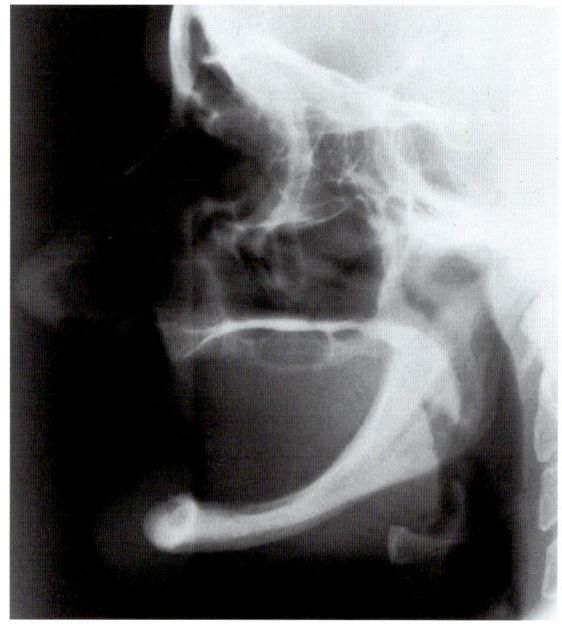

Fig. 6.20 The relation of atrophic jaws shown in a lateral skull radiograph. This is useful for planning.

relations for edentulous patients. These views identify the antra, inferior dental canal and incisive foramen, and confirm the absence of retained roots, etc. (Figs 6.19, 6.20).

Complex scanning and analysis are more likely to be necessary in the presence of atrophy and where an edentulous jaw is opposed by natural teeth in order to consider the relative positions of the implants and restored arch, including the option of bone grafting.

Preparing and planning with a diagnostic set-up

Both the patient and the dentist benefit from seeing the potential arrangement of the restored occlusion, including its relations to the surfaces of the edentulous jaw(s). If the intention is to avoid prosthetic replacement of the alveolus, then the arch should be set up without a labial flange. The extent of cantilevering and divergence between the long axis of the teeth from the projected positions of the implants may be even more obvious if the arch is indexed and the trial prosthesis is removed from the articulated study casts.

Any problems of potential space for the abutments and adequate bulk of the metal framework, sufficient to avoid fracture either of the frame or teeth from the frame, must be envisaged by the dental team. The likely position of the emerging abutments, use of angulated components and space between the occlusal table and edentulous ridge should be discussed. This is especially important where natural teeth will oppose a restored arch producing constraints on the design. Finally, the form of the surgical template and positions of the implants to be marked on the cast(s) must be agreed when the details of the clinical and radiograph examination are present (Fig. 6.21). Modern computer planning may make this process easier, but the patient's understanding and consent may be more easily achieved by the use of a diagnostic wax-up of a trial prosthesis which they can see inserted in their mouth.

Construction of complete dentures

Many patients seeking implant treatment present with unsatisfactory dentures that are inadequately designed or 'worn out'. It is often desirable to construct and fit

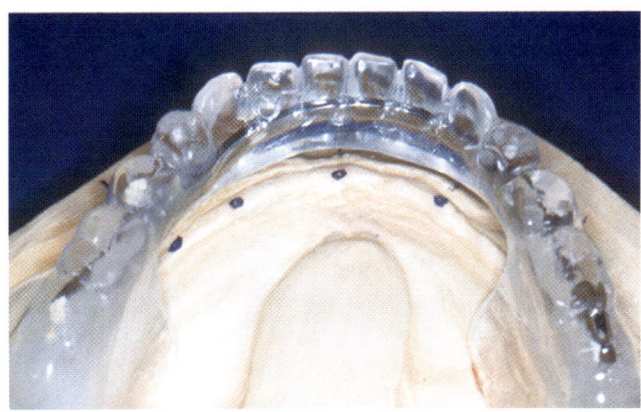

Fig. 6.21 A surgical template prepared for assisting implantation.

new conventional dentures for two reasons. During the period of osseointegration when immediate insertion has not been planned, the patient's complete denture must be adapted. Failure arising through fracture or discomfort and looseness of an old denture evokes doubt and disquiet about the intended outcome. Also wearing new dentures can be appropriate to assess whether or not implant treatment is really needed.

The agreed treatment plan

Consent must be obtained from the patient regarding the type of treatment, with full understanding of its duration and costs, including follow-up and maintenance. A written statement will make clear which one of three options is appropriate:

- a removable implant-supported prosthesis without or with additional zygomatic implants to enhance the maxilla;
- a fixed-implant prosthesis without jaw augmentation or one constructed after an autogenous bone graft;
- an immediate complete fixed-implant prosthesis secured to mandibular implants placed immediately.

Further discussion can be found in Chapters 4 and 9.

TREATMENT OF THE EDENTULOUS JAW

Surgical treatment: inserting and activating the implants in an edentulous jaw

The surgical procedures are usually accomplished under local analgesia, often with intravenous sedation, in order to provide controlled operating access in the oral cavity and reduce the awareness of the patient. Full nasotracheal intubation with obturative throat packing, required with general anaesthesia, is likely to be selected for autogenous bone grafting and the placement of zygomatic implants or other auxiliary surgical manoeuvres. Prior to elevation of the mucoperiosteal

flap it is necessary to ensure that the surgical template can be stabilized in the correct position on the jaw with good access for the drills. Also, it is advisable to make a small puncture through the mucosa and dimple the surface of the jaw where each bony canal is to be prepared. This is particularly important where fixed prostheses are to be constructed so that each implant is correctly aligned with the future arch and appropriately spaced, permitting wide distribution of occlusal load and the correct emergence beneath, rather than between artificial teeth. If CT scanning has been used with data downloaded to a rapid process-modelling machine it is possible to construct a customized surgical template. Its surface is prepared to fit the exposed bony surface of the jaw, and it includes appropriately sited channels that accept the surgical drills, enabling each implant to be positioned predictably. The techniques of implant insertion have been fully described in Chapter 5.

It is important to stress that two approaches exist in postsurgical management. Originally it was advised that a complete denture should not be worn for 2 weeks where it is intended to submerge implants for a period of 4–6 months. This advice was based on the need to allow the extensive flap to heal. Using a crestal incision and careful positioning of the implant heads, complete dentures can be inserted postoperatively without the risk of loading the implant bodies. Some adjustment of the base may be necessary where a resilient lining is to be added in order to cover the site. If relief is likely to precipitate fracture, the denture should be thickened or reinforced, e.g. with a fibre mesh, avoiding the fit surface, before reducing the denture base. This is particularly important in the mandibular prosthesis. Where immediate insertion is intended to be used with direct exposure of abutments at a single surgical stage then it is essential to adjust the complete denture to minimize the risks of immediate loading. This procedure is also adopted after a second stage and the fit surface over each healing abutment is relieved correctly in order to seat the denture. To do so, either a thin alginate wash is applied before the denture is partially seated, or the tops of the healing abutments are marked with a tracing pencil, so that contacts with the temporary lining are identified. Each contact that inhibits seating is penetrated with a denture trimming bur until adequate relief is achieved and more lining is then added.

The likelihood of successful integration can be assessed before the second surgical phase of adding the healing abutments, by recording a local intra-oral or panoral radiograph to detect any lack of intimate contact between the implant and the bone or a loss of crestal bone at the implant head. A conventional complete denture can usually be reinserted after 1 week or even earlier if access has been gained with a biopsy punch rather than by raising a flap. After a further interval of about 4 weeks to allow full healing of the mucosal cuffs, prosthetic treatment may continue.

Postsurgical prosthetic procedures

Recording impressions

Prior to recording an impression a decision should be made regarding the type of permanent transmucosal abutments to be placed (Box 6.6). In the case of removable overdentures and most mandibular complete fixed prostheses, a multi-unit abutment or a standard abutment is used which will protrude about 2 mm above the mucosal cuff. Topical anaesthetic is applied to each cuff before releasing the healing abutments. It is then possible to measure the depths to the implant heads with a graduated probe and choose the appropriate lengths. Each new abutment is screwed into position with the appropriate torque, e.g. 25 N cm, avoiding rotational forces on the implant/bone interface. Securing the abutment onto a protruding hex head linkage is occasionally difficult. A local intra-oral radiograph should be taken to ensure the correct seating. The abutment screw is next sealed temporarily with a plastic cover screw to avoid damage (Fig. 6.22).

A primary impression is then recorded of the jaw surface, enclosing appropriate landmarks as well as the area containing the abutments. In the case of removable implant and mucosa-borne overdentures it is essential to cover the tissues within the functional depth of the sulci. This usually necessitates adapting the stock tray appropriately with impression compound or silicone putty before applying a wash to provide the detail in the impression. Where an existing well-made complete denture has been adapted to accommodate the healing abutments the fit surface may be recorded in silicone putty. The model is very suitable for producing a special tray with the desired extension within a known prosthetic space.

The special trays used for fixed prostheses are designed differently from those for removable overdentures. The latter can be built with access holes or tubes of an appropriate diameter to allow impression material to surround transfer impression copings that are to be screwed onto the abutments (Fig. 6.23). In the case of fixed-implant prostheses an open-topped box

---

Box 6.6 Abutment selection for complete fixed implant prostheses

PREMACHINED

Standard abutments

- Appropriate for 'oil rig' design, typically in mandible
- Aesthetics not significant
- Minimum of 4 mm spacing between each one
- Easy to clean

Wide platform abutments

- Meet criteria for standard abutments
- Enhance loading potential in molar areas of jaws

Multi-unit abutments

- Alternative to standard abutment
- Appropriate for optimal emergence profile from good ridge forms, e.g. maxilla
- Facilitate siting of cylinder component in the 'prosthetic envelope'

Angulated abutments

- Necessary where long axis of implant body and tooth crown are divergent, e.g. Class II div ii incisor pattern
- Compensates for differences in implant/posterior arch alignment
- Avoid perforating buccal/labial tooth face with a channel for access to the prosthesis screw

CUSTOMIZED

- Individually fabricated by casting onto a gold alloy abutment post, milling a precision abutment (clinic/laboratory)/CADCAM produced by scanning, milling/spark erosion of a titanium block
- Optimize emergence profile of the unit
- Optimize superstructure form in relation to the restored arch

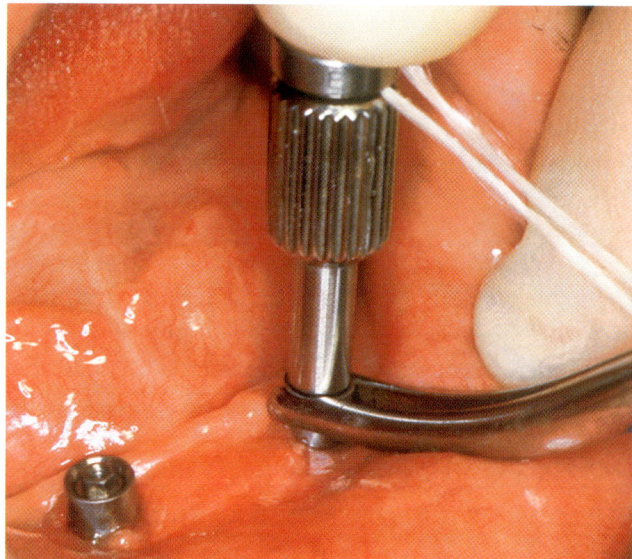

Fig. 6.22 Healing abutments are replaced by standard abutments at stage 2.

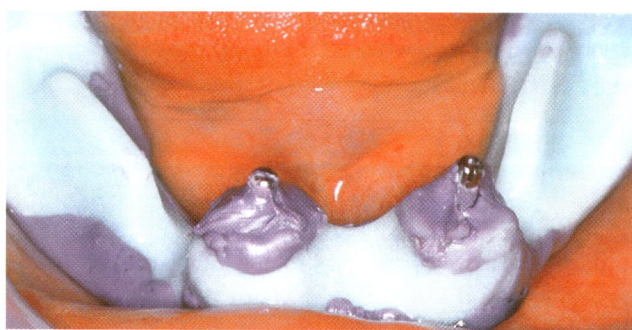

Fig. 6.23 An impression of the mandible is recorded with transfer impression copings screwed to the abutments.

is formed in the resin tray to enclose the transfer copings in much the same way as natural teeth. The edentulous ridge mucosa is either covered by a closely fitting tray surface or one that is slightly spaced by 1–2 mm, incorporating stops to assist its correct seating. The top of the open box should just cover the top of the transfer impression copings when the impression is made (Fig. 6.24).

However, when constructing a fixed maxillary prosthesis a choice must be made between using a standard abutment and either an angulated abutment or a tapered shouldered abutment which provides a specific emergence profile. The choice depends on (1) how much clearance for cleansing is to be provided beneath the prostheses, (2) coincidence between the alignment of artificial teeth in the residual arch and the long axis of the implants and (3) the appearance of the dental arch when alveolar 'gum work' is not required (Figs 6.25, 6.26).

Many dentists prefer to delay this choice and so record the master impression using transfer im-

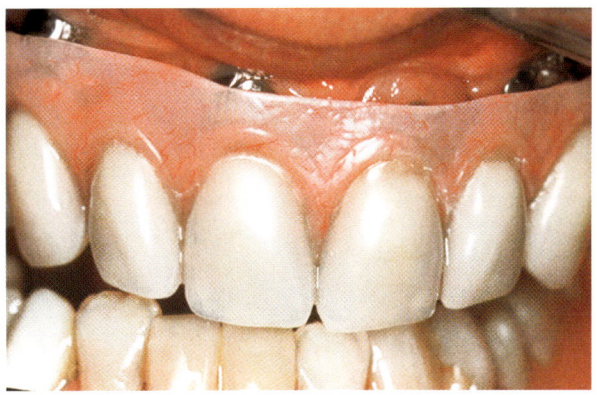

Fig. 6.26 The use of a spaced flange to mask the abutments.

pression copings positioned on the head of the implant bodies. This allows the choice of abutments to be made later in the dental laboratory from a selection of dummy abutments, or by laser scanning the cast and fabricating a CADCAM design. Some dentists choose to make an impression from the implants immediately they have been inserted, before the surgical flap is sutured. It is then a much more rapid procedure to construct the prosthetic frame. This procedure relies on the certainty of osseointegration and normal healing. Hence it is most likely to be used when implanting a well-formed edentulous mandible.

Whichever approach is adopted, a stiff elastic impression material should be selected with a single sequence of insertion and removal. A polyether artificial rubber is recommended for ease of handling and providing accuracy of the cast. It is possible to position tapered impression copings, allowing the impressions to be withdrawn while they remain secured in the mouth. This is useful when access is poor but the authors prefer those which are located with fixing screws that protrude through the impression surface above the tray, because these screws can be released when the impression is set, leaving the copings within the impression (Figs 6.27–6.29).

It is important for the patient to have border moulded the impression when complete overdentures are made. This involves raising the floor of the mouth in simulated swallowing, etc. Some over-displacement of the border tissues is not important when a fixed mandibular implant prosthesis is to be made.

After this procedure healing caps are placed on the abutments so that the existing denture can be inserted.

Recording jaw relations

A jaw registration will have been made previously in planning the treatment. A further recording is now made at the same vertical dimension and in a similar horizontal retruded position. This may be achieved using an orthodox base and wax rim which is appropriately extended and fits over the abutments. It is usually unnecessary to screw this in position since adequate stability is provided by the protruding abutments.

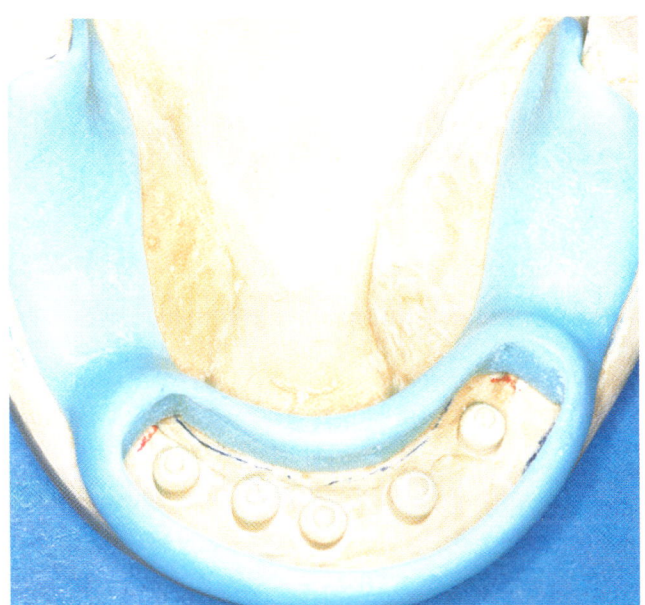

Fig. 6.24 An open-topped special tray is prepared for recording the master impression of a fixed prosthesis.

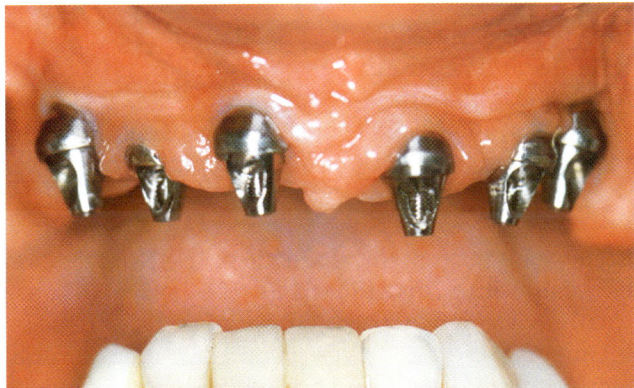

Fig. 6.25 Angulated abutments may be used to correct the alignment of the arch to the dental implants.

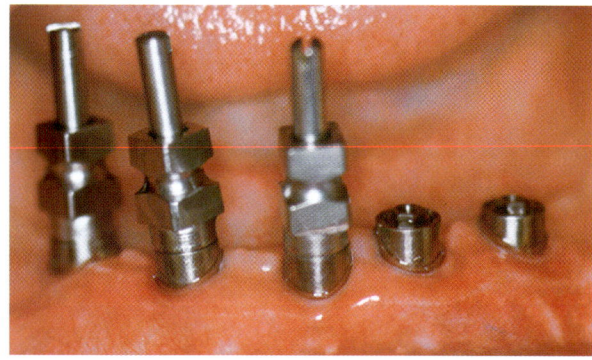

Fig. 6.27 Transfer impression copings are screwed to the abutments.

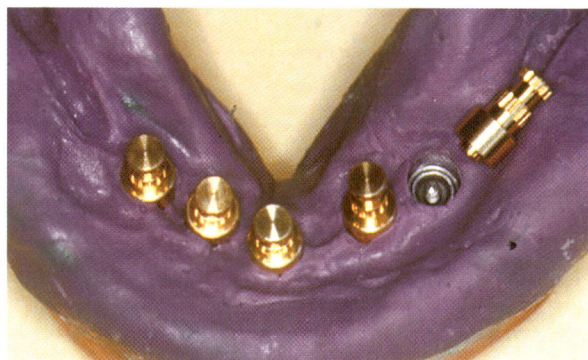

Fig. 6.28 Dummy abutments are screwed onto transfer impression copings before pouring the master cast.

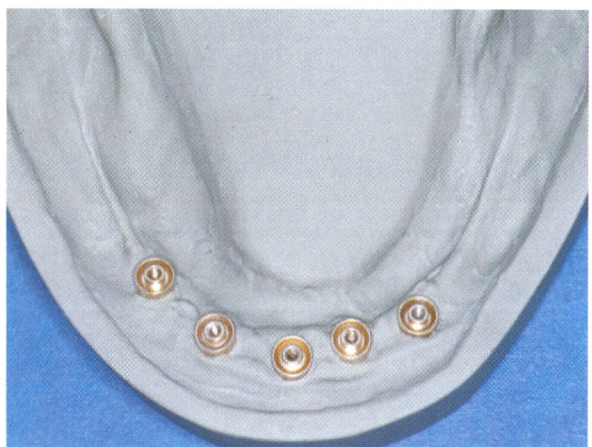

Fig. 6.29 The master cast shows appropriately spaced abutments in an arc.

An alternative approach whereby the adapted complete denture is duplicated and poured in wax has its advantages for producing complete removable overdentures. Often in the presence of atrophy the use of the denture space is critical in creating stability.

Having adapted the duplicate to the master cast containing abutments, recording an appropriate jaw relation is easier and the overall shape is known for setting up the trial denture. Registration with a wax wafer or registration paste is appropriate.

Trial prostheses

It is usual to set up artificial teeth on a temporary base, or in the duplicated denture for all complete over-dentures and most fixed prostheses, in order to assess the appearance and occlusion at a trial insertion. Where little alveolar resorption has occurred it is more appropriate to prepare an acrylic resin and wax diagnostic set-up since the prosthesis will finally comprise a metal frame veneered in composite resin without 'gum work'. However, many technicians prefer to work with a temporary trial arch with teeth gum fitted over the abutments, and set on a temporary base, to verify the tooth arrangement before proceeding to a diagnostic wax-up.

Greater lattitude exists in selecting the mould of tooth and positioning the arch for the removable overdenture or Zarb ('oil rig') style fixed prosthesis, whereas the diagnostic wax-up for a fixed maxillary prosthesis usually requires a choice of mould that will obscure the abutment and, with some components, create the correct emergence profiles.

An occlusal scheme embodying balanced articulation is employed when both jaws are edentulous. When a natural arch opposes the implant prosthesis group, function should be achieved. In either situation, the retruded contact position of the jaw should coincide with maximum intercuspation of the teeth.

Particular attention must be paid to the arch form and lip support given by the prosthesis. It is inappropriate to provide a flange where none is intended in the completed prostheses. Any conflict between the position of the abutments and the intended shape of the prostheses may become apparent at this stage, e.g. inadequate space for teeth set against the abutments.

When the trial insertion has been approved it is returned to the articulator so that the arch can be indexed with silicone putty on both the buccal and lingual aspects. The teeth can then be separated and assessed for position in relation to the abutments.

Fixed prostheses (Box 6.7) and removable ones are prepared differently and so are discussed separately.

PREPARATION OF REMOVABLE PROSTHESES (Box 6.8)

In preparing a removable prosthesis a decision will have been made to use either several anchorages on isolated implants or a linked anchorage spanning across two or more implants. When using isolated implants retentive caps can be positioned on ball anchorages screwed into analogue implant bodies set into the dental cast. Cylinders may be screwed to the standard dummy abutments when bars will be used for retention between several linked implants. The amount of space existing around these components can then be identified with the indices prepared around the trial overdenture (Fig. 6.30). When the thickness of acrylic resin will be inadequate to resist fracture it is appropriate to design an external metal strengthener. Hence it is

Box 6.7 Important features in designing a fixed implant-supported prosthesis

TOOTH RETENTION
- Framework should have retention tags and backing for anterior teeth

OCCLUSION
- Loads should be spread widely, avoiding local high concentration
- Avoid canine guidance
- Optimize the number and position of implants with heavy loads, provide biteguard for night wear

OCCLUSAL MATERIAL
- Modified acrylic resin material for artificial teeth or composite veneering most commonly used. (Porcelain teeth may be used for overdentures)

STRENGTH
- Superstructure frameworks require adequate cross-sectional form, e.g. 8 mm × 5 mm in cast type iv gold alloy, cantilever lengths of typically 10 mm (maxilla) and 13 mm (mandible)

SCREW ACCESS
- Channels of precise diameter with good access assist screw manipulation
- Avoid labial/buccal access

ORAL HYGIENE
- The inferior surface of prosthesis to be convex or flat, minimizing food impaction
- Access for spiral brushes/superfloss is required for plaque removal
- Irrigation with water removes debris (e.g. Water Pik)

Box 6.8 Essential features for planning an implant-supported complete overdenture

JAW VOLUME V. IMPLANT BODIES
- Mandible: minimum width 5 mm, depth 7 mm
- Maxilla: minimum width 5 mm, depth 10 mm

APPROPRIATE SITES OF AVAILABLE BONE
- Canine, incisor, first premolar using two in the mandible, four in the maxilla

DENTURE SUPPORT TISSUES
- Favourable maxillary ridge/palate
- Adequate mandibular foundation
- No evidence of fibrous ridge, prominent mylohyoid ridge and genial shelf or enlarged torus

DENTURE SPACE V. IMPLANT BODY ANGULATION
- Normal: aligns arch with implants
- Abnormal: limits implant position

JAW RELATION
- Normal: prosthesis with favourable volume
- Abnormal: instability, leverage on the implants, restraint on the components

OCCLUSAL RELATION
- Complete denture: balanced occlusion
- Natural arch: avoid canine guidance

POSITION OF RIDGE V. PROPOSED DENTAL ARCH
- Gross resorption: increases instability
- Implant components may increase denture bulk

WELL-DESIGNED EXISTING COMPLETE DENTURES
- Capable of modification

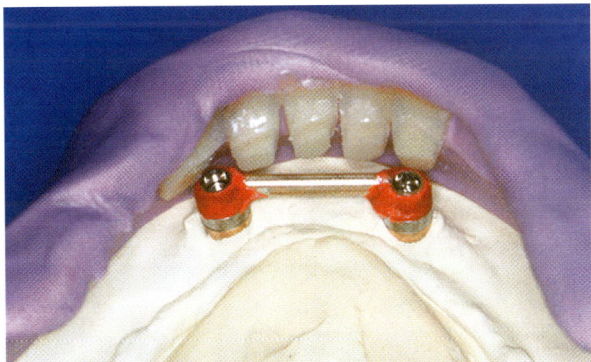

Fig. 6.30 A master cast shows the positioning of a Dolder bar between the cylinders in the correct relation to the incisor and canine teeth supported in an index.

crucial to be certain of the exact denture space, because once the metal strengthening frame is part of the completed denture any significant adjustment is difficult to achieve. A failure to consider the required denture space may result later in complaints of (1) difficulty in tolerating the denture and (2) instability of the mandibular denture and phonetic problems with the upper one.

When bars and sleeves have been chosen it is appropriate to select an oval cross-sectional form with a matched sleeve when two implants are used to create stability. In this design the denture will be permitted small vertical and rotational movements around the fulcrum. This design is commonly used in the mandible with implants positioned in the canine/first premolar areas of the jaw so that the bar is positioned parallel with the hinge axis (Fig. 6.31). Some authorities argue that when a mucodisplasive impression has been employed to relate the denture-bearing area to the implants a resilient joint is unnecessary and a parallel-sided bar can be used. There is no research evidence to support either contention. When four widely spaced abutments are used in the maxilla, a parallel-sided bar is soldered to the gold cylinders secured to the abutments. The use of cantilever bar extensions to increase the retention is recommended by some

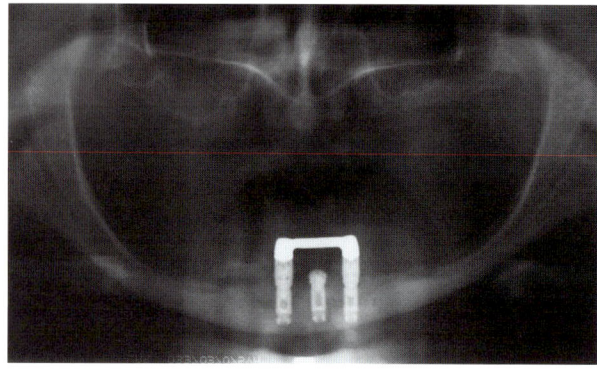

Fig. 6.31 The OPT identifies the alignment of the bar with the condylar hinge axis.

in order to perfect balance in the occlusion (Table 6.2). Failure to achieve this will exert unfavourable stress on the implants and may result in trauma to the mucosa or instability of the implant-supported overdenture. Edentulous patients may also complain of instability of the opposing complete denture. After this laboratory procedure it is usually necessary to improve retention by activating the male component (cap or sleeve) with a specific tool provided by the manufacturer.

Alternative procedure: relining/adapting a denture

There is an alternative approach when a well-designed complete denture is to be converted to an implant-stabilized prosthesis. This is usually adopted when two implants have been inserted in the anterior mandible.

Assuming the denture has been adapted to fit over two healing abutments then these may be exchanged for standard ones that project 1–2 mm above the mucosal cuffs. The lingual surface of the denture base is perforated above the abutments with sufficient access to allow transfer impression copings to be added. The tapered pattern allowing the copings to remain in the mouth is preferred as this shape is less bulky, requiring removal of less acrylic resin. When isolated balls are to be used these specific abutments can be positioned on the implant heads and this produces sufficient detail in the recorded impression. After applying a bonding agent to the denture base, a polyether wash impression is recorded, covering the entire fit surface of the denture with sufficient material to localize the transfer impression coping or two male ball attachments and abutments. When using this internal impression technique it is important to establish the occlusal contact in the retruded jaw relation.

authorities, who limit the extension to 10 mm from the centre of the cylinder because of the risk of fracture of these components. It is usual practice to try-in the linked bars after soldering to confirm the exact fit of the cylinders on the abutments or of the attachment in the implant body where certain 'low-profile' components are used.

In the final phase of finishing the denture, the alignment of the cylinders and abutments must be examined with a dental surveyor so that undercuts can be removed by blocking out with dental plaster. This also applies to the space inferior to a bar. Likewise the leaves of a cap or sleeve require relief in order to permit them to expand when seating the overdenture onto the male attachments.

Insertion of the prosthesis

When the complete overdenture is finally inserted it is very desirable to remount it with a check record against the opposing complete denture or natural arch

Table 6.2 Complete over-denture anchorage to dental implants

Implant component	Denture component	Application
Isolated implants		
Patrix ball (stud) Screwed into implant body Integral/separate abutment e.g. Dalbo type	Matrix cap Processed into fitting surface of denture	Well-aligned implants
Matrix abutment Screwed into implant body e.g. Zaag	Patrix nylon stud Processed into fitting surface of denture	Malalignment of implants Limited vertical space
Keeper Screwed into implant/abutment e.g. Zaag	Magnet Processed into fitting surface of denture	Malaligned implants
Linked implants		
Patrix	Matrix	
Round, oval Dolder bar soldered to cylinder	Clip/sleeve processed into fitting surface of denture	Adequate vertical space
Zaag 'low-profile' bar Soldered to abutments	Nylon clip Processed into fitting surface of denture	Reduced vertical space

Before pouring the master case in improved die stone, matching dummy abutments can be located in the impression. It is then mounted against a replica of the opposing arch. The complete denture is then removed and cut back to allow the caps or bar and sleeve to be positioned prior to waxing up and finishing the case.

The authors do not recommend this treatment when the conventional denture fits poorly or if the artificial teeth are severely abraided after several years of wear. Nor is it appropriate when a newly fitted denture fails to meet the patient's needs, in the expectation that increased stability will cure unsolved problems.

Some dentists use magnets and keepers as an alternative anchorage. However, although the maintenance subsequently required has been shown to be no more than when using other attachments, corrosion and wear resulting from continuous making and breaking of the force can result in more frequent replacement of the components. Loss of retention cannot be corrected by adjustments which can be achieved with a cap or sleeve. Some evidence from the literature indicates that patients claim that magnetic retention functions less satisfactorily.

Preparation of fixed implant prostheses

In recent years the production of a metal superstructure to support the dental arch has been undertaken in two different ways (Box 6.9).

Originally the framework was waxed up around gold alloy cylinders secured to the abutments and then invested and cast using the lost-wax process (Figs 6.32, 6.33). Where the superstructure is extensive it has proved difficult to compensate for thermal changes created in the casting process, so that an exactness of fit (so-called passive fit) has not been achieved between each of the cylinders and the abutments. To minimize the distortion larger superstructures have been cast in two parts and then soldered in order to improve the desired clinical fit. CADCAM systems using laser scanning, spark erosion and milling have enabled the pattern to be recreated as a titanium superstructure that fits each abutment to which it is screwed. The process, named Procera, originally welded blocks of titanium into a beam that was milled/spark eroded to a defined shape (Figs 6.34–6.36).

Whichever method is used it is critical to control the length, width and depth of the cantilever, so that

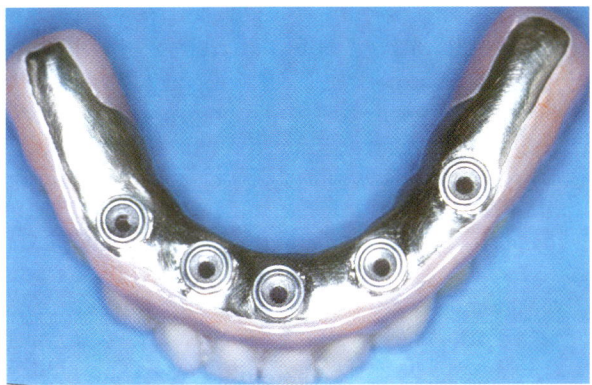

Fig. 6.33 A cast alloy superstructure showing the cantilever extensions and the enclosed gold alloy cylinders.

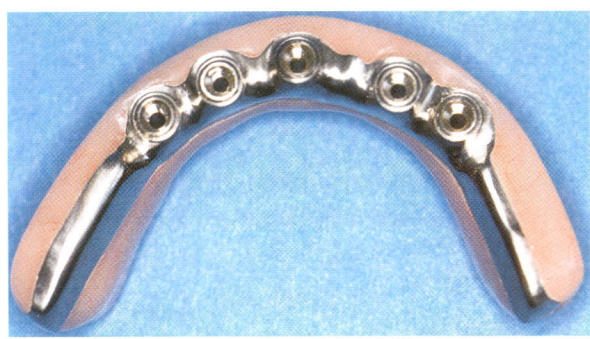

Fig. 6.34 A superstructure can be constructed by the Procera™ technique of milling.

Box 6.9 Choices in superstructure construction for fixed complete implant prostheses

- Cast gold alloy superstructure with gold alloy cylinders
- CAD/CAM: laser-scanned pattern and milled titanium superstructure
- Prematched titanium components secured to immediately inserted implants (see Ch. 9)

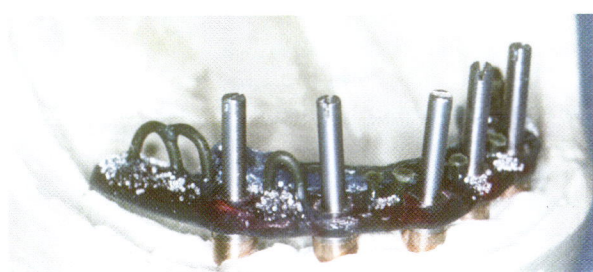

Fig. 6.32 The wax pattern prepared for the cast alloy superstructure.

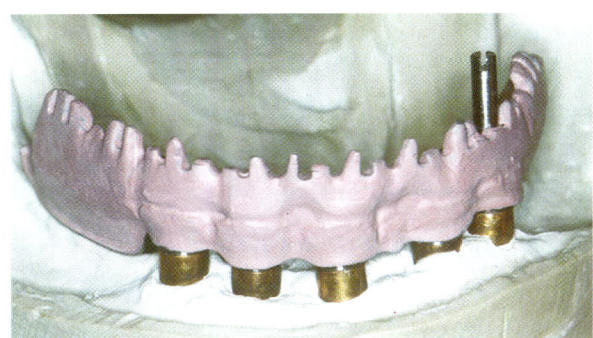

Fig. 6.35 Masking is applied to the titanium beam.

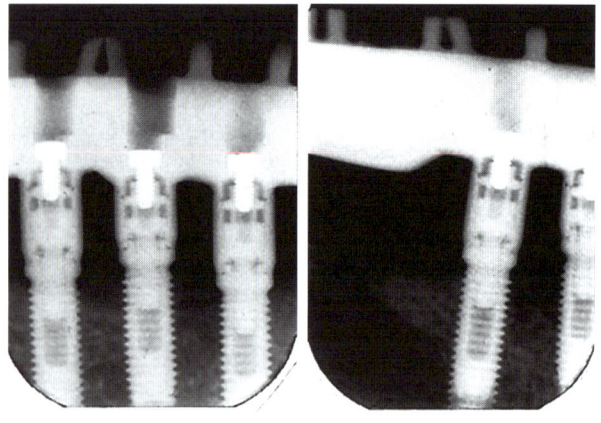

Fig. 6.36 Intra-oral radiographs of the Procera™ prosthesis sited on the implants.

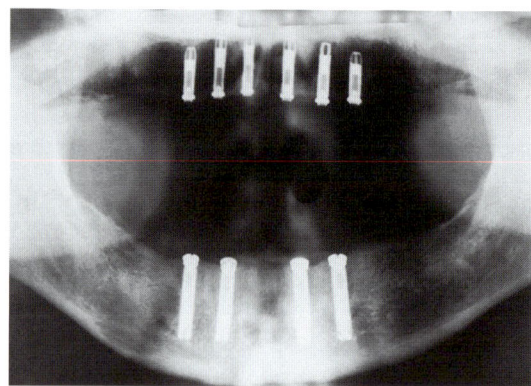

Fig. 6.37 Implants placed for the provision of fixed prostheses.

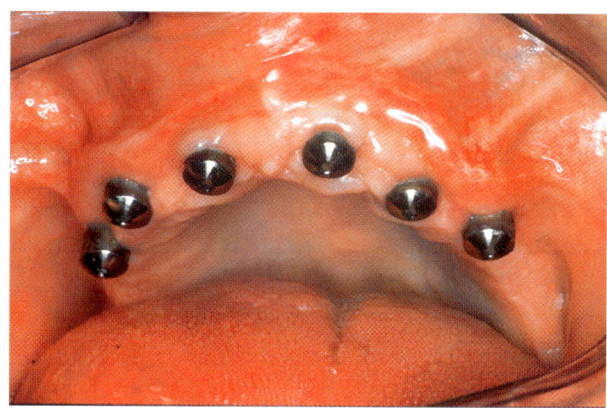

Fig. 6.38 Healing abutments will be removed and replaced by standard or multi-unit components.

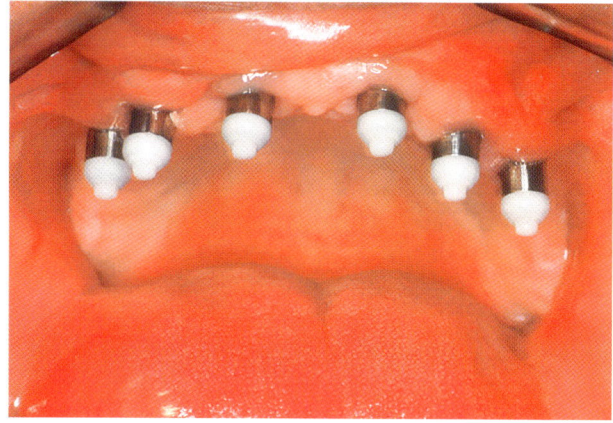

Fig. 6.39 Healing caps have been placed on standard abutments and the patient's denture modified to clear them.

sufficient bulk provides rigidity and avoids the risk of fatigue failure. One factor affecting the design is the level of the occlusal plane and therefore space in which to develop the correct dimensions. It is also important to consider the distribution of forces to the implants remote from the cantilever that are affected by the length of the distal extension of the occlusal table (Figs 6.37–6.39).

It is crucial to try-in the metal superstructure and apply the 'one-screw test' to ensure an even contact with all the abutments when only one gold cylinder is screwed into place. A misfit of the framework requires it to be sectioned into one or more parts so that all cylinders fit accurately on all the abutments. The divided parts are then linked with resin. The united frame is unscrewed and soldered or welded, depending on the material. Adequate mechanical retention should be provided to attach acrylic resin teeth. Similarly, the pattern will have been cut back sufficiently to allow for adequate bulk of an appropriate composite to be bonded, where this is the choice. Most anterior teeth are retained on posts with a metal backing in order to prevent them fracturing from the framework.

If the implants have been correctly positioned, the access holes for securing the framework to the abutments will be placed in posterior teeth to ensure axial loading and on the palatal aspect of the prosthesis with regard to the anterior teeth (Fig. 6.40).

Greater difficulty in the design arises when:

• there is significant resorption especially in the maxilla;

• with Classes II and III jaw relations;

• where an opposing natural arch has several overerupted or tilted teeth.

In the anterior mandible resorption of the alveolar process can be compensated by increasing the extent of the body beneath the arch. This is satisfactory provided the direction of the implants is not greatly different from the perimeter of the arch, so avoiding excessive labial cantilevering (Figs 6.41, 6.42).

Moderate resorption of the maxilla, however, may create a problem because of the need to replace part of the ridge with acrylic resin of the prosthesis. In order to mask the abutments during smiling and avoid the display of titanium and a space above the prosthesis, a short flange must cover the site. This makes access difficult for cleaning in order to remove plaque or food debris.

The design becomes even more difficult where (1) the arch is set labially to the ridge and (2) the artificial crowns are not set in the same vertical axis as the

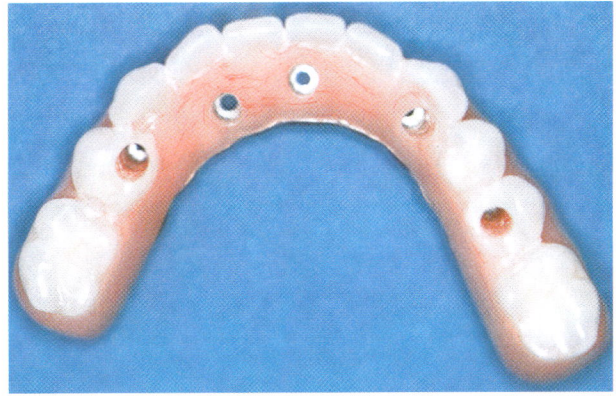

Fig. 6.40 Access holes enable placement of the gold screws, which secure the prosthesis to the abutments.

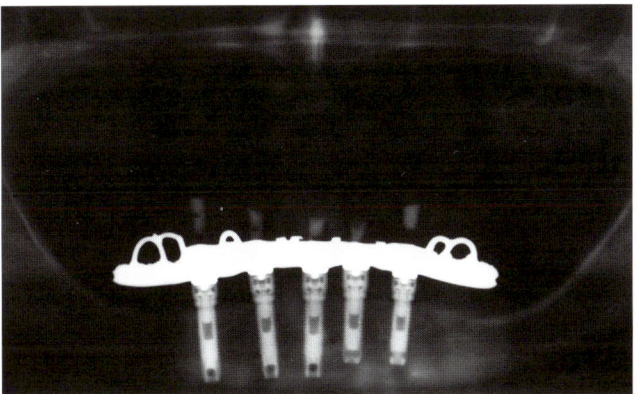

Fig. 6.41 Radiograph showing a fixed mandibular prosthesis.

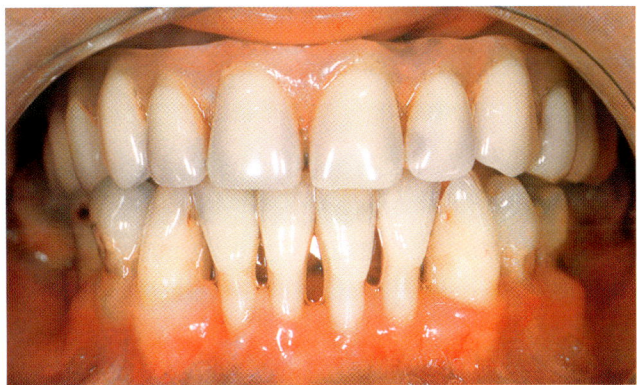

Fig. 6.42 A functioning maxillary prosthesis after 5 years.

implants, e.g. in a Class II division ii incisor relationship. The flange must be extended to cover angulated abutments that are needed to position the screw access holes on the palatal aspect of the prosthesis.

Box 6.10 Patient complaints of new implant prostheses

LOOSENESS/INSTABILITY OF REMOVABLE PROSTHESIS
- Ensure correct fit and retention of anchorage
- Assess base extension, body/arch shape with disclosing medium
- Confirm correct jaw relation and occlusion

DIFFICULTY WITH ORAL HYGIENE
- Disclose, and demonstrate plaque accumulation
- Observe cleaning/brushing techniques of patient.
- Are mucosal cuffs inflamed?
- Arrange repeated hygiene instruction

FOOD ACCUMULATION
- Encourage patient to rinse after a meal
- Use water jet

SPEECH IMPAIRMENT
- Persistent complaint may be solved with flexible obturator inferior to fixed prosthesis, or adjustment of prosthetic space for overdenture

MONITORING AND MAINTENANCE

A regular programme of monitoring patient complaints of new implant-supported prostheses is required in order to avoid unexpected difficulties arising from mechanical failure or patient neglect (Box 6.10). Artificial tooth wear may promote undesirable loading of screw joints, leading to looseness of the prosthesis, or fracture of the fixing or abutment screws; also, because of abutment looseness, inflammation of the mucosal cuff can occur, with resultant swelling and pain. Similarly, poor standards of oral hygiene may promote erythema, oedema and hyperplasia of the cuffs. The dentist should set down a specific programme of inspections for the patient that are more frequent initially and arrange for hygiene assessments, with appropriate guidance for each patient. Initial baseline radiographs are usually followed by one annual and then biennial records to determine the level of bone surrounding each implant body. An appropriate diagnosis should be made where bone levels are not stable and the action to be taken explained to the patient.

See Chapter 10 for more information.

FURTHER READING

Abdel-Latif H H, Hobkirk J A, Kelleway J P 2000 Functional mandibular deformation in edentulous subjects treated with dental implants. Int J Prosthodont 13(6): 513–9

Adell R, Lekholm U, Rockler B, Brånemark P I 1981 A 15 year study of osseo-integrated implants in the treatment of the edentulous jaw. Int. J Oral Surg 10: 387–416

Albrektsson T, Dahl E, Enblom L, Engvall S 1989 Osseo-integrated oral implants: a Swedish multi-centre study of 8139 consecutively inserted Nobelpharma implants. J Periodontol 59: 287–296

Blomberg S, Brånemark P I, Carlsson G E 1984 Psychological reactions to edentulousness and treatment with jaw bone anchored bridges. Acta Psychiatr Scand 68: 251–262

Chan M F, Nähi T O, deBaat C, Kalk W 1998 Treatment of the atrophic edentulous maxilla with implant-supported overdentures. Int J. Prosthodon 11: 7–15

Davis D M, Packer M E P 1999 Mandibular overdentures stabilized by Astra Tech implants with either ball attachments or magnets: 5 year results. Int J Prosthodon 12: 222–229

Gotfredsen K, Holm B 2000 Implant-supported mandibular overdentures retained with ball or bar attachments: a randomised prospective 5 year study. Int J Prosthodon 13: 125–130

Kiener P, Oetterli M, Mericske E, Mericske-Stern R 2001 Effectiveness of maxillary overdentures supported by implants: maintenance and prosthetic complications. Int J Prosthodont 14: 133–140

Sethi A, Kaus T, Sochor P 2000 The use of angulated abutments in implant dentistry: five year clinical results of an on-going prospective study. Int J Oral Maxillofac Implants 15: 801–810

Watson R M, Jemt T, Chai J et al 1997 Prosthodontic treatment, patient response and the need for maintenance of complete implant-supported overdentures: an appraisal of 5 years of prospective study. Int J Prosthodont 1997 10: 345 –354

7 The partially dentate patient

INTRODUCTION

The provision of dental implants for the partially dentate patient may be the preferred option where:

- certain key teeth have been extracted from the arch;
- a traditional dental bridge abutment has failed and cannot be replaced by another natural tooth;
- a localized fixed structure would reduce the coverage of a removable partial denture.

Before implant surgery is contemplated the team must have agreed with the patient on the detailed treatment objectives. These will be based on potential solutions to their complaints, using a thorough history and examination and relevant special investigations. Use will invariably be made of mounted study casts, radiographs, a diagnostic wax-up and a surgical stent. The number of implants and their distribution may be complex and variable, and will then require more detailed planning than simpler single-tooth cases. Factors of importance include the extraction of key teeth from the arch, such as the remaining distal abutment on a bounded saddle, where a traditional dental bridge abutment has failed and cannot be replaced by another natural tooth, or where a localized fixed structure would reduce the tissue coverage of a removable partial denture.

Such treatment must be based on a comprehensive history, thorough clinical examination, careful diagnosis and agreed treatment plan. Effective and close teamwork is therefore, essential between those providing the surgery and those responsible for the construction of the prosthesis, which of course, includes the dental technician.

The partially dentate patient

Case assessment

While the modern development of dental implants was spurred by the problems of the edentulous patient, it soon became evident that this technique had a significant role to play in the treatment of the partially dentate. This partly reflects the potential of the procedure, and partly shifts in patterns of tooth loss in many countries, with falling numbers of edentulous citizens and an increasing population who are partially dentate. In many societies it is considered important to be dentate, with an acceptable appearance and function. Thus the absence of anterior teeth, evident loss of posterior teeth, or a severe reduction in masticatory efficiency are considered unacceptable by most of our patients. In the edentulous patient, this necessitates the use of complete dentures, which, in some situations, fail to meet the patient's needs. If these problems relate to looseness or sensitive denture-bearing tissues, then major improvements can often be produced by using dental implants. The partially dentate patient, on the other hand, may have little or no motivation to replace their missing teeth, and there is often a wider range of treatment options available to them compared with the edentulous person. Motivation, expectations and treatment alternatives are therefore particularly important in this group.

SYSTEMIC FACTORS
Patients' desires and needs

Patients' desires reflect their perceptions of their oral problems, while their needs reflect the professional assessment of their oral health and function as compared with normative values, which may be little appreciated by the patient. The severity of the impact of missing teeth on the patient's life will vary with their location and number, and the patient's expectations, as well as sometimes their occupation.

Professional views concerning the need to replace missing teeth have evolved from the era when it was considered essential for all patients to have complete dentitions, whether natural or artificial. The more modern approach is to make individual decisions to replace teeth on the basis of research evidence.

The patient's expectations

It is most important when preparing a treatment plan to verify the patient's expectations. These are often unrealistic, or based upon inadequate or inaccurate information. Since it is the patient's expectations of outcomes which are the driving force behind most dental treatment, it is essential that a thorough assessment be made of these, the problems that exist and the likely outcomes of the various treatment alternatives. These can then be used as a basis for explaining matters to the patient, and producing a suitable treatment plan based on informed consent.

Commitment

Treatment with dental implants, particularly in its more complex forms, requires significant commitment from the patient in terms of regular attendance, the ability to accept the limitations of interim phases of treatment and the maintenance of high standards of oral hygiene.

Resources

Complex restorative dental treatment is inherently expensive, although its relative lifetime costs may be more modest. While the dentist has a duty to explain to the patient the range of available treatment options, together with their advantages and disadvantages, it is prudent when considering extensive therapy such as that with dental implants to ascertain whether the relevant resources are likely to be available.

Residual life expectancy

While there is thought to be a lower age limit for implant treatment, reflecting the cessation of facial growth, there are no absolute upper age limits, although the increasing numbers of very elderly in many communities, often with multiple disorders, may in itself place restrictions on implant treatment. Every patient must be treated as an individual and their rights respected when jointly reaching treatment decisions.

Ability to cooperate

Where a patient is unable to cooperate with the complexities of implant treatment then this should be avoided and consideration given to more straight-forward procedures.

Ability to undergo surgery

Reference has been made earlier to the significance of a patient's ability to undergo implant surgery for whatever reason; however, where this is not possible then by definition the treatment becomes unsuitable.

LOCAL FACTORS

There are a number of local factors of particular importance when deciding on a treatment plan for the partially dentate. These include periodontal status, endodontic considerations, conservation status, the occlusion and the appropriateness of restoring the space in the arch.

Treatment alternatives

The treatment alternatives available for replacing missing teeth have been discussed in Chapter 2 and are outlined here for completeness. They include the following.

Orthodontic treatment

This can be employed to eliminate or redistribute space in the dental arch so as to produce a better appearance, or to realign teeth to facilitate implant placement, both in terms of the dimensions of any superstructure and the appropriate location of the implants themselves in relation to the roots of adjacent teeth. An example of this is the decision to realign maxillary central incisors and canines to permit the insertion of implants to replace missing lateral incisors.

Removable partial dentures

These can have a valuable role to play as a diagnostic or interim procedure, or when restoring extensive defects that are not amenable to other procedures, for example when replacing multiple missing teeth in the dental arch.

Resin retained bridges

These have transformed the management of missing teeth and can provide an aesthetically satisfactory outcome in many circumstances. They are, however, limited in their application by the size and location of the adjacent teeth, the occlusion and the contours of the residual alveolar ridge.

Conventional bridges

These are often viewed as an alternative to a resin-retained bridge; however, they do require significant tooth preparation and are not suited to many situations. Neither type of bridge will preserve alveolar bone and therefore compare unfavourably with dental implants in this respect.

Implant-based treatment

Where treatment with dental implants is being considered, local factors of importance include the bony and prosthetic envelopes and their relationship, the contours of the bone and adjacent soft tissues at the ridge crest, where they will influence the appearance of the implant-stabilized prosthesis, and the dynamic and static relationships of the prosthetic space with the opposing teeth.

Missing posterior teeth

The most frequently encountered partially dentate situations are those with missing posterior teeth with either bounded or free-end edentulous spaces. These

---

Box 7.1 Methods for replacement for edentulous spaces in the arch

- Observation
- Removable partial denture
- Adhesive bridgework
- Conventional bridgework
- Implant-stabilized prosthesis

may be difficult to treat because of limitations caused by anatomical structures such as the maxillary sinus in the upper jaw and the mandibular canal in the mandible. A severely resorbed alveolar ridge or a large maxillary sinus may preclude the placement of dental implants or demand complex bone grafting.

In the most posterior part of the maxillary arch, the tuberosity may have a sufficient quantity of bone for implant placement but its quality may be poor; more dense bone may be found in the pterygoid process and the vertical part of the palatine bone.

The difficulty in placing implants in posterior regions is often one of access, limiting the length of devices that may be inserted.

Anterior spaces

The clinical situation when replacing missing anterior teeth with implants may place very demanding requirements on the operator to achieve an aesthetic result. In the anterior edentulous maxilla the position of the incisive canal and the midline suture may affect the implant positioning. Owing to the pattern of bone resorption in both a labial and vertical direction the maxilla effectively becomes smaller. As a result, it becomes difficult to place artificial crowns in the positions of their natural predecessors while achieving a natural appearance. The influence of the lip position (Figs 7.1, 7.2), which can screen or highlight the anterior maxillary zone, is very important, as is the jaw relationship. In the anterior edentulous mandible the loss of the incisors may lead to significant vertical loss or narrowing of alveolar bone, making the replacement of teeth with implants difficult.

Clinical examination

Extra-oral examination

The most important and significant factor to be considered in the extra-oral examination will be the effect of the missing teeth on the aesthetic zone. How much of the intra-oral cavity does the patient display on talking or laughing? Examination of any previous prosthesis will aid in judging the need to replace not only the teeth but also hard and soft tissues. This prosthesis may support the lip and therefore influence the decision on the type of prosthetic replacement. Is a flange essential for positioning the artificial teeth correctly with the appropriate length of crowns? Might it be possible to make suitable adjustments to the overbite and the level of the occlusal plane to avoid using excessively long anterior teeth, resulting in an unnatural appearance? The range of jaw opening will be important, and may restrict access to the posterior part of the mouth so as to preclude implant placement.

Intra-oral examination

Oral hygiene assessment

Evidence of poor plaque control, bleeding on probing and increased pocket depths around natural teeth are

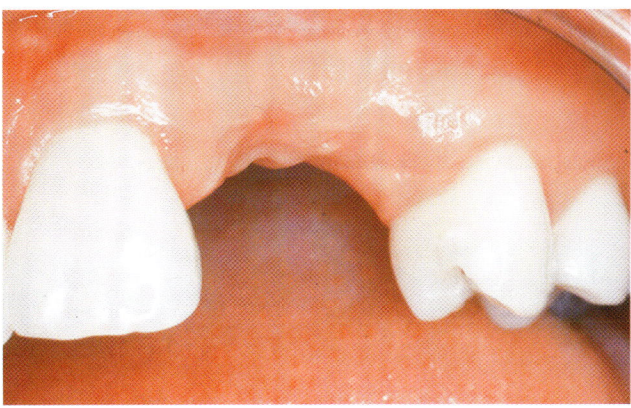

Fig. 7.1 Missing 22, 23 showing extensive soft and hard tissue loss in the aesthetic zone, in a patient with a high lip line. This is a very demanding case, which would be difficult to restore directly with either an implant-stabilized or conventional fixed prosthesis.

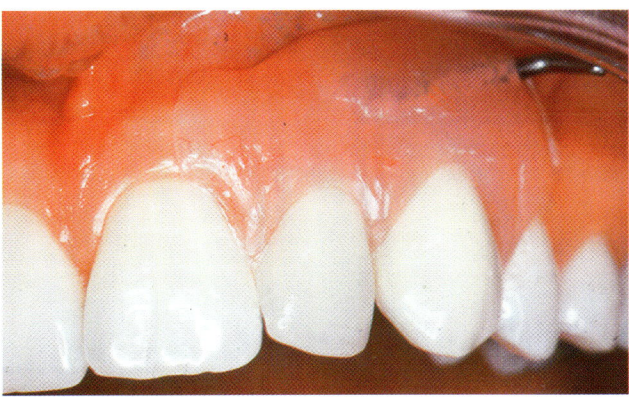

Fig. 7.2 The same case shown in Figure 7.1, demonstrating use of a two-part partial denture, which replaces the missing hard and soft tissues.

unsatisfactory and indicative of uncontrolled periodontal disease. Implant treatment in these situations is susceptible to failure, whereas a history of regular periodontal maintenance and monitoring of bone levels, and evidence of good patient motivation may warrant further consideration of implant treatment.

Careful examination of all the soft tissue in the edentulous spans is important. The presence or absence of papillae around adjacent teeth will influence not only the aesthetic outcome but also the necessity to regenerate these structures surgically. Ridge mapping may be helpful to determine thickness of the mucosa covering the potential areas for implant insertion.

If the patient has been edentulous for a long time, a shallow vestibule may make it difficult for them to maintain their final prosthesis and to achieve an aesthetically acceptable result. The position and attachment levels of any frena should also be noted, as these can create problems in soft tissue management adjacent to implants.

The underlying bone must also be assessed by palpation for resorption and the presence of any bony concavities, sharp contours and restricted width, which may affect the positioning of implants.

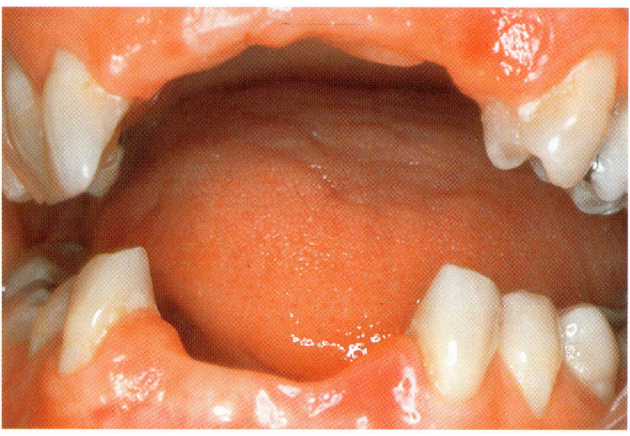

Fig. 7.3 Extensive loss of both upper and lower teeth together with marked loss of the alveolus. This case is complicated by the obvious parafunction, and therefore may not be suitable for restoration with dental implants.

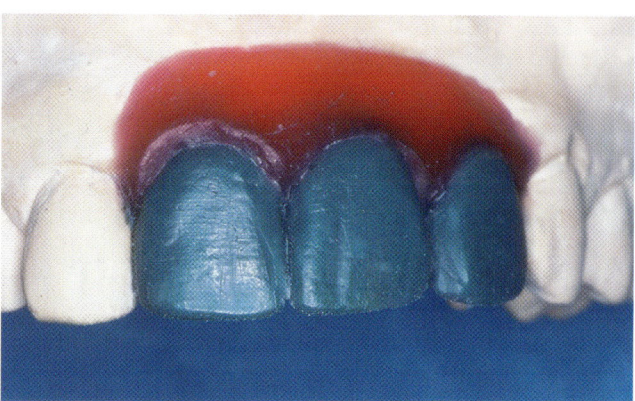

Fig. 7.4 The diagnostic wax-up demonstrates not only the final tooth positions but also the hard and soft tissue loss. These factors may have an impact on the choice of restoration.

Occlusal examination

A diagnosis of parafunctional habits such as bruxism and tooth clenching can often be made from the clinical findings of abrasion, attrition and wear facets (Fig. 7.3). Parafunction may lead to increased tooth mobility, fracture and even loss of teeth. Although parafunction may itself not be a contraindication for implant placement, it can, if uncontrolled, cause problems due to overloading of the final prosthesis and its supporting implants. Risks range from fractured porcelain/artificial teeth to screw loosening or fracture of the implant bodies.

All lateral and protrusive jaw movements should be examined carefully. A more detailed examination of these and their influence on the final prosthesis will be discussed later.

The inter-arch relationship should be examined to determine available occlusal space; tooth movement and over-eruption might have occurred over time. Anteroposterior or lateral discrepancies need to be recorded, as these will influence the form and positions of the crowns, and hence the occlusion on the final prosthesis.

Special tests

All remaining teeth should be assessed for their restorative, endodontic and periodontal status. A decision on their individual prognosis may influence the overall plan and decisions regarding planning for future implants.

Articulated diagnostic casts

Carefully articulated study casts, mounted with the aid of a face-bow transfer, and an inter-occlusal retruded contact record are an important treatment planning aid. Casts may be mounted in the retruded contact position (RCP) on an articulator, which will help in the assessment and planning of the treatment options.

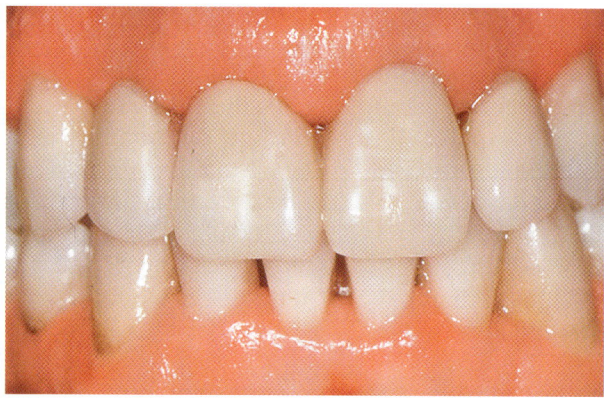

Fig. 7.5 A tooth try-in gives both the clinician and patient evidence of the position and appearance of the intended final restoration.

Where implant treatment is contemplated the diagnostic casts may be used for:

- a general occlusal examination over the full range of mandibular movements, and an assessment of their potential effects on an implant retained prosthesis;
- diagnostic wax-up or tooth set-up. (Fig. 7.4);
- construction of a radiographic stent;
- sectioned casts in conjunction with ridge mapping;
- construction of a surgical stent.

Owing to the pattern of bone loss, especially in the maxilla, it may be necessary to prepare a diagnostic wax-up using denture teeth set in wax and tried in the mouth, as a planning aid (Fig. 7.5).

This is especially important where there has been loss not only of teeth but also of the associated hard and soft tissues. When placed in the anterior part of the mouth, this may show the position of the teeth on the final prosthesis and their influence on appearance, phonetics and lip support. It is preferable to avoid the use of a flange, unless it is intended to incorporate this in the design, e.g. as with a partial overdenture. If the previous prosthesis had a flange, removal of this may reduce the lip support, which will affect the nature of the final design of the prosthesis.

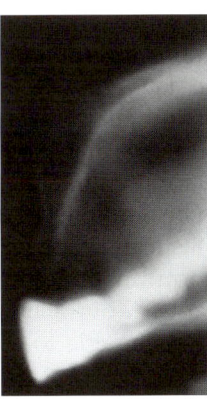

Fig. 7.6 This tomograph of the upper anterior incisor region demonstrates the outline of the proposed tooth position in relation to the existing bone, available for possible implant placement. Lack of bone may have an impact on the position and angulation of the implant.

Radiographic template/stent

Various forms of radiographic templates have been described using acrylic stents incorporating metal markers, coated with metal foil or made from a radio-opaque resin.

The ideal form should be one which, in combination with a suitable radiograph, such as a spiral or computed tomograph (CT), will show the ideal final tooth position and its relationship to the remaining bone (Fig. 7.6).

Surgical stent

A surgical stent that fits correctly on the natural teeth adjacent to the edentulous space is an essential aid to positioning implants. The stent design should be agreed by the team and has been discussed in Chapters 3 and 4.

Sectioned duplicate casts used in conjunction with ridge mapping

Ridge mapping may be also used to assess the topography of the alveolar bone in cross-section at potential implant sites. This method is relatively easy, especially in the maxilla, and requires no special equipment. After the appropriate area is anaesthetized with a local anaesthetic, measurements of the soft tissue thickness to the underlying bone at each implant site are obtained by 'sounding down' to bone with a sharpened periodontal probe. If a simple grid of sounding points is marked with an indelible pencil on the disinfected mucosa, then a simple contour map can be produced.

The recorded measurements are transferred to duplicated casts of the patient's mouth, which have been trimmed to expose the edentulous ridge in cross-section at each planned implant site. A dot is marked on the trimmed surface of the cast at each sounding point on that section, to indicate the mucosal thickness at that point. A line connecting the marks is then drawn to indicate the topography of the bony ridge in the plane of the section.

HOW MANY IMPLANTS SHOULD BE SELECTED AND WHAT SHOULD BE THEIR DISTRIBUTION IN THE EDENTULOUS SPAN?

Planning implant numbers and distribution

Historically implant placement tended to be overly influenced by surgical considerations, with particular respect to the amount of available bone in a given location. The current concept is one of a 'top down' approach in which the starting point is the planned prosthetic reconstruction, which is then used as a basis for planning the preparatory procedures. Based on the diagnostic wax-up, and utilizing the radiographs, the surgical placement must be designed so as to ensure optimal appearance, phonetics, loading and masticatory function, while facilitating home oral hygiene.

There are no set rules but only guidelines as to the number of implants required to restore a partially dentate arch, but a good understanding of implant biomechanics makes it possible to optimize the treatment plan for each case to reduce the risk of functional failures.

Utilizing the diagnostic wax-up, it is possible to formulate a view on the optimal number of implants for each case, which will be partly limited by the available space. While this is a subjective decision, the following points are currently believed to be relevant.

Mechanical considerations

- Longer implants are to be preferred to shorter ones, provided that excessive heat is not generated during their insertion.
- Bicortical fixation is to be preferred.
- Implant placement in denser, but not highly dense, bone is to be preferred.
- High occlusal loads indicate the use of more implants. History and examination can provide clues to this, e.g. tooth wear, a history of bruxism or tooth clenching, bulky masticatory muscles and fractured restorations or teeth.
- Loads are best directed down the long axes of the implants.
- Cantilevers should normally be shorter than the separation of the closest two implants.
- Implants should not be angulated towards each other to the extent where restoration is precluded.

Aesthetic considerations

- Implants should be in alignment with the overlying crowns.
- Implants should not be closer than 3 mm, where they are parallel.
- Implants and their projected connecting components should be contained within the prosthetic envelope.

- Implants and their projected connecting components should not prevent oral hygiene.

The optimal number of implants is a function of all these factors.

Posterior region

As a guide, in the posterior part of the mouth it is recommended that when possible there should ideally be one implant for each tooth being replaced. A diagnostic wax-up, together with the relevant radiographs, will facilitate a decision concerning the positions and angulations of the implants (Fig. 7.7). From a biomechanical view it is suggested that implants should not all be placed in a straight line, but with a slight offset in the vertical plane. This variation in orientation creates a tripod effect, and so increases the biomechanical stability of the bone–implant–prosthesis complex. A minimal distance of 3 mm should be maintained between implants in order not to compromise the soft tissue. A greater separation may be needed if the implants are converging, to permit the seating of the prosthetic components.

Anterior region

Within the anterior part of the mouth it may not be necessary to have one implant for each tooth replaced, and the utilization of pontics between implants may produce a more natural appearance.

The type of anterior guidance to be constructed in the final prosthesis should be determined at this stage as implant placement may influence this.

Linked units or individual crowns?

It would seem logical to replace each tooth with one implant in the posterior part of the mouth, and then restore the implants with individual crowns. In most clinical situations, this theoretical ideal is often challenged by the lack of available bone due to alveolar resorption and anatomical structures such as the inferior alveolar nerve and the maxillary sinus. As a result, implant placement may be precluded or only shorter devices can be employed. An additional factor is the increase in masticatory forces which occur more distally and can form an unfavourable combination with shorter implants. From a biomechanical standpoint it is therefore preferable to consider linking the implants to gain increased stability and spread occlusal loads. The role of occlusal contacts will be discussed later in this chapter.

Anterior restorations

Depending on the number of teeth to be replaced both linked units and individual crowns should be considered. If a spaced dentition were previously present, then individual crowns would be the treatment of choice. However, due to the pattern of bone loss in the maxilla, it may be difficult to place implants with at least 3 mm spacing between them while achieving an acceptable appearance. Linking the implants may allow the use of artificial gum work made from pink porcelain or acrylic resin, so as to improve the appearance, which is rarely possible with single crowns (Fig. 7.8).

Linking teeth to implants

There is much discussion as to whether implants should be joined mechanically to natural teeth and, if so, what form of attachment should be used. There are concerns that combining two systems with a great difference in rigidity may result in unbalanced load sharing between implant and tooth; nevertheless, there are reports of shorter-term prospective studies which suggest that in suitable circumstances the technique can be successful. It should, however, be approached with caution, since these reports should be set against reported failures of the linkages in such designs.

A typical scenario would be an edentulous span bounded mesially by a natural tooth and distally by a single implant.

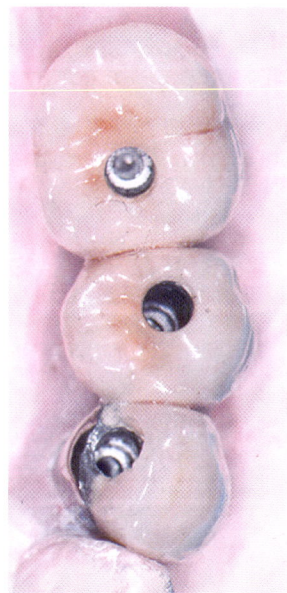

Fig. 7.7 Laboratory model demonstrating the offset position of the implants in the premolar regions in relation to the occlusal table.

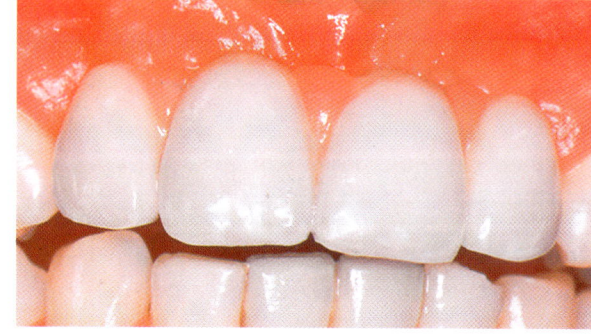

Fig. 7.8 A four-unit implant-retained bridge demonstrating pink porcelain to mask soft tissue deficiency.

The various options for attachment of the prosthesis are:

- a fixed linkage between implant and tooth;
- a fixed–movable design with the movable joint on the distal aspect of the tooth;
- a fixed–movable design with the movable joint on the mesial aspect of the implant;
- a fixed-movable design with the movable joint integral to the implant body and connecting components.

The vertical and lateral movement of an integrated dental implant in function is typically < 5 μm, while comparable figures for healthy natural teeth are of the order of 50–100 μm. As a result, if such a linkage is contemplated then there should be some form of full occlusal coverage on the abutment tooth to minimize the risk of dislodgement of the retainer.

When using a fixed–fixed type of linkage with a multi-unit rigid framework joining the implant to the tooth, there is a risk of the movement of the tooth under load creating what in effect is a cantilevered superstructure. As a result, the forces on the implant may be excessive. Lateral forces on the prosthesis may also cause rotational and bending movements, creating a similar effect. Over time these can cause loosening of screwed joints, cement failure in joints of that type, fracture of the prosthesis or failure of the patient–implant interface.

It has therefore been suggested that one method of overcoming these problems would be to place a small movable attachment between the abutment tooth and the bridge.

With occlusal loading the tooth may move in both a lateral and vertical direction, and if this is the case, especially with vertical movements, then the attachment will disengage. Over time this can result in gradual intrusion of the tooth, as a result of a ratchet effect, even with relatively short bridges.

Placing the attachment on the implant

It has been suggested also that the movable attachment within the bridge should be reversed and placed on the proximal aspect of the implant. With vertical occlusal forces some intrusion on the natural tooth could then place undue forces on the attachment as it 'bottoms out', possible leading to cementation failure or fracture of the bridge.

Intramobile element in the implant

Some implant systems allow for the use of an integral movable component or 'intramobile element' to permit some micro-movement of the implant prosthesis. Unfortunately these can require frequent replacement and may lead to increased screw loosening.

On the basis of current knowledge it is recommended that wherever possible in partially dentate cases the implant prosthesis should not be linked to adjacent teeth, whatever form of attachment or connector might be employed.

Where are cantilevers permissible?

The presence of any cantilever will increase the potential loads on the supporting implants, and where leverages are unfavourable can result in forces being experienced by the implants that are greater than those applied. They should therefore be avoided where possible and only employed when necessary; for example, a distal extension to avoid the need for a sinus lift procedure to permit the placement of a distal implant. Cantilevers should, however, be employed with due regard to the biomechanics of the situation, longer implants and shorter cantilevers being preferred.

What space is required for placing implants?

With all systems there will be a minimum space required from the head of the implant to the opposing tooth in the opposite arch. This intra-occlusal space is important, and will have minimum dimensions depending on the type of prosthesis and abutment; it is typically 7 mm. The occlusal material used on the final prosthesis will be influenced by the available space. When assessing this it should be borne in mind that the prosthetic space envelope is partly defined by the relative functional movements of the opposing dentition.

In the anterior part of the mouth, especially in the maxilla, where aesthetics may be especially important, if the implants are too close to each other then this may

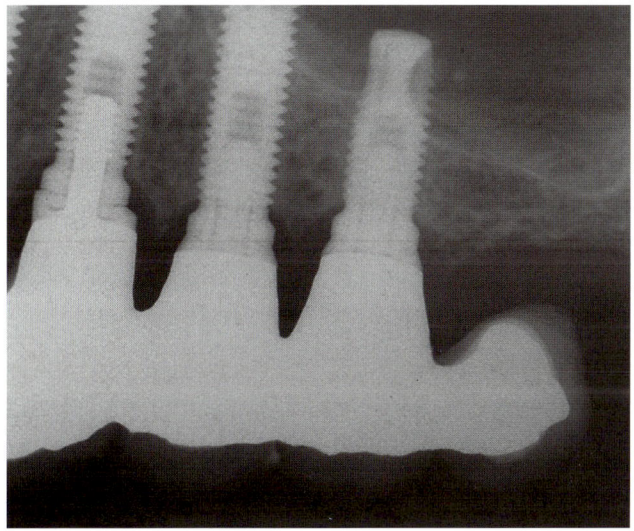

Fig. 7.9 At the 1-year review the radiograph demonstrates the expected bone remodelling to the first thread on this four-unit implant bridge.

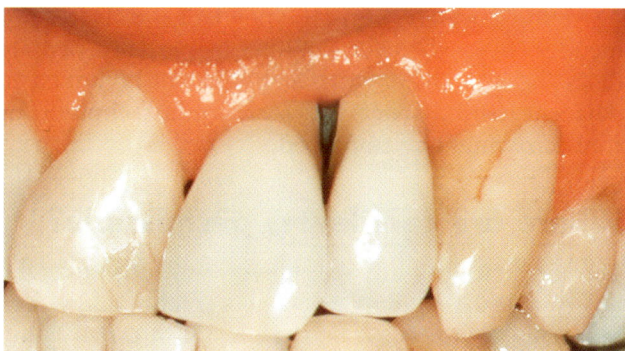

Fig. 7.10 Implant replacement of 21 and 22. The implants have been placed too close, resulting in the loss of the papilla between them and the artificial crowns.

lead to a poor appearance (Fig. 7.10). It is recommended that the minimum interproximal distance between implants should be 3 mm, in order to maintain a satisfactory soft tissue profile between them. In some circumstances it may well be better to place implants in alternative sites and link the implant crowns with pontics, so as to produce a better appearance.

Occasionally, for example in the anterior mandible, better positioning can be achieved with narrow-diameter implants, especially if the occlusal load is not likely to be excessive.

Both the surgeon and the prosthodontist should be fully conversant with the different type of abutments available for the system they are using and have made a clear decision on what type of prosthesis is to be finally used before the surgery is undertaken.

HOW SHOULD SECOND-STAGE SURGERY BE PLANNED FOR PARTIALLY DENTATE CASES?

The aim of second-stage surgery is to uncover the implants and place healing abutments, which will:

- facilitate gingival healing;
- allow easy access to the implants following healing.

There are two types of healing abutments:

1. Conventional axisymmetrical healing abutments. These are cylindrical in design, of varying diameters depending on the size of the implant, and of various lengths depending on the thickness of the soft tissue. The disadvantage of this type of healing abutment is that it does not follow the outline or emergence profile of the teeth to be replaced.
2. Custom-made anatomical abutments. Customized healing abutments, which are in two parts, can follow the root outline of the teeth being replaced. This has the advantage of facilitating the re-formation of the soft tissues to improve the form of the 'interdental' and other soft-tissue contours. The methods for reconstructing

interdental papillae have been discussed in Chapter 5.

Healing times

Following second-stage surgery the authors recommend that the area be left to heal for a minimum of 4 weeks to establish 'gingival maturity'. Early intervention may result in further soft-tissue changes around the final prosthesis. If it is necessary to place a prosthesis in these circumstances, then a temporary device may be used.

PROSTHESIS FIXATION: SCREW OR CEMENT RETAINED?

The next decision for the prosthodontist in treatment planning concerns the use of screw- or cement-retained prostheses.

There are three types of screw-retained prosthesis:

- Prosthesis screw retained direct to the implant body.
- Prosthesis screw retained direct to an abutment.
- Prosthesis screw retained with a lateral screw on a custom abutment.

Cement-retained prostheses may be placed on pre-manufactured or custom-made abutments.

Screw-retained prostheses: advantages

- Ready retrievability.
- Machined component interfaces.
- No cement to break down or extrude from the joint during placement. This can be difficult to remove and may irritate the soft tissues.
- They provide a defined and controlled failure point if overloaded, which can aid repair/retrieval. Screw loosening can also warn of mechanical overload.
- They permit the use of a sequence of contoured components to modify soft-tissue contours.

Retrievability

Probably the main advantage of having a screw-retained prosthesis, whether it is directly linked to the implant itself or to overlying abutments, is the ability for the prosthodontist to retrieve the prosthesis easily and predictably. This may be necessary to change contours, e.g. where artificial teeth have worn, to repair the prosthesis if any damage has occurred and to replace the screws.

Machined component interfaces

A screw-retained prosthesis will have machined components at various levels, and will therefore require an accurate fit. This places demanding requirements on the surgeon, prosthodontist and technician. While a totally passive fit is viewed as the ideal, it is probably not achievable owing to the practicalities of screw mechanics, limitations of the production process and functional jaw deformation.

Loss of cement

Cement can be difficult to control during implant placement, and its subsequent loss will increase the gap between the prosthetic components. If it remains in the peri-implant soft tissues it can act as an irritant and initiate peri-implant mucositis.

Fail-safe mechanism

In addition to acting as a predicable failure point in response to overload, it has been suggested that if excessive forces were generated within the prosthesis then loosening of the screws would occur and provide early warning of the overload. It has been suggested that this is particularly the case with the small gold, prosthesis-securing screws inserted in the abutments. Careful examination may then give a clue as to the reason why the screw has loosened. Untoward screw loosening should always be investigated; common causes are under-tightening, failure to achieve a near passive fit, excessive cantilevering and increased occlusal loads due to poor design.

Modification of soft tissue contours

By far one of the most predictable aspects of the screw-retained prosthesis is the ability to help to modify and form the soft-tissue contours using temporary crowns (Fig. 7.11). This is extremely difficult with some forms

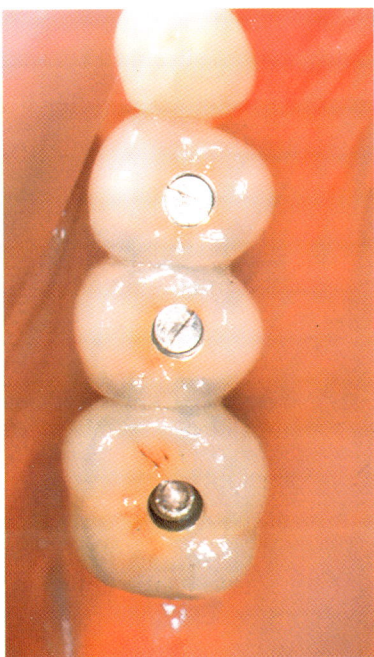

Fig. 7.11 A three-unit screw retained fixed implant prosthesis in a free-end saddle. Screw retention allows for retrieval if necessary. A hexagonal screw head is placed more deeply in the molar crown.

> **Box 7.2** Screw-retained implant prosthesis
>
> Advantages
> - Easily retrievable
> - Precise fit of manufactured components
> - No risk of excess cement in soft tissues
> - Decrease in clinical and laboratory time
>
> Disadvantages
> - Access holes need to be in the long axis of the implant
> - Access holes may be visible on occlusal surfaces
> - Increased technical skill needed to achieve passive fit
> - Increased bulk of material in the cingulum areas of restorations placed in the anterior dental arch

of cemented temporary prosthesis, while the risk of excess cement extrusion into the soft tissues may lead to subgingival inflammation.

Screw-retained prostheses: disadvantages

Access holes

The major disadvantages of having a screw-retained prosthesis are the requirement for access holes, which of necessity must lie in the long axis of the implant or abutment. This may well mean that in the anterior portion of the mouth there will have to be an enlarged cingulum. The choice of screw or cement fixation may influence the orientations and positions of the implants. There will no doubt be some access holes, which will be visible, and these will need to be filled with a permanent filling material at the end of treatment, e.g. a resin-based material. It has been suggested that differential wear of these materials may lead to occlusal instability.

A one-piece casting or CADCAM-designed frame where screws hold the prosthesis directly on the implant will result in much larger access holes to accommodate the greater diameter of the screws used at the level of the implant body. Using intermediate abutments will reduce their diameter since narrower screws are used with these.

More complex technique

A screw-retained prosthesis will often be more complex mechanically to allow for the various components.

Cement-retained prostheses: advantages

Access holes

Avoidance of the need for access holes on the occlusal or labial surfaces can result in an improved appearance. This can be particularly beneficial anteriorly.

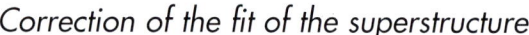

Box 7.3 Cement-retained bridges

Advantages
- No access hole on occlusal surface
- Use of techniques similar to conventional bridgework
- Passive fit not as critical as for a screw-retained bridge

Disadvantages
- Retrieval more difficult
- Increase in both clinical and laboratory time
- Cementation needs to be controlled
- Increased costs of production

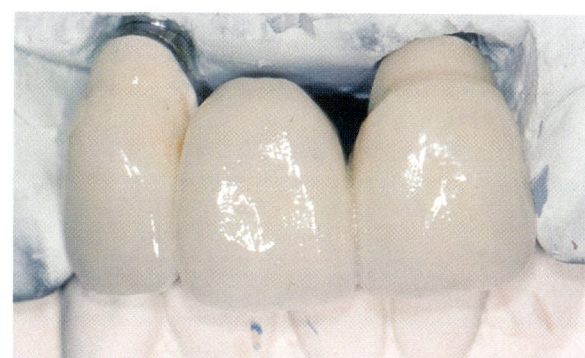

Fig. 7.12 Laboratory model with the soft-tissue mask removed, showing a three-unit cement-retained fixed implant prosthesis replacing 12, 11 and 21. Constructed on customized abutments.

Correction of the fit of the superstructure

Deficiencies in the fit of the superstructure are corrected. It could be argued that the superstructure does not need to fit as well when cemented since deficiencies will be made good by the layer of cement. Set against this are the occlusal errors introduced by incorrect seating during cementation. These can be very difficult or impossible to correct without removing and recementing the prosthesis, which is sometimes impossible without damaging it.

Familiar technique

An undoubted attraction of the cemented prosthesis is its ready familiarity to those experienced in conventional crown and bridge technology.

Cement-retained prostheses: disadvantages

Removal problems

A major disadvantage is that it may be difficult to remove the prosthesis, as even temporary cements may harden over a period of time (Figs 7.12, 7.13).

Cement extrusion

On cementation excess cement can sometimes be extruded deep into the adjacent soft tissues, with significant repercussions to the health of the mucosa and alveolar bone.

Relocation errors

It is extremely difficult to accurately relocate the prosthesis in a identical position to that used on the master cast during fabrication. As a result, more extensive occlusal adjustments may be needed.

ABUTMENT SELECTION

The decision as to whether to use abutments or fit the prosthesis direct to the implants has been discussed in the previous section. A one-piece superstructure may

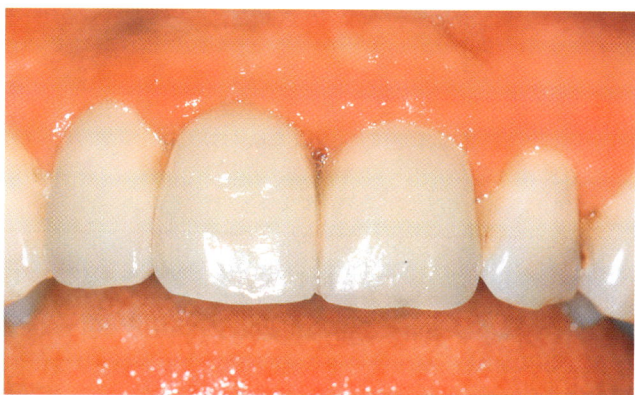

Fig. 7.13 Three-unit cement-retained implant-stabilized prosthesis, cemented in place (see also Fig. 7.12).

sometimes be made to fit straight on to the implants where it is screw retained and the implants have a high degree of parallelism. Abutments can be used to correct lack of parallelism in the implants, and are necessary with some systems where cement fixation is to be used. The range of available abutments includes:

- standard preformed machined abutments;
- abutments designed for custom modification ('prepable');
- customized laboratory abutments, produced using CADCAM techniques or customized casting procedures.

Each of these has its advantages and disadvantages.

Standard pre-formed machined abutments

Generally used in screw-retained prostheses, these are commonly manufactured in titanium as two pieces with an abutment, which fits on top of the implant, and an intermediate screw, which links the abutment to the implant body (Fig. 7.14). They are usually provided in a range of lengths and sometimes different collar heights.

The major advantage of these is that they are simple, and can be selected from both clinical and laboratory

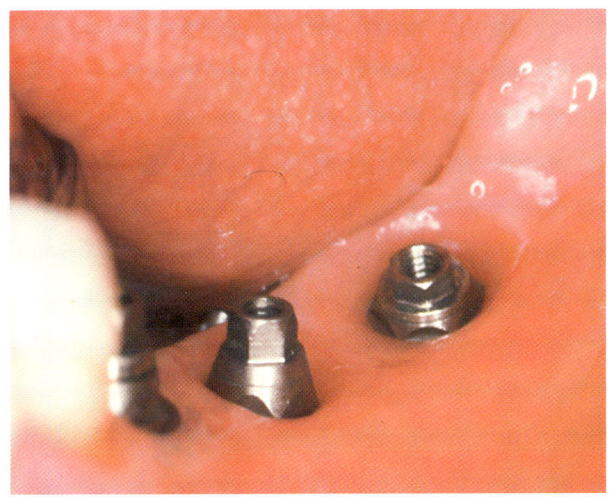

Fig. 7.14 Three precision manufactured abutments in place.

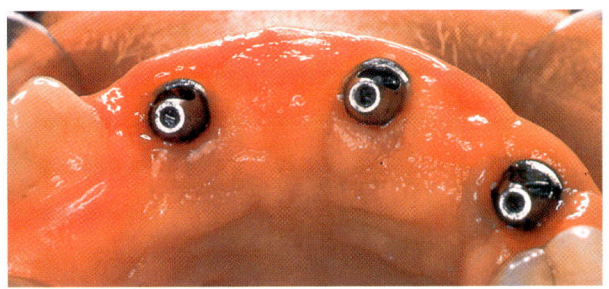

Fig. 7.15 Standard precision machined angled abutments placed to compensate for the divergence and locations of the implant bodies.

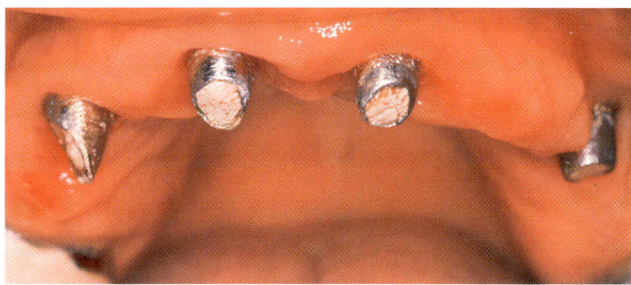

Fig. 7.16 Four custom-modified abutments in position. The final prosthesis will be cemented in place.

data, be it chairside assessment or examination of a study model. The relative ease of use of these devices decreases both the clinical and laboratory time. They can also produce a very predictable fit. Their major disadvantage is that the margin of the crown does not follow the gingival contour, as in most cases the shoulder on the abutment is parallel with its end faces.

Standard preformed machined angled abutments (Fig. 7.15)

Angled abutments are designed to compensate for divergence between the long axes of the implants and the abutment. They can enable a rigid prosthesis to be removable by compensating for divergences between implants. They can also facilitate the location of the access hole for a screw-retained prosthesis within the central region of the occlusal or cingulum surface of the restoration. They also have the advantage of enabling the prosthesis to remain screw retained, the advantages and disadvantages of which have been discussed in the previous section.

Preparable abutments

These are supplied as stock shaped abutments, which can be placed directly on the implants and prepared directly in the mouth or laboratory. They provide for flexibility of use, and have the advantage of a similarity of technique for conventional crown- and bridgework. Since they are usually fabricated in titanium or a ceramic they are difficult to prepare and adjust in the mouth.

An alternative technique is to record an impression from the head of the implant and prepare the abutments subsequently in the laboratory. They are placed on the analogue in the master cast and prepared to follow the orientation of the soft tissue and future arch.

The disadvantage of this technique is that both the clinical and laboratory time are increased, with the additional requirement of recording a second working impression within the mouth after the abutments have been placed on the heads of the implants. While in theory the abutments may be placed on a master cast produced from an impression of the heads of the implants, this technique is prone to inaccuracies due to vertical and rotational location errors when placing the abutments on the master cast. This problem may be overcome by preparing a customized acrylic jig to locate the abutments accurately on the implant bodies.

Customized laboratory abutments

These can also be utilized for cement-retained prostheses. Again this will necessitate recording an impression from the heads of the implants and then waxing up and casting the customized abutments. These are then replaced on the implants and a working impression made from which the final master cast is prepared. The major advantage of the prepable and customized abutments is that the clinician is able to control the orientation of the prosthesis if the implants have been placed in positions that do not allow access holes through the occlusal or cingulum surfaces (Box 7.4).

IMPRESSION PROCEDURES

Impression procedures for dental implants usually make use of manufactured impression transfer copings. These are designed to fit on either the implant body, sometimes called fixture head copings, or the implant abutment, sometimes called abutment copings. The impression procedures associated with these are often referred to colloquially as fixture head impressions and abutment impressions.

Box 7.4 Abutment selection for fixed partial prostheses

- Pre-machined manufactured titanium abutments
  - Simple to use
  - Minimal chairside and laboratory time
  - Predictable fit
- Customized abutments
  - Gold/titanium/ceramic
  - Suitable for all cases
  - Can allow for angulation changes
  - Modifications promote good gingival contours
  - Increase in clinical and laboratory time needed

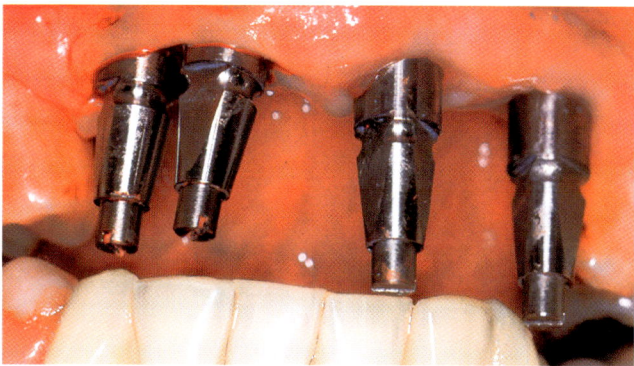

Fig. 7.17 Impression technique to record the positions of the implant heads using manufactured impression copings.

In addition, the copings may remain in the impression when it is removed, being secured to the implant or abutment with a screw so that they may be disengaged before the impression is removed. These are often called pick-up copings and the impression is called a pick-up impression. Where this is not technically feasible then the coping remains fixed to the implant or abutment and is subsequently removed and reseated in the impression.

Where abutments have been individually prepared, then impression procedures similar to those used in conventional fixed prosthodontic techniques may be employed.

Primary impressions

Following second-stage surgery, and as gingival maturity is taking place, the prosthodontist may record primary impressions on the healing abutments using an alginate impression material in a stock impression tray. A primary cast can be constructed in the laboratory on which a special tray may be made. This can be constructed with an open window where the impression copings are to remain in the impression, or in a closed design if they are to be reseated in the impression after its removal from the mouth.

Selection of impression material

An elastomeric impression material must be used in implant dentistry to ensure the necessary accuracy. The polyether or polyvinylsiloxane impression materials are well suited to this purpose since they have superior dimensional stability and accuracy.

Impression recorded at the level of the top of the implant

A working impression of the implant at a fixture level may be taken for one of three reasons (Fig. 7.17):

- To delay the decision on the type and size of the abutments. This decision may then be made in the laboratory after construction of a master model.

- To provide a master impression for constructing a one-piece prosthesis designed to fit directly on the implants.

- To construct a master cast for the use of prepable abutments or custom-made abutments.

Most implant systems utilize machined impression copings, usually made in two pieces. Typically one part seats onto the implant head and is retained with a guide pin or screw. A carefully aligned radiograph is sometimes necessary to confirm that the copings have been fully seated on the heads of the implants. The coping may be designed either to remain within the impression when the screw is released, or to allow the impression to be withdrawn while it remains secured to the implant. Often the latter are less bulky and may be appropriate for well-aligned implants within a small span.

Either custom or rigid disposable trays may be used. These should have holes for access to the guide pins, which locate the impression copings, so that these can remain in the impression when it is removed. It is important that all the surfaces of the impression copings are thoroughly dry before the impression material is gently syringed around them, and the loaded tray then fully seated. Following complete setting of the impression material the guide screws are loosened and the impression, complete with copings, removed from the mouth. Where there are spaces between the natural teeth into which the impression material may lock, these should be blocked out prior to recording the impression. This may be done either with soft wax or a proprietary light-polymerizing elastomer.

The impression should be cleaned and disinfected before being transferred to the laboratory.

Abutment-level impressions

Impressions may be recorded following abutment selection and placement. Measurement from the head of the implant to the margin of the mucosal cuff will aid in determining the height of the necessary abutments to be used. This may be done at the

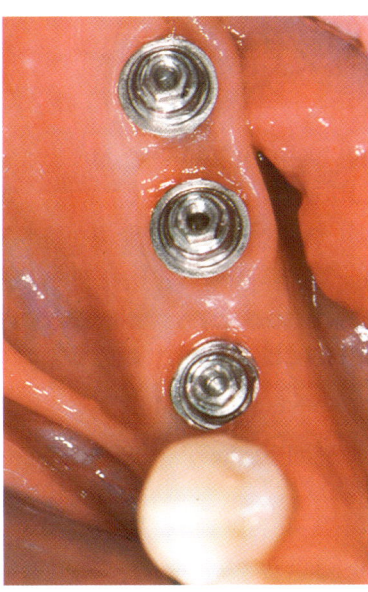

Fig. 7.18 Manufactured conical abutments in position for restoration of a free-end saddle with implants.

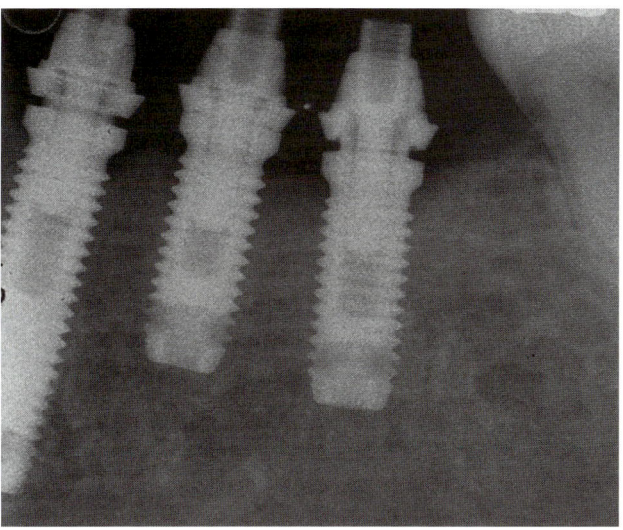

Fig. 7.19 Radiograph showing poor seating of two manufactured abutments for a partially dentate patient. This may be due to soft- or hard-tissue entrapment.

chairside or in the laboratory on a primary cast. The objective is to produce a submucosal margin of 1–1.5 mm from the crest of the 'gingival' tissue, and to provide sufficient interocclusal distance from the head of the abutment to the opposing teeth to place the prosthesis. Most machined abutments are supplied in various heights, and these can be tried to determine the optimal positioning. Following placement, a long cone periapical radiograph may be taken to ensure correct seating of the abutments, where this is unclear from clinical observation.

Following confirmation from the radiograph of complete seating, they are then definitively secured by tightening the retaining screws with a torque device, ensuring that the manufacturer's recommendations for this are followed (Fig. 7.18).

Incorrect seating may be due to:

- failure to ensure that the abutment correctly engages an anti-rotation feature, such as an external hexagonal projection;
- the presence of soft tissue or bone encroaching on the head of the implant (Fig. 7.19).

There are two different methods available to record abutment impressions.

Pick-up impression coping technique at abutment level

This technique is similar to a fixture-level impression technique, as it utilizes a machined impression coping, which is seated on the abutment where it is retained with a screw or 'guide-pin'. This is accessed via a hole in the impression tray. Following setting of the impression material the guide-pin is unscrewed, releasing the coping, which is designed with retention and anti-rotation features to secure it in the impression material (Fig. 7.25).

Reseating technique

Where lack of space makes access to the screw-retained copings impossible, a non-retentive, usually tapered coping may be employed. This utilizes a one-piece machined impression coping, which screws directly on the abutment and remains in the mouth when the impression is removed. It is then unscrewed from the abutment and reseated in the impression. This must be done carefully, as it is a common source of inaccuracy if care is not taken and the coping incorrectly seated. For these reasons the procedure should only be used when necessary.

Careful inspection of the impression will confirm the key features:

- Stability of the impression copings can be tested with tweezers. If movement is present in the impression, it is recommended that the impression be retaken.
- An accurate record of all hard and soft tissues including the teeth.

At this stage the impression is disinfected and sent to the laboratory.

LABORATORY PHASE

The appropriate laboratory analogue is attached to the impression coping, and a cast is then prepared in two stages, using silicone elastomer to represent the soft tissues and dental stone the remainder of the record, so as to produce a master model reproducing the position of the implant and the contours of the soft tissues (Figs 7.20, 7.21). The silicone elastomer permits placement of abutments on the cast for planning purposes, and their simulated expansion by the emerging profile of the prosthesis.

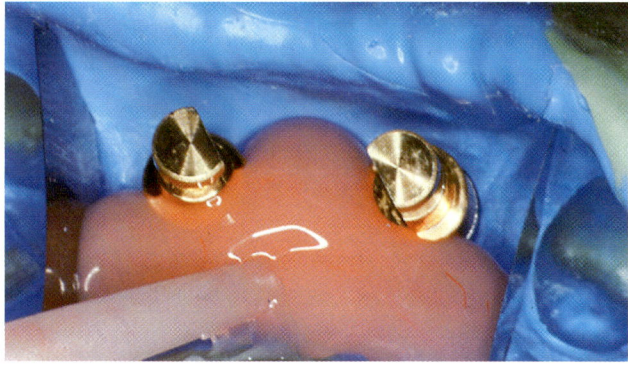

Fig. 7.20 Following the removal of an impression the abutment analogues are attached to the impression copings, and a master cast is constructed, usually beginning with the soft-tissue mask, as seen here.

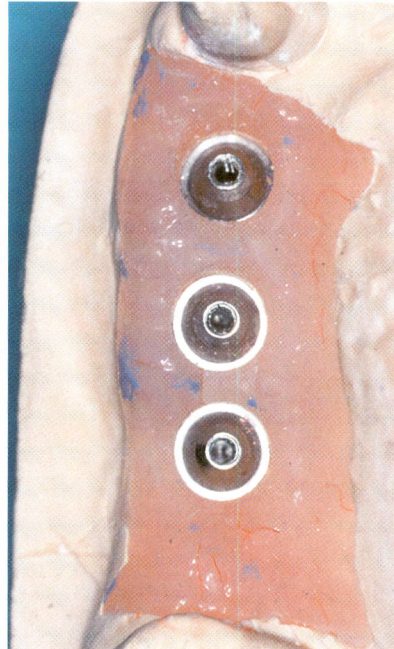

Fig. 7.21 A master cast is constructed with the abutment analogues in position for a partially dentate patient. A soft gingival mask has been constructed to reproduce the partially dentate patient mucosal cuffs.

Construction of a removable soft-tissue replica model is essential for access to either implant analogue head or abutment analogue. The gingival replicas can be removed to check the marginal fit and ensure that the final restoration has the optimal contours.

The type of definitive prosthesis will now influence the next stages.

One piece screw-retained prosthesis secured direct to the implants

The sequence of stages in construction is as follows:

- fixture-level impression;
- master cast construction;
- occlusal registration;

- try-in of trial prosthesis;
- full-contour wax-up;
- try-in and verification of metal framework;
- try-in with teeth on framework;
- final insertion;
- review.

Screw-retained prosthesis on manufactured abutments

The sequence of stages is as follows:

- (fixture level impression, select abutment(s) in the laboratory: optional stage);
- placement of abutments in the mouth;
- abutment-level impression;
- occlusal registration;
- insertion of temporary prosthesis;
- full-contour wax-up;
- try-in and verification of metal framework;
- try-in with teeth on framework;
- final insertion;
- review.

Cement-retained prosthesis on custom abutments

The sequence of stages is as follows:

- fixture-level impression;
- occlusal registration;
- construction of abutments in laboratory;
- placement of abutments in mouth;
- abutment level impression;
- occlusal registration;
- insertion of temporary prosthesis;
- full-contour wax-up;
- try-in and verification of metal framework;
- try-in with teeth on framework;
- final insertion;
- review.

As can be seen from the above lists, there are some common features regardless of the nature of the final prosthesis.

Occlusal registration

It is recommend that the casts for all partially dentate cases should be mounted on a semi-adjustable articulator. This will require appropriate occlusal records and a face-bow transfer for mounting the maxillary cast. Where there is an insufficient number of occlud-

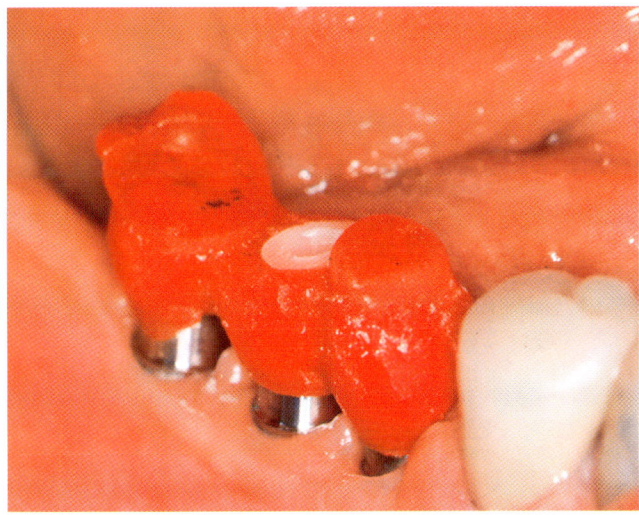

Fig. 7.22 Duralay occlusal record previously constructed on a master cast, and seated in the mouth to record the correct occlusal vertical dimension.

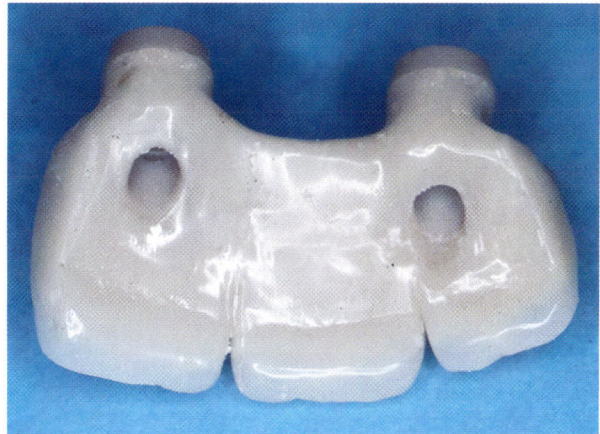

Fig. 7.23 A screw-retained temporary partial prosthesis can be custom made to achieve ideal soft-tissue contours before the final implant bridge is constructed.

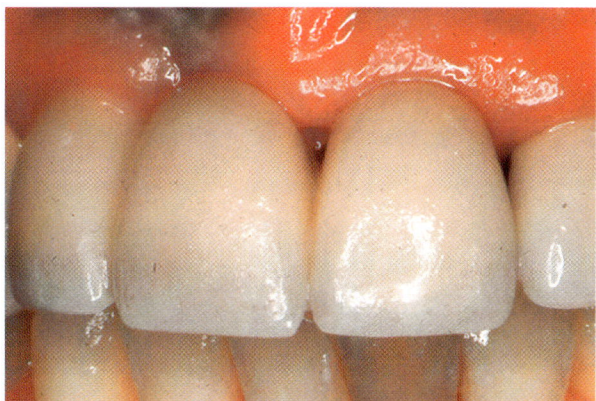

Fig. 7.24 A temporary partial prosthesis screwed in position.

ing teeth to permit freehand location, then records suitable for mounting the casts in the intercuspal position (ICP) will be needed. This usually requires a technique that utilizes some form of occlusal platform to obtain an occlusal record at the working vertical dimension of occlusion. This can be made so as to fit the implants either directly or via abutments, in order to maximize the accuracy of the record. For these reasons the occlusal jig should be made in a relatively rigid material such as an acrylic resin, rather than wax, which is not recommended (Fig. 7.22).

The 'registration device' is then secured intra-orally on either the abutments or the implants, ensuring that it is carefully adjusted to have no deflecting contacts with the opposing teeth. A fluid interocclusal recording material is then placed between the opposing teeth and the occlusal jig to record the desired jaw relationship. Where this is coincident with ICP, then neither the jig nor a bulk of registration material should intrude between the opposing natural teeth in this position.

Utilization of temporary prostheses

It may be decided that because of the position of the mucosal cuffs, or in cases where aesthetics or phonetics are particularly important, a temporary prosthesis should be used. This may be adjusted clinically by the addition and removal of material to provide the optimum contours, and can help in achieving the optimum shape for the prosthesis before making the final version (Fig. 7.23). Such temporary prostheses are frequently made using manufactured polymeric components, some patterns of which can be placed directly on the head of the implant. It is recommended that these be screw retained, since this permits repeated removal and replacement, which can facilitate incremental modification (Fig. 7.24). This can be valuable where it is desired to gradually modify the

contours of the adjacent soft tissues. If the prosthesis is made of acrylic resin it is frequently necessary to incorporate a strengthening device.

Laboratory phase

When using screw-retained definitive abutments, it is recommended that they should be secured with the screws tightened to the correct torque, and not repeatedly removed. Thereafter the temporary prostheses should be secured using polymeric analogues of the gold cylinders.

Indexing the definitive shape of the temporary prosthesis

Preparation of the definitive prosthesis

A full-contour wax-up of the final prosthesis should be prepared, following successful loading of a temporary one (Fig. 7.26).

Gold cylinders are placed on the laboratory analogues, and conventional waxing procedures used to form the framework, taking note of the design of the type of veneering material that will be used. This will enable the technician to develop the appropriate

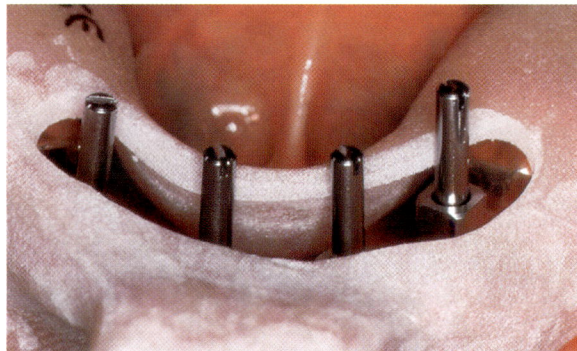

Fig. 7.25 An open-topped custom made impression tray with screw-retained impression copings.

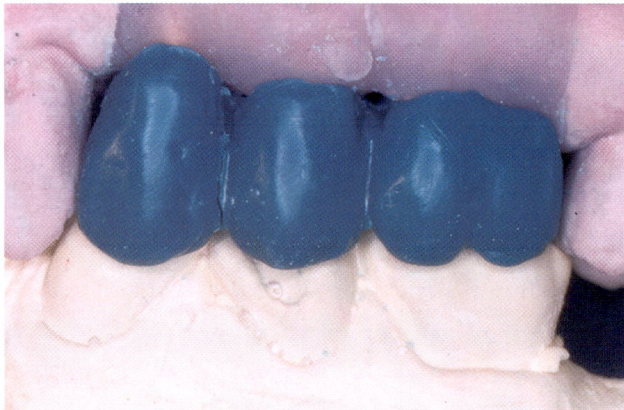

Fig. 7.26 A full contoured wax-up of the final tooth position on the master cast.

occlusal contacts and occlusal scheme. It is recommended that wherever possible a mutually protected occlusion should be provided. That is a scheme in which there are stable occlusal contacts in the posterior part of the mouth in ICP, and where possible no non-working contacts on the implant-retained prosthesis.

Canine guidance, if present on the natural teeth, should be accommodated on the implant-stabilized prostheses. If canine guidance needs to be provided by the fixed implant prosthesis or denture, then, wherever feasible, this should be as shallow as possible, achieving clearance on both the non-working and working sides.

In replacing anterior teeth there should be multiple light occlusal contacts in the ICP, while in protrusive movements there should be smooth, shallow anterior guidance to achieve posterior disocclusion, wherever possible, on all posterior teeth. An index may then be produced in the laboratory, which will permit trimming of the wax-up to facilitate substructure production and subsequent occlusal reconstruction using the material of choice.

Material for the prosthesis

The substructure can be made from either type IV gold alloy or gold bonding alloy, utilizing standard lost-wax techniques or from titanium employing a CADCAM method.

Box 7.5 Sequence of events for treatment with a screw-retained prosthesis in a partially dentate patient

- Removal of healing abutment
- Fitting of standard abutment
- Recording a radiograph to check fit of the abutment
- Making an impression (Fig. 7.25)
- Fitting a temporary prosthesis
- Recording jaw relationships
- Fabrication of the prosthesis in the laboratory
- Try-in of prosthesis
- Placing of the finished prosthesis
- Final radiograph for monitoring bone levels

Box 7.6 Sequence of events for treatment with a cemented implant prosthesis in a partially dentate patient

- Removal the healing abutment
- Record an implant-level impression
- Record a radiograph to confirm fit
- Record an impression
- Place a temporary prosthesis
- Record the jaw relationship
- Fabricate the prosthesis in the laboratory
- Fit the prepared abutments
- Record a radiograph to confirm the abutments are fully seated
- Preload the abutments
- Place a temporary prosthesis
- Record an impression
- Fabricate the crown in the laboratory
- Try-in of prosthesis
- Insertion of the finished prosthesis
- Record a radiograph to establish baseline bone levels

In the former technique, the wax pattern is reduced to allow for the addition of the teeth ('cutback'), and then sprued, invested, cast and reseated on the master cast for verification of its fit (Fig. 7.27).

Checking cast metal frameworks for screw-retained prostheses

It is recommended that the metal framework be tried in the mouth before any veneers are added, so as to confirm that it fits satisfactorily. The final occlusal veneer may be made from porcelain, a filled resin-based material or acrylic resin.

The metal framework is placed in the mouth and can be assessed clinically by tightening and then loosening each gold screw in turn, while checking visually for discrepancies (Fig. 7.28). All screws should then be tightened, and the patient asked about any sensations of pain or pressure around the implants, which can indicate an unsatisfactory fit. When the margins are

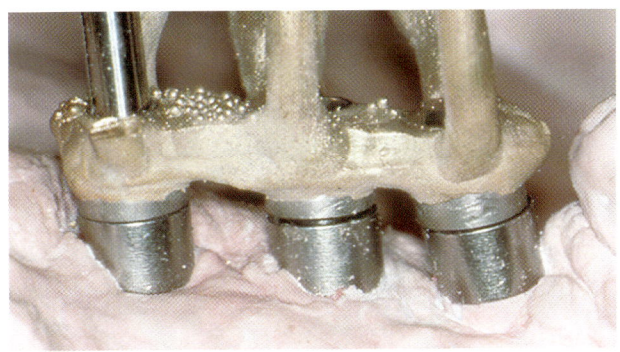

Fig. 7.27 Following failure of the casting process this framework does not fit the abutment analogues in the master cast. This may be managed either by sectioning the casting and re-soldering it or making a new framework.

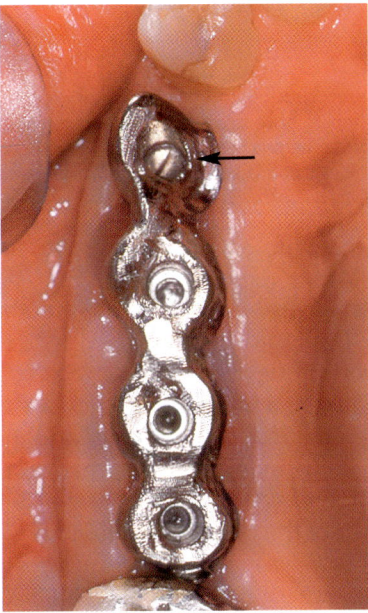

Fig. 7.28 The metal framework is tried in the mouth by securing one end of the framework with the appropriate screw. Any gaps or movement between the framework and the abutments will be easily seen if there is not a passive fit.

subgingival it may be necessary to check the final seating with a radiograph.

If there is a satisfactory fit on the working cast but not in the mouth, then it can be concluded that the working cast is inaccurate, and will require replacement. Where the framework is at fault, it may be sectioned with a carborundum disk, and resoldered. Sometimes this is best achieved by reseating the sectioned framework in the mouth and recording a locating impression, for which plaster is often suitable.

The occlusion

The design of the occlusion in the partially dentate case requires careful consideration. As discussed before, the normal physiological mobility of natural teeth is absent in the implant. Therefore the occlusion of an implant-retained prosthesis should be adjusted so that a single layer of 10 µm shimstock is not gripped securely by the implant-stabilized occlusal contacts, especially if these are in both opposing arches, since if this is present it indicates preferential loading, resulting in transfer of excessive forces to the implants.

To minimize lateral loads on posterior implant-stabilized prostheses, disclusion should occur in lateral and protrusive movements. This may not be possible when a natural canine is to be replaced with the prosthesis; however, it is recommended that there should be shallow disclusion, and that group function should be avoided.

Posterior implant-stabilized prostheses where a canine is not to be replaced

In these situations the occlusion should be arranged where possible to provide:

- contact of opposing natural teeth;
- multiple light contacts in ICP;
- no working or non-working interferences.

Posterior implant-stabilised prostheses where a canine is to be replaced

In these situations the occlusion should be arranged where possible to provide:

- opposing natural teeth;
- multiple light contacts in ICP;
- shallow canine disclusion;
- no working or non-working interferences.

Anterior bridgework

In these situations the occlusion should be arranged where possible to provide:

- multiple light contacts in ICP;
- shallow anterior disclusion shared by the prosthetic teeth.

Which material should be used for the occlusal surfaces of an implant bridge?

The occlusal surface for the prosthesis may be made of:

- porcelain;
- acrylic resin;
- composite resin;
- metal.

The decision on which material to employ should be made while planning the prosthesis with the aid of a diagnostic wax-up (Fig. 7.29).

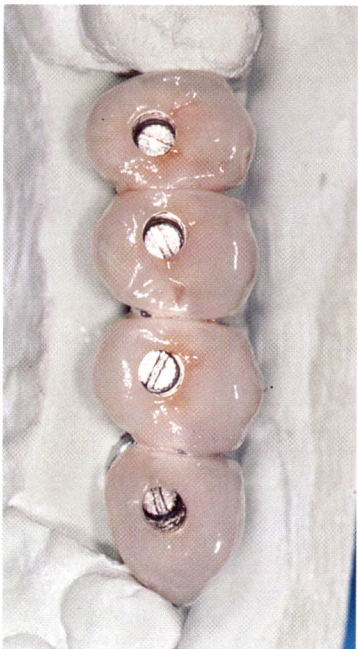

Fig. 7.29 Once a passive fit of the framework is achieved the final veneering material may be added and the prosthesis completed.

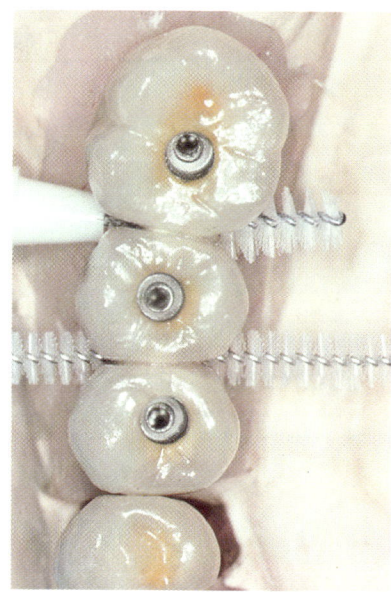

Fig. 7.30 Correct spacing and positioning of implants must be made to allow the patient to have access below the prosthesis for easy oral hygiene. Otherwise there is conflict between the appearance of the units in the prosthesis and access for proxy brushes or dental floss.

Four factors influence the choice:

- space restrictions;
- number of implants in the construction;
- amount of hard and soft tissue to be replaced by prosthesis;
- evidence of parafunctional activity.

Space restrictions

Limited interocclusal space between the head of the implant and the opposing arch may require the use of a metallic occlusal surface.

Number of implants in the construction

In a large reconstruction using more than four implants, if the final prosthesis has a porcelain veneer then any damage or fracture of the prosthesis after it has been fitted would result in a costly repair. The use of a polymeric material, however, would make repair and maintenance simpler.

Amount of hard and soft tissue to be replaced by prosthesis

A large, bulky prosthesis replacing both hard and soft tissue becomes difficult to fabricate using porcelain, and the resultant device is heavy and difficult to repair if a fracture occurs. In these situations veneering with a modified acrylic resin is to be preferred.

Evidence of parafunctional activity

From the initial occlusal examination it may be considered that a more resilient material should be used on the occlusal surface of the prosthesis, such as acrylic resin, which can also be more readily refurbished than porcelain.

Insertion of the prosthesis

After the final veneering material has been placed, the prosthesis should be rechecked in the mouth. At this stage soft-tissue contours can be confirmed, and occlusal anatomy and contacts checked both in ICP and protrusion, and on working and non-working sides. Any adjustments can be made at this stage. Carefully aligned check X-rays may also be taken to confirm the fit of the prosthesis, which is then returned to the laboratory for final staining and glazing. Following completion the prosthesis is replaced and the retaining screws, if used, fully secured. The fit of the superstructure should not be dependent on the tightening of the screws. The screw holes are then obturated with a temporary material such as gutta percha or an elastomeric impression or registration material. This can be conveniently done with a self-mixing syringe and a fine-tipped nozzle.

In the case of cement-retained prostheses there are various temporary cements that can be used. All excess cement should be removed.

Two-week review

It is suggested that the prosthesis be reviewed after 2 weeks, when the occlusion should be checked. Patients who have evidence of parafunctional activity should have a nocturnal occlusal night guard, firstly to potentially decrease parafunctional activity and secondly to protect the prosthesis.

For a screw-retained prosthesis, the screws should be checked to see if any are loose. This is not uncommon; however, they should then be retightened and checked again 1 week later. If screws are loose at the first or subsequent reviews then there should be a careful reassessment of occlusal contacts. If the screws

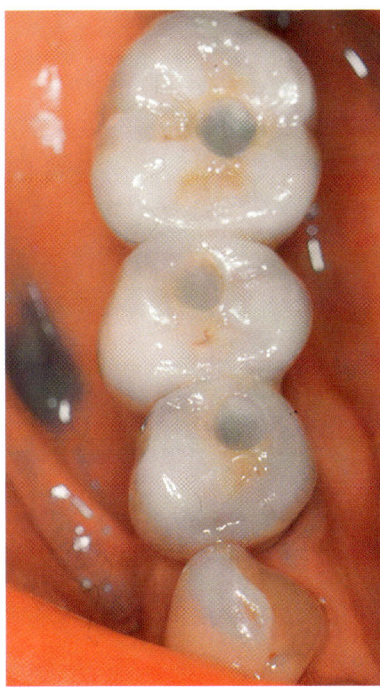

Fig. 7.31 The access holes in the prostheses have been sealed with a composite resin.

remain tight then a temporary seal can be placed directly over the screw, and the hole obturated with a more permanent composite resin restoration (Fig. 7.31).

In a cemented prosthesis a final X-ray will help to confirm that all excess cement has been removed.

What are the danger signs at review appointments?

The following is a list of some of the key problems that may be encountered when reviewing implant-retained prostheses:

- loosening of retaining screws (screw-retained prosthesis);
- cement failure (cement-retained prosthesis);
- loosening of abutment screws;
- fracture of veneering material, ceramic or resin;
- fracture of retaining screws;
- fracture of abutment screws;
- increased bone loss around an implant;
- fracture of the implant.

If any of the above has occurred, a diagnosis should be made of the cause. Repeated failure to diagnose the problem will lead ultimately to failure of the prosthesis or implant.

The most common causes are as follows.

Occlusal overload

Careful review of all occlusal contacts in all patterns of mandibular movement and their refinement may be needed. Reduction of occlusal loading can also be achieved if a cantilever is present, by its removal or reduction. Check patient compliance with the use of the nocturnal occlusal guard where one has been provided.

Poor fit of the final prosthesis

Radiographic or clinical examination may reveal that the final prosthesis does not fit correctly. Resolution of this problem may require remaking the prosthesis or its sectioning and resoldering after removing any veneering materials.

Evaluation of marginal bone levels

It is important to establish baseline radiographs when the prosthesis is inserted. Repeated long-cone periapical radiographs on an annual basis will demonstrate marginal bone heights in the radiographic plane.

Most implant systems appear to be associated with a small amount of bone loss in the first year after insertion, after which loss of marginal bone height becomes minimal. If an implant is associated with an increase in bone loss then this may be a sign of overloading, and a thorough review of the occlusion will be required.

Oral hygiene

As with patients with a natural dentition, the patient with an implant-retained prosthesis should follow a strict oral hygiene programme. Many of the patients who have been wearing a removable prosthesis may need further instruction to maintain good hygiene around their prosthesis. This can be achieved by routine tooth brushing and flossing. Angled and single-tufted brushes may be useful to clean around posterior abutments, although in some circumstances poorly contoured prostheses, resulting from inappropriate positioning of an implant, may require modification to aid oral hygiene measures. Electric toothbrushes are not contraindicated and can be recommended.

Professional scaling may be required in cases where supragingival calculus is seen; this should be removed from titanium abutments with non-metallic instruments, which will minimize damage to the surfaces. Ultrasonic instruments are contraindicated for this purpose. After the removal of hard deposits, the prosthesis and abutments may be selectively polished with a rubber 'prophy' cup. Aluminium oxide polishing paste is recommended to avoid unnecessary scratching of the titanium abutments and the prosthetic superstructure.

Maintenance intervals

Maintenance intervals are determined by several factors, such as the amount of plaque and calculus formation, the condition of the soft tissues, the status of the prosthesis and the patient's commitment to meticulous home care. Appropriate recall intervals are therefore best determined on an individual basis.

FURTHER READING

Belser U C, Mericske-Stern R, Bernard J P, Taylor T D 2000 Prosthetic management of the partially dentate patient with fixed implant restorations. Clin Oral Implants Res 11 Suppl 1:126–45

Hobkirk J A 2002 Advances in prosthetic dentistry. Prim Dent Care 9(3):81–5

Hultin M, Gustaffosn A, Klinge B 2000 Long-term evaluation of osseointegrated dental implants in the treatment of partly edentulous patients. J Clin Periodontol 27(2): 128–33

Meredith N, Book K, Friberg B, Jemt T, Sennerby L 1997 Resonance frequency measurements of implant stability in vivo. A cross-sectional and longitudinal study of resonance frequency measurements on implants in the edentulous and partially dentate maxilla. Clin Oral Implants Res 8(3): 226–33

Ortop A, Jemt T 1999 Clinical experiences of implant-supported prostheses with laser-welded titanium frameworks in the partially edentulous jaw: a 5-year follow-up study. Clin Implant Dent Relat Res 1(2): 84–91

Single-tooth implants

INTRODUCTION

An artificial tooth crown supported by a dental implant is an extremely attractive option for a patient who has a missing tooth, and for the dentist seeking to replace it. As a cosmetic replacement, especially for an incisor or canine tooth, or the functional restoration of a single posterior unit, it has the advantage of limiting the treatment to the span while avoiding preparation of the abutment teeth or contact with others in the dental arch. Risks to the pulp, and facilitation of recurrent caries or periodontal disease are therefore much reduced. Furthermore, it may seem a natural progression in the practice of implantology for a dentist who has experience of treating the anterior mandible. However, the opportunity to create an ideal aesthetic solution to tooth loss is not commonly found, and the need for a careful evaluation of the patient's problem as well as knowledge of those auxiliary procedures that are needed to achieve an acceptable result must be understood.

The first objective is for the clinician to assess, compare and contrast the various merits of the treatment options for a single-tooth replacement. The aesthetic challenge of the missing upper labial tooth may be extremely demanding, and careful assessment, both clinical and radiographic of each case, will be necessary.

There are of course many reasons for the absence of a tooth creating a space in the dental arch.

CAUSES OF THE MISSING SINGLE TOOTH

1. Failure to develop.
2. Removal of teeth due to:
   - a gross carious lesion;
   - advanced periodontal disease;
   - iatrogenic damage;
   - pulp death, failed endodontic therapy, perforation of the root, a fractured post;
   - trauma/sequelae of trauma (Fig. 8.1);
   - avulsion, fracture of the root, internal/external root resorption.

THE DECISION TO REPLACE A MISSING ANTERIOR TOOTH

The decision on the appropriate treatment, including the option to replace a single tooth, will depend on a number of factors. It is extremely important for the clinician to spend time gathering all the relevant information, both from the patient and from clinical assessment. Mounted study casts and diagnostic wax-ups will always assist in deciding upon the best treatment modality to replace a single tooth space.

The clinician will have two principal options:

- whether or not to replace the tooth;
- to select, when appropriate, which treatment modality should be used for tooth replacement.

A number of general factors will be involved:

1. The patient's attitude. The patient must perceive the need to eliminate the space or have the tooth replaced. Aesthetics may be the most important factor to the patient and their demands affect the decision concerning the method of treatment.

2. The timing of tooth replacement. If a missing single tooth has been lost during adolescence, the decision of what treatment to use may change. For example, the clinician may not consider placing implants in a patient under the age of 16. Another treatment option may be more appropriate until jaw and dental development are largely completed. Orthodontic space closure or a transitional denture may be appropriate alternatives.

3. The patient's desire to have some form of fixed prosthesis as opposed to a removable prosthesis. This may be a supporting factor if the patient's

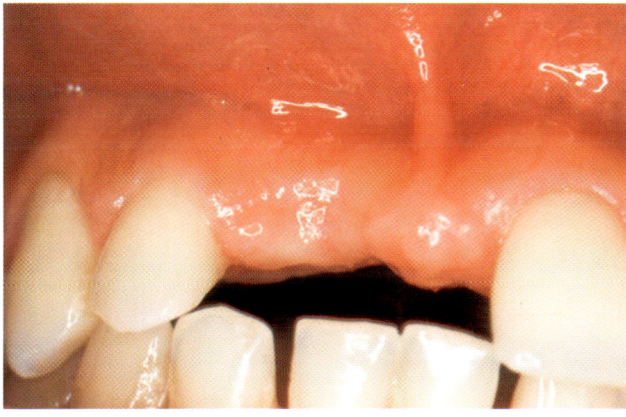

Fig. 8.1 Traumatic loss of 11 in an arch with a large diastema on either side of this tooth has complicated the options for replacement with a fixed prosthesis.

occupation involves public speaking or playing certain musical instruments. However, the decision may be different if the patient is involved in any form of contact sport that risks further tooth loss or damage to expensive and complex treatment.

Specific dental factors, which should be assessed during careful clinical examination, are:

- The patient's oral hygiene. Is there an absence of gingivitis and a low incidence of plaque accumulation?

- Previous dental disease. Is there an absence of recurrent caries and few instances of extensive restorations liable to failure?

- The periodontal health of the remaining teeth. Is there evidence of local bone loss or progressive periodontal disease affecting the dental arches?

PATIENT EXAMINATION

There are specific factors to be assessed in making the definitive treatment decision.

Extra-oral examination

The pattern of the jaw relationships and the form and function of the lips have a significant effect upon the aesthetic zone. Hence, the area of the dental arch and surrounding gingivae that is displayed when the patient smiles, laughs and speaks will have great importance in deciding on treatment. Generally, where there is a low lip line, any compromise in the form of the single crown or in the position of the surrounding soft tissues is more readily accepted by patients.

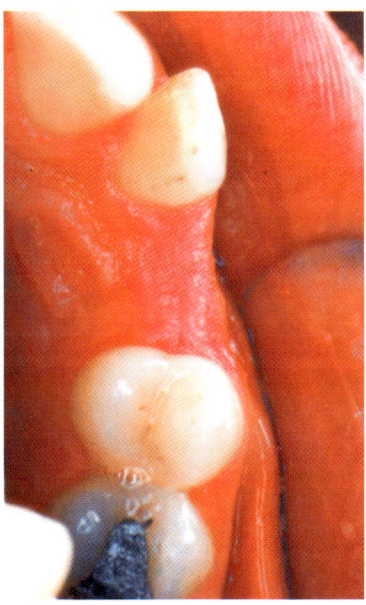

Fig. 8.2 The canine (23) is missing and the crowns of 22 and 24 are short and unrestored. These teeth are not therefore well suited to act as abutments for conventional or adhesive bridgework, making an implant a preferable option.

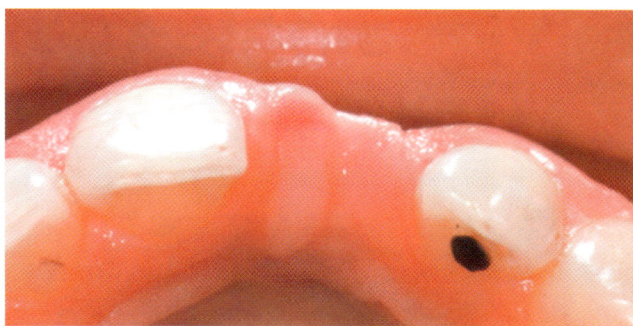

Fig. 8.3 Missing 21 in this site with extensive loss of both hard and soft tissue.

However, in the case of a tooth missing in the aesthetic zone, for example an upper incisor tooth, the evidence of the position of the lip line and smile line along with that from a careful intra-oral examination should be combined before deciding on the final treatment.

Intra-oral examination

Soft tissues

The gingival tissues surrounding the natural teeth adjacent to the space and the mucosa covering the edentulous ridge must be examined (Fig. 8.3). Evidence of bleeding and increased probing depths in the gingival crevices should not be present. The position of the gingival margins and of the papillae will indicate if recession is present and therefore likely to affect the emergence profile of the crown. Comparison should also be made with other teeth in the aesthetic zone.

Both palpation and ridge mapping are helpful in determining the thickness of mucosa covering the ridge. Increased thickness will influence unfavourably the depth of the mucosal crevice of the intended crown. It is also necessary to record sites of racial pigmentation, since gingival augmentation or flap transfer may be adversely affected. Obviously, there should be no sign of a sinus as this may indicate the retention of a root fragment. Inspection will also show if the level of the ridge crest or form of the buccal mucosa is indicative of resorption. If central incisors, canines or premolars have been lost it is important to assess the form and position of the frenum as this may influence the health of the gingival crevice of the abutment tooth, or the mucosal cuff formed around the single crown and its abutment.

Hard tissues

The teeth on either side of the edentulous space and the alveolar span should be examined in a logical sequence (Fig. 8.4).

1. Are the abutment teeth restored (in particular with a post crown, since their prognosis is poorer)?

2. Is there exposure of the root surface or evidence of tooth surface loss?

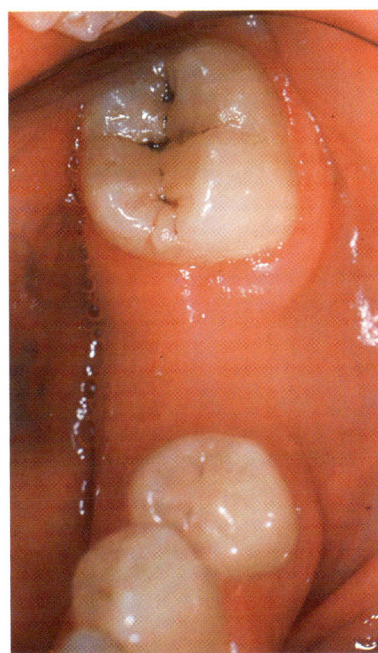

Fig. 8.4 Missing 36. The short, natural clinical crowns on 35 and 37 removing the option for adhesive or conventional bridgework makes an implant the preferred treatment.

3. Does the crown-to-root ratio of either abutment tooth appear unfavourable?

4. Is either abutment tooth abnormally mobile and are there wear facets on the enamel of the tooth?

5. Do the clinical crowns occupy an irregular position in the arch and is there obvious cervical convergence of the abutment teeth? (This may make it difficult to restore the space effectively with a single tooth implant.)

Palpation of the edentulous span will indicate the likely form of the underlying alveolar ridge, in particular its width and presence of natural concavities, which are likely to influence the position of the implant body. (This may suggest that the artificial crown and implant body may need to have divergent long axes). Both trauma and hypodontia, as well as normal resorption after tooth loss, may reduce the bone volume available for implantation below that which is desirable, so that grafting will need to be considered in assessing potential implant treatment.

Assessment of the occlusion

Two aspects of the occlusion require consideration. These are the reference position to be selected for restoration of the arch, and the specific relation of the abutment teeth and the edentulous space to the opposing arch. Examination will reveal if maximum interdigitation (ICP) is the same as, or close to the retruded contact position (RCP), in which case it is appropriate to select ICP for planning. However, where there is a major discrepancy between the positions, consideration must be given to the need to eliminate deflective contacts before further planning of the restorations.

When considering restoration of the space it is important to identify if the abutment teeth or others in the arch will provide guidance in eccentric occlusion or if the single-tooth crown will be the only site of guidance, such as occurs often when the maxillary canine is replaced with an implant. The crucial point is whether sufficient space exists for the single-tooth crown and its abutment or, conversely, if resorption or a malocclusion has produced a major discrepancy between the arches that will be difficult to restore. As a guide, the minimum vertical space required for an implant crown restoration is 7 mm from the head of an implant to the opposing tooth.

A diagnosis of parafunctional activity may be made from clinical examination. Evidence of a tooth lost due to attrition and abrasion and wear facets may be evidence of parafunction. This may also lead to increased tooth mobility and fracture of the restorations and teeth themselves. Parafunction, if not controlled, may cause overloading of the final prosthesis, leading to fracture of porcelain, screw loosening or fracture of the implant itself.

Special tests

The adjacent teeth should be assessed for their restorative, endodontic and periodontal status. A decision on their individual prognosis may influence the treatment plan for the individual space.

Radiographic assessment

It will be necessary to have a detailed radiographic assessment of the following:

- The area of the missing tooth.
- The adjacent and surrounding teeth.
- The position of any vital structures such as the mental foramen, mandibular canal, incisal canal and the positions of the nasal and sinus floors.

All can be assessed with a variety of different radiographic procedures. The radiographic views commonly employed are as follows:

- Long-cone periapical radiograph. This will provide a minimally distorted image of the edentulous space and adjacent teeth.
- Orthopantomograph (OPG). This provides an overall image of the whole mouth, positions of the teeth and vital structures, but commonly provides variable magnification in the vertical plane of ×1.25 to ×1.75.
- Tomographic scans. It may be necessary to supplement intra-oral radiographs with these views to assess the position of anatomical structures such as the mandibular canal, or where there is doubt about the thickness of the jaw in areas where a conventional two-dimensional view is not sufficient.

- CT scans. Even though these can provide a very accurate and detailed image of areas with missing teeth, except in unusual circumstances they result in an unnecessarily large radiation dose for preoperative assessment of a single-tooth implant.

Mounted study casts

The importance of the use of mounted study casts cannot be overemphasized. These should be mounted on an arcon type of articulator, using a face-bow transfer record. The RCP should be employed where the ICP is considered inappropriate. This will simulate movements similar to those of the actual jaw and confirm the findings of the clinical examination. It is therefore necessary to have good irreversible hydrocolloid or silicone elastomeric impressions of both arches, and a retruded jaw record using a wax or silicone elastomer material. The use of a face-bow will facilitate correct mounting of the upper cast.

The mounted study casts have a number of further uses:

- To prepare a wax-up with the diagnostic position of the missing tooth, its relationship to the adjacent teeth and opposing arch, and its occlusal contacts both in the intercuspal position and in retruded contact and lateral excursions (Fig. 8.5).
- To make a radiographic stent, if necessary.
- To fabricate a surgical stent.
- The preparation of sectioned casts used in conjunction with ridge mapping.

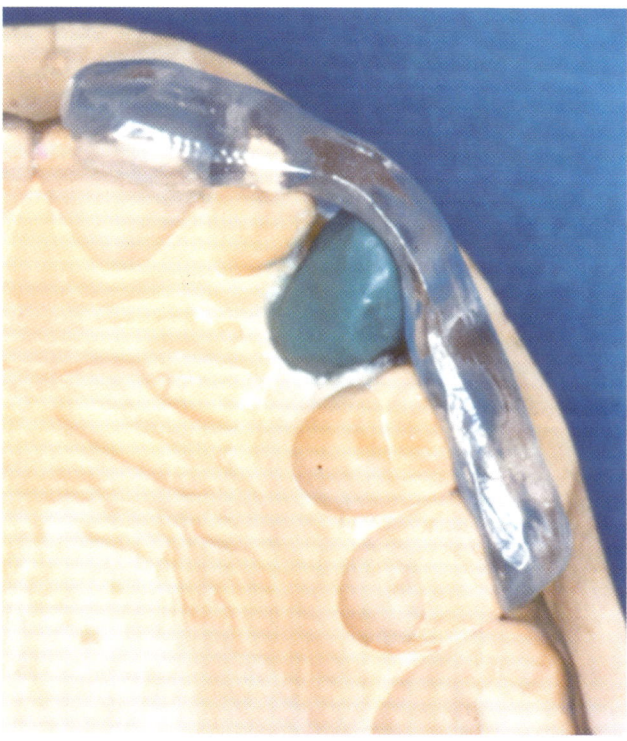

Fig. 8.5 Diagnostic wax-up with prepared surgical stent in position.

Treatment options

Following information gathering, the various treatment options to replace a single tooth may be considered. These are as follows:

Observation

If the tooth is not in the aesthetic zone, and the patient has no desire to replace the tooth for aesthetic or functional reasons, then a careful assessment should be made of the necessity to restore the space. This will largely depend on the degree of stability of the adjacent and opposing teeth, and the likely effects on masticatory performance. If there are stable opposing contacts, there has been no drifting of the teeth on either side of the space and the occlusion appears adequate for masticatory function, then it may be deemed unnecessary to replace the missing tooth.

Partial denture therapy

Where assessment has revealed large soft-tissue or osseous defects then it may be very difficult to replace the missing tissues with a fixed prosthesis, and the use of a removable partial denture may be preferable.

Adhesive bridgework

Adhesive bridgework may be used in situations where adequate retention may be provided by adjacent teeth. It may be necessary to consider bridgework as an option where there is limited mesial and distal space between the natural abutment teeth.

Where limited space exists between the roots of adjacent teeth, it is particularly important to check whether converging roots encroach on the edentulous space, as it may be extremely difficult or even impossible to place a single-tooth implant in these circumstances.

There may be situations where anatomical features make it impracticable to place an implant; for example, a large incisive canal or limited bone in both the vertical and horizontal planes.

The main advantages of the adhesive bridgework are that:

- it can be placed fairly quickly;
- no, or minimal tooth preparation is required;
- a predictable appearance may be achieved with the pontic;
- it is relatively inexpensive compared to other options.

The major disadvantage of an adhesive bridge is that occasional debonding may occur. Aesthetics can also be poor, especially where the abutment teeth are thin as the metal retainers may result in apparent tooth discoloration (Fig. 8.6).

Conventional bridge

This may not be suitable in cases with dental arches where diastemas are required. Depending on which

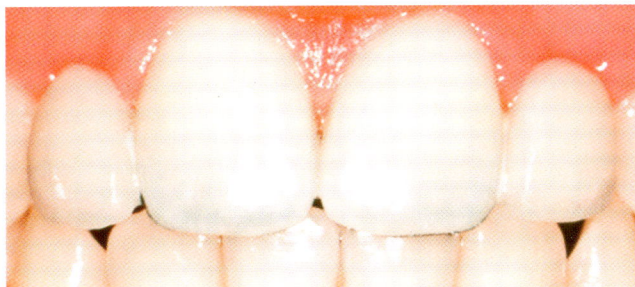

Fig. 8.6 Missing 12 and 22 replaced with a Maryland bridge seen on 11 and 22. The metal on the palatal aspect of these abutment teeth has caused the teeth to appear discoloured.

tooth is involved it may be difficult to replace the missing unit:

- when the adjacent teeth are unrestored;
- where the abutment teeth have smaller clinical surface areas than the tooth being replaced, i.e. a missing upper canine.

Careful assessment of the adjacent teeth to assess whether they require full or partial coverage restorations may also influence a decision on the use of a conventional fixed bridge.

Orthodontic treatment

Careful consideration of the orthodontic aspects of treatment of the arch is important. It may be possible that this treatment modality can be used to close the space, depending on the root morphology and the position of adjacent teeth. In cases of limited space, orthodontic procedures may be used to increase the separation between the crowns and/or the roots of the adjacent teeth so as to permit the safe placement of a dental implant.

Autotransplantation

In some situations, e.g. a missing upper anterior tooth, it may be worth considering extraction of one of the premolars and its insertion into the space. This is limited to the younger patient, but has been shown to be a successful option in some cases, particularly patients who are due to have a premolar extracted for orthodontic reasons. Recent work suggests that the single-tooth implant option may be more suitable, since it has a better long-term prognosis, as transplanted teeth are prone to root resorption and often provide an inferior appearance.

Armed with a complete view of all diagnostic aspects it is now possible to select the treatment of choice.

Minimum requirements for the single tooth implant

Standard implants (3.75 mm diameter)

While different manufacturers use a range of diameters for their implants, these are typically about 3.75 mm

in diameter. This width of implant is ideally suited for replacement of upper central incisors, upper and lower canines and upper and lower premolars, and the minimum recommended space between adjacent crowns and roots for its safe placement is 7 mm. The minimal vertical space between the head of the implant and the opposing dentition for placement of a fixed restoration is also 7 mm.

Narrow implants (3.3 mm diameter)

Most manufacturers produce a narrower implant, which would typically have a diameter of 3.3 mm. This facilitates insertion into a reduced space, at the expense of a weaker structure and a smaller potential area of bone–implant contact. The minimum separation between the adjacent crowns and roots for safe placement of a narrow implant is 5 mm, and the minimum space between the head of the implant and the opposing dentition 7 mm. This implant is well suited for replacement of upper lateral incisors and lower incisors.

Wide implants (5 or 5.5 mm diameter)

Implants with a wider diameter are also available. These are intended to maximize potential bone–implant contact, and enable primary stability by engaging the buccal and lingual cortical plates, while using shorter devices as dictated by the bony envelope. Their long-term success has yet to be established, although some early reports have suggested that this may be less than for standard-sized implants. Whether this reflects an inherent property of the design or the use to which it lends itself is yet to be clarified. The minimum space between adjacent crowns and roots for safe placement of a wide implant is 9 mm; however, the vertical space between the head of the implant and the opposing dentition remains 7 mm. This diameter is ideally suited for replacement of single molar teeth.

Wherever possible the longest feasible implant should be selected in order to develop the maximum contact with bone and optimize cortical stability during initial healing.

The surgical aspects of single-tooth implants have been covered in Chapter 5, which includes particular comment on the surgical procedures that may be required to adapt the 'gingival tissues'.

The clinical examination, radiographs and diagnostic wax-up are all important in formulating an optimal plan for implant treatment. Basic principles include the following:

- Use the longest implant that is possible without interfering with key anatomical structures.
- Have an implant length to crown height ratio of greater than one.
- Loads are best directed down the long axes of the implants and should be aligned with the overlying crowns.
- Single implants should not be used to support cantilevers.

What are the prosthetic stages of treatment with single-tooth implants?

The prosthetic stages of single tooth implant treatment can be divided into seven aspects:

1. Timing of prosthetic treatment.
2. Selection of the type of restoration.
3. Abutment selection.
4. Impression techniques.
5. Laboratory fabrication.
6. Try-in of the prosthesis.
7. Delivery of the final prosthesis.

Timing of prosthetic treatment

It is generally recommended that wherever possible it is better to leave the healing abutments in place until the gingival tissue around them has matured (Fig. 8.7). A minimum of approximately 4 weeks from the time of second-stage surgery is recommended. Where the implant has been inserted with a single surgical phase sufficient time should pass to allow the gingival tissue to mature.

Type of restoration

The next decision for the prosthodontist is how the final prosthesis is to be secured to the implant. There are two principal alternatives:

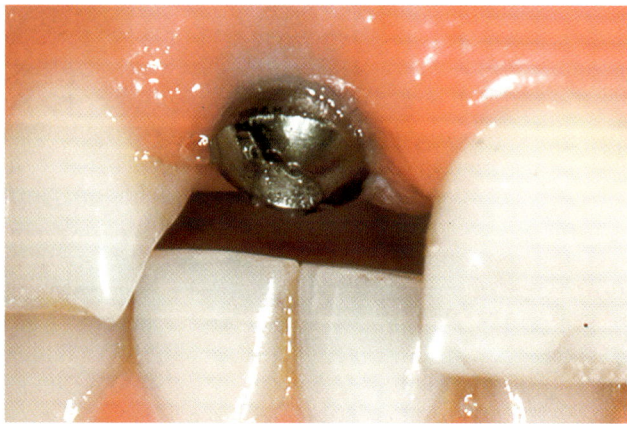

Fig. 8.7 Healing abutment in place in the 11 region. The gingival tissues show full maturation.

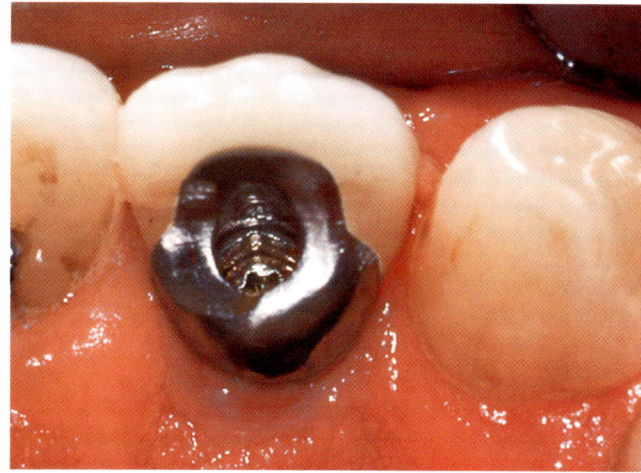

Fig. 8.8 Single-implant replacement of 22 using a porcelain fused to metal crown with access to the retaining screw.

1. A screw-retained prosthesis secured direct to the implant.
2. A cement-retained prosthesis secured direct to an abutment.

Both options have advantages and disadvantages. A screw-retained prosthesis can be retained directly on the implant, which will provide the advantage of retrievability (Fig. 8.8). The abutment to implant interface is premachined, providing optimal fit. The major disadvantage of this is the requirement for an access hole to pass through the occlusal or palatal/lingual surface of the crown and the need to ensure that the implant and prosthesis are not so angulated as to dictate a buccal/labial access hole in the artificial crown. Unfortunately, in an anterior tooth the accommodation of the access hole may result in an expansion of the cingulum. The access hole will usually need to be restored with some form of permanent filling material at the end of treatment, e.g. a resin-based material.

Retrievability may be required for changes to the restoration or to repair breakages of the restoration. In this case, all that would be required is to simply remove the material from the access hole to unscrew and remove the prosthesis.

The cement-retained implant prosthesis has the same advantages as those of cementing a standard crown and bridge prosthesis. In particular, it has the benefit of compensating for a change in alignment between the long axes of the implant body and the artificial crown. Unfortunately, if the margins of the abutments are subgingival, excess cement may lodge within the gingival tissue. This can lead to gingival inflammation, bone loss and loss of the implant (Figs 8.9, 8.10).

In addition, retrievability of the cemented prosthesis may be extremely difficult even with the use of some form of temporary or soft cement.

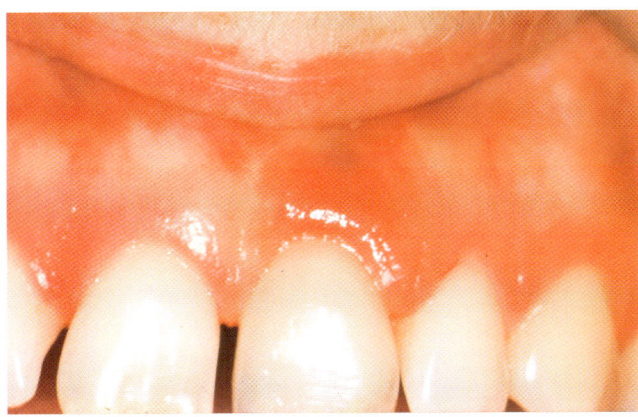

Fig. 8.9 Recently cemented implant crown on a standard manufactured abutment. The gingival inflammation is due to excess cement, as seen in Figure 8.10.

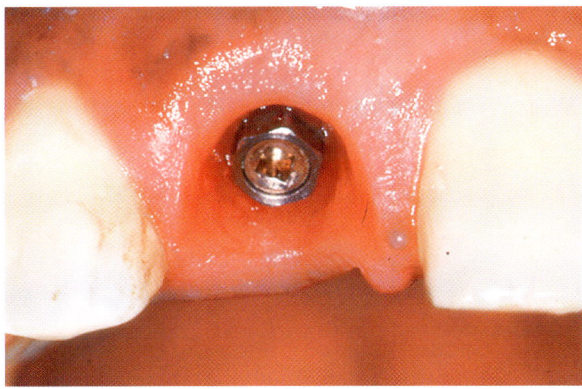

Fig. 8.11 A manufactured abutment in position. The 'CeraOne' design does not follow the natural gingival contour.

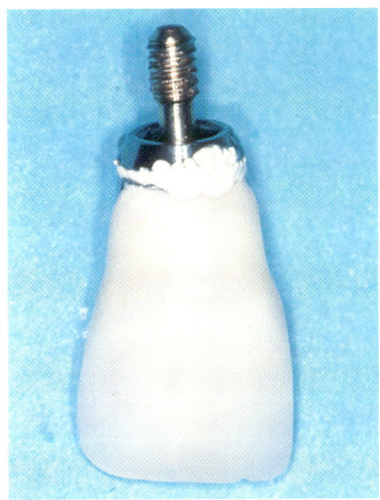

Fig. 8.10 A disadvantage of a cement-retained crown is that deep subgingival margins may lead to poor seating and retention of excess cement.

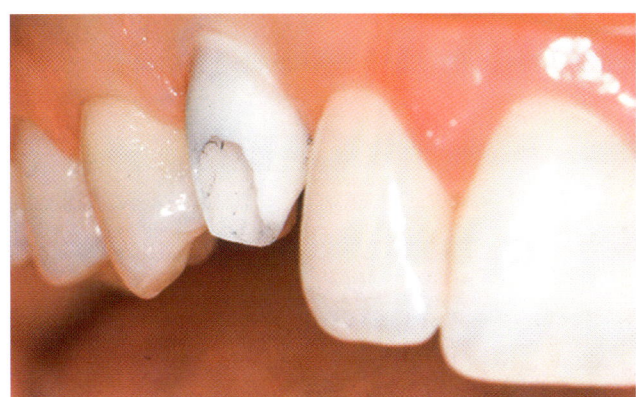

Fig. 8.12 An all-ceramic abutment has been prepared in the mouth for 13. The margins have been prepared to follow the gingival contour.

Abutments

The role of the abutment is to connect the final prosthesis to the implant body. Most manufacturers provide a range of designs; however, these are usually product specific.

Standard preformed abutments

These are usually premachined abutments supplied by the manufacturers. The decision on when they can be used will either be made at the chairside or in the laboratory, after the impression of the implant head within the arch has been recorded. Premachined abutments have the advantage of a precision fit, usually with an anti-rotational feature on the head of the implant body, and are manufactured with a range of collar sizes to match different depths of mucosal cuff. They are usually fairly uncomplicated and used in simple cases. A major advantage is the decreased time required for clinical and laboratory procedures. The disadvantages of many of these types of abutment are that they do not follow the gingival contour, and cannot be customized to compensate for poor placement of an implant (Fig. 8.11). Realistically, they should only be used when the implant is in the ideal position.

Prepable abutments

These are usually supplied by the manufacturer as blank abutments, which fit accurately on the implant, but have excessive bulk to permit modification by the clinician at the chairside or by the laboratory technician. They are made in a variety of materials such as alumina, zirconium and titanium. The major advantage of these abutments is their flexibility of use. There is also a similarity for the clinician to conventional crown and bridge construction, so preparation can be carried out directly in the mouth. This will allow the margins of the abutment to follow the gingival contour, and they usually permit sufficient angulation changes to overcome most alignment problems and poor implant positioning (Fig. 8.12).

The major disadvantage of prepable abutments is the increase in both clinical and laboratory time and, therefore, the possible increase in cost to the patient. If the preparation of the abutment has been done in the laboratory, a second clinical visit and clinical impression to record the final contours may be required in

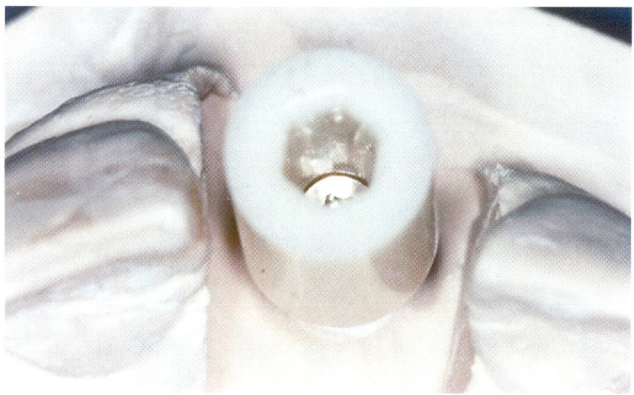

Fig. 8.13 An all-ceramic abutment ('CerAdapt') in place on the fixture analogue situated in the master cast.

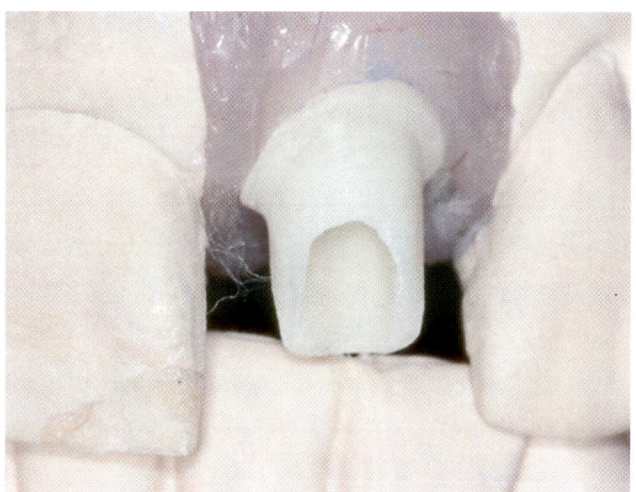

Fig. 8.14 Preparation of an all-ceramic abutment in the laboratory is done with a high-speed turbine using copious irrigation to achieve the appropriate contours.

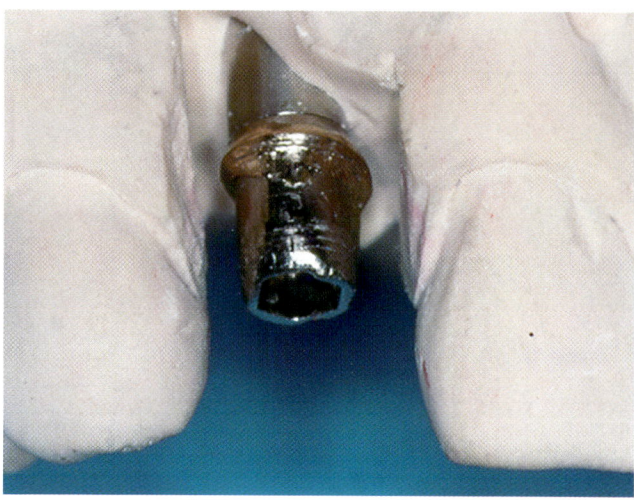

Fig. 8.15 Following wax-up and casting on to a manufactured gold cylinder ('Auradapt'), a custom-made abutment is produced in gold alloy.

CADCAM-derived abutments

This relatively new development is likely to assume increasing importance as manufacturers develop the technique. These abutments have the advantage that the design is carried out using specialist software. It has the disadvantage that at present it has no three-dimensional orientation with the opposing or adjacent teeth. It is possible to make the abutments in titanium or a ceramic, which is considered by some to be a more biocompatible material.

Assessment of abutment choice

The decision on the type of abutment will depend on a number of factors related to the clinical situation. Following second-stage surgery and complete healing of the soft tissues, removal of the healing abutment will show the position of the head of the implant, which will help in abutment selection (Fig. 8.16).

Consideration should be given to the following:

- The height from the head of the implant to the opposing teeth, i.e. the interocclusal space.
- The amount of soft tissue from the head of the implant body to the gingival margin of the mucosal cuff (both in depth and thickness).
- The aesthetic requirements of the patient.
- The orientation of the implant body to the proposed prosthetic crown.
- Preference for cement- or screw-retained prosthesis.

Certain abutments will require a minimum height from the head of the implant to the opposing tooth. Careful clinical assessment of all these factors will lead to correct abutment choice. It may be preferable to record an impression of the top of the implant body (implant head), and thus allow for the decision on the abutment to be made in the laboratory.

some situations. It may also be desirable where the abutment does not have a clearly defined location on the implant around its long axis to construct an abutment locator in order to ensure the correct orientation on the implant head.

Custom laboratory-made abutments

These can be used for cement-retained prostheses. The use of these abutments will necessitate recording an impression of the head of the implant. After the construction of a master cast the abutments can be custom made in the laboratory, usually by casting onto a gold alloy platform (Fig. 8.15). Precision fit and customized abutment support are their principal advantages. While maintaining a premachined fit to the implant head, the technician is still able to customize the contours of the abutment to support the final prosthesis. The main disadvantage of this technique is that both the clinical and laboratory time are increased, with the additional requirement of recording a second working impression within the mouth after the abutments have been placed on the head of the implant.

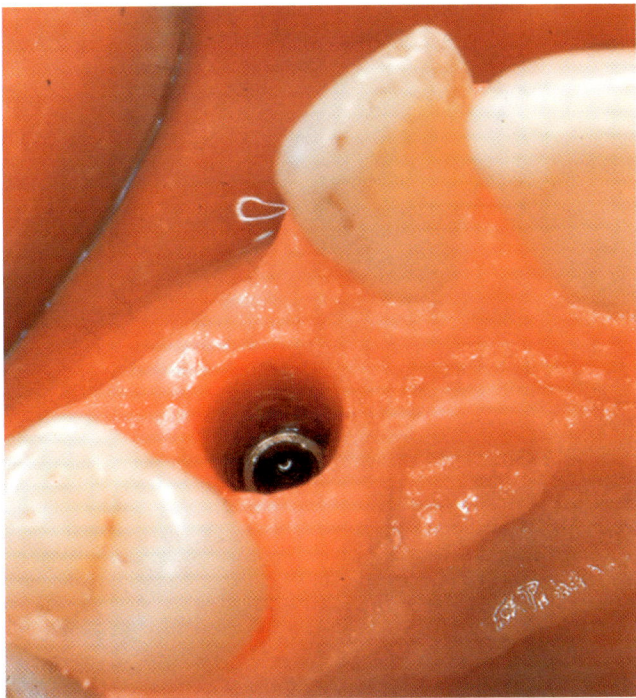

Fig. 8.16 Following removal of the healing abutment the head of the implant is clearly seen, together with an outline of a mature gingival cuff.

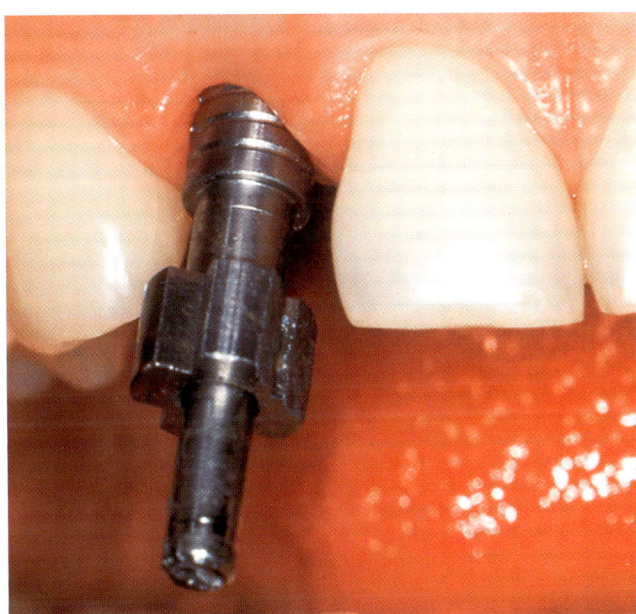

Fig. 8.17 Using an impression coping to the fixture level a clear outline of the implant and surrounding hard and soft tissues will be gained in the working impression.

Impression of the implant head

Most implant systems provide a premachined impression coping for recording an impression of the head of the implant. This is usually made up of two pieces: the impression coping and the guide pin. The impression coping seats directly onto the implant head and is retained with the guide pin (Fig. 8.17). A long-cone radiograph is almost always necessary to confirm that the impression coping is fully seated and to

---

Box 8.2 Abutment selection

MANUFACTURED PRECISION ABUTMENTS

Material of manufacture
- Titanium

Advantages
- Simple to use
- Minimal chairside and laboratory time
- Predictable fit with implant–prosthesis components
- Good retention

Disadvantages
- Design may increase bulk, limiting aesthetic outcome

PREPABLE ABUTMENTS

Material of manufacture
- Titanium
- Gold alloy
- Ceramic

Advantages
- Suitable for all cases
- Allows for angulation changes
- Modification allows for good gingival contour

Disadvantages
- Increases clinical and laboratory time

CUSTOMIZED ABUTMENTS

Material of manufacture
- Gold alloy
- Titanium
- Zirconium
- Ceramic

Advantages
- Suitable for all cases
- Allow for angulation changes
- Modification allows for good gingival contour

Disadvantages
- Increases clinical and laboratory time
- Material choice influenced by occlusal loads

---

ensure absolute accuracy before any construction of the crown begins.

A polymeric standard stock tray may be used and modified so that the guide pin projects beyond the adjacent teeth and through the impression tray. A polyvinyl silicone or polyether impression material can be used; when set, the guide screw is loosened and the impression tray removed from the mouth with the coping picked up in the impression.

Careful inspection of the impression will confirm the stability or otherwise of the impression coping, and reveal if an accurate record of all hard and soft tissues has been made (Fig. 8.18). The impression is then disinfected and sent to the laboratory.

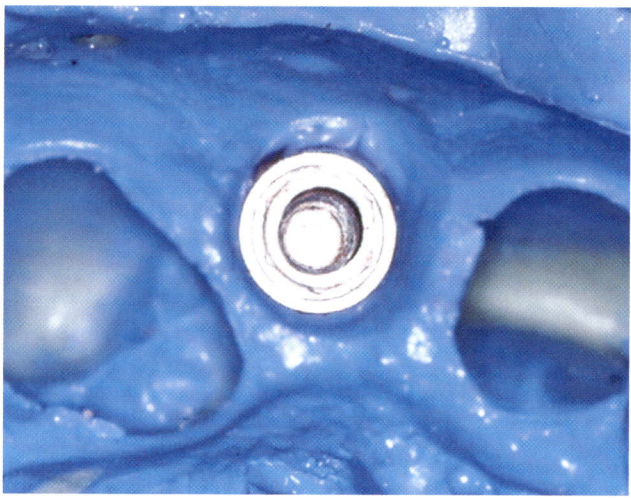

Fig. 8.18 Following an impression using the fixture-level impression coping, a clear view of the position of the implant in relation to surrounding teeth and the contours of the soft tissues are recorded.

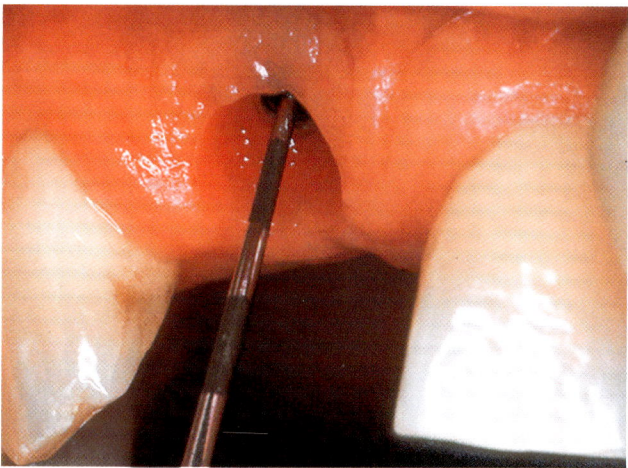

Fig. 8.19 Use of a periodontal probe to measure the depth of the gingival cuff in preparation for abutment selection.

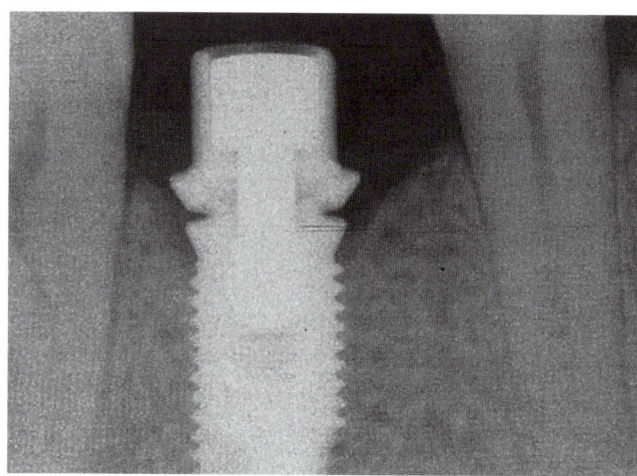

Fig. 8.20 A long-cone radiograph to check proper seating of the premachined abutment onto the head of the implant is required before final tightening and recording of the impression. Soft tissue or bone entrapment, or failure to engage the hexagon of the implant with the premachined abutment, may prevent seating.

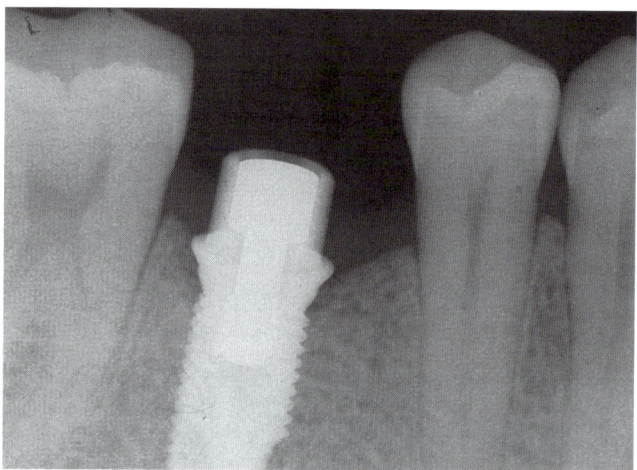

Fig. 8.21 A clear long-cone radiograph shows correct seating of the abutment onto the head of the implant.

Impression of a preformed machined abutment

Following removal of the healing abutment, measurements from the head of the implant to the margin of the mucosal cuff will help determine the height of the final abutment to be used in the restoration (Fig. 8.19). This can be done at the chairside. The objective is to produce a submucosal margin of 1.5–2 mm from the crest of the 'gingival' tissue, and to provide sufficient interocclusal distance from the top of the abutment to the opposing tooth. Following correct placement of the definitive abutment, a long-cone periapical radiograph may be taken to ensure that it is correctly seated (Figs 8.20, 8.21). Following confirmation from the radiograph that this is the case, the retaining or abutment screw should be tightened to the manufacturer's recommended torque using a torque device. This may reduce the risk of loosening of the abutment screw at a later stage.

An impression is taken using a machined plastic or metal impression coping that is placed over the abutment. A standard stock tray may be used and modified so that the impression coping projects beyond the adjacent teeth and through the impression tray (Figs 8.22, 8.23).

A polyvinyl silicone or polyether impression material can be used and following complete setting the impression tray is removed from the mouth with the impression coping picked up in the impression. Careful inspection of the impression will confirm the stability of the impression coping, and an accurate record of all the relevant hard and soft tissues.

At this stage the impression is disinfected and sent to the laboratory.

Impression of prepable abutments

Prepable abutments are usually supplied in various materials such as alumina, zirconium and titanium. The manufacturer typically supplies these as stock shaped abutments, which can be placed directly on the implants and modified by the clinician in the mouth.

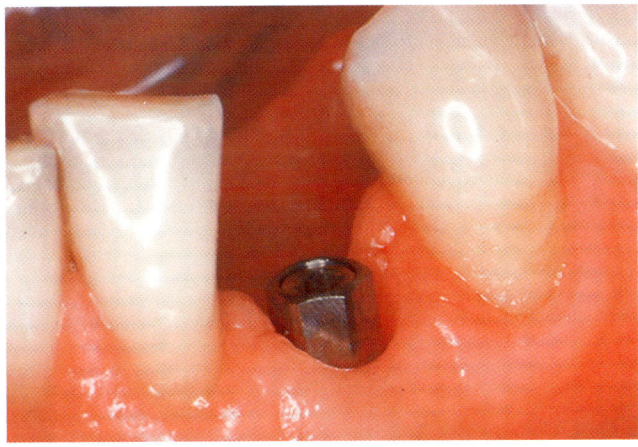

Fig. 8.22 Single-tooth replacement of 33 using a premachined 'CeraOne' abutment.

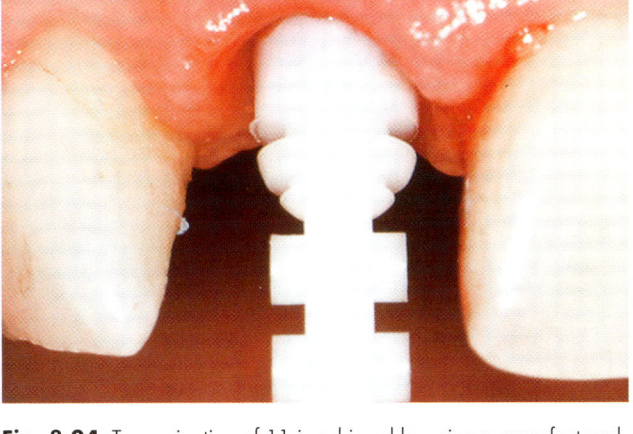

Fig. 8.24 Temporization of 11 is achieved by using a manufactured coping for the 'CeraOne' abutment.

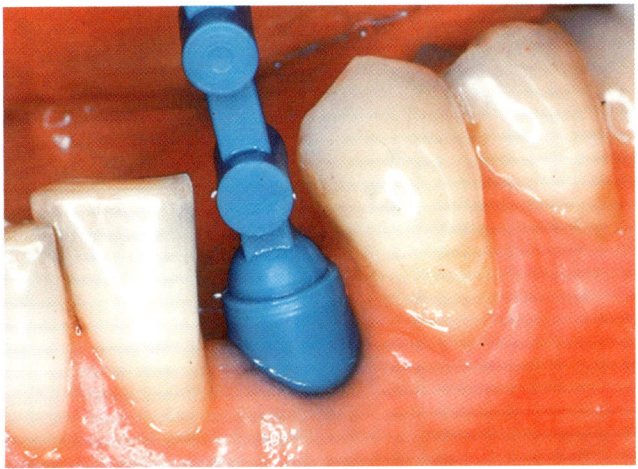

Fig. 8.23 Using a preprepared impression coping, an impression is recorded of the manufactured single-tooth abutment ('CeraOne').

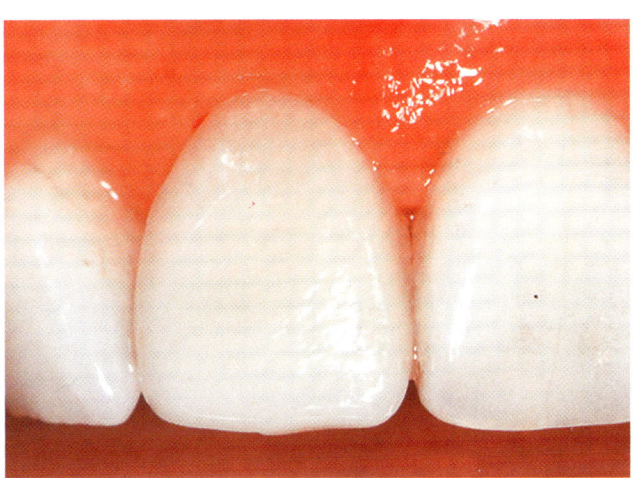

Fig. 8.25 Using acrylic resin bonded to the temporary coping, a temporary tooth replacement can provide the optimum soft-tissue contours.

The major advantage of these is their wide range of use in varying situations. The technique of preparing them is similar to traditional crown and bridge techniques, and allows for preparation to be carried out directly in the mouth. This will allow the margins of the abutment to follow the gingival contour.

Utilizing standard crown and bridge principles, an impression can be recorded of the prepared abutments directly in the mouth.

Temporization following the recording of impressions

Fixture head

Following the recording of an impression of the fixture head the healing abutment that had been previously in place can be repositioned on the implant. Note that the healing abutment should be cleaned to remove any dried blood or saliva as this may affect proper seating. Chlorhexidine is the solution of choice for this purpose.

Preformed machined abutment

Following placement of the preformed, machined abutment, the abutment screw is tightened to the correct torque as the abutment may be left in position. A manufactured protective cap may be placed over this and a temporary crown constructed (Figs 8.24, 8.25).

Prepable abutments

Following the impression of the prepared abutments, conventional temporary crown and bridge materials may be used to make temporary restorations for use between appointments.

Laboratory phase

The appropriate laboratory analogue (abutment replica) is attached to the impression coping for the first two techniques, and a cast then prepared in two stages. The soft tissues are reproduced using a silicone elastomeric material, and finally dental stone is used

Box 8.3 Sequence of events for treatment with a single-tooth 'prepable' abutment

- Remove healing abutment
- Position fixture-level impression coping
- Record radiograph to confirm fit
- Make impression
- Complete temporization
- Prepare laboratory component
- Try-in abutment
- Record radiograph to confirm fit
- Undertake laboratory phase of construction of crown
- Try-in prosthesis
- Cement finished prosthesis
- Record final radiograph for monitoring

Box 8.4 Sequence of events for treatment with a single-tooth manufactured precision abutment

- Remove healing abutment
- Fit standard abutment
- Record radiograph to confirm fit
- Preload abutment
- Record impression
- Complete temporization
- Undertake laboratory phase of construction of crown
- Try-in prosthesis
- Cement finished prosthesis
- Record final radiograph for monitoring

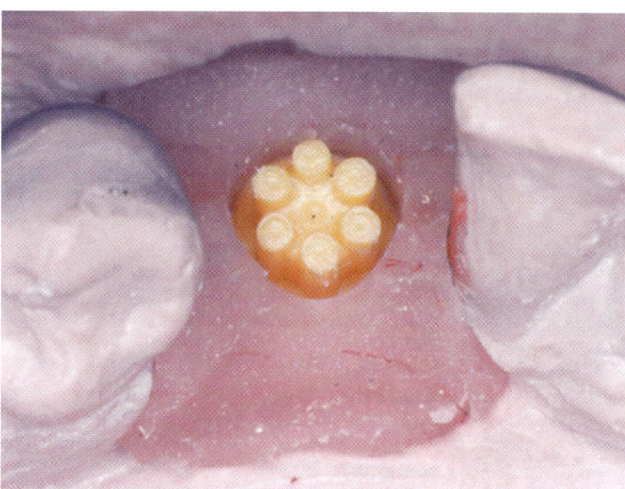

Fig. 8.26 A 'CeraOne' abutment analogue with a soft-tissue gingival mask provides the basis for final tooth reproduction.

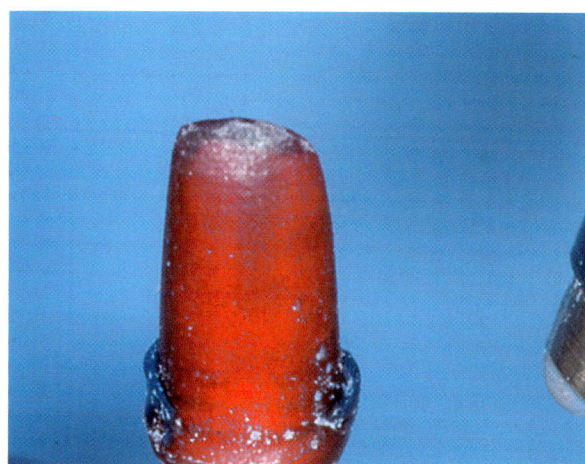

Fig. 8.27 A waxed outline of an abutment is scanned using a Procera™ scanner.

for the remainder of the record to provide a master cast to mirror the position of the implant and related soft-tissue contours (Fig. 8.26). The silicone elastomer permits placement of abutments on the cast and expansion by the emerging profile of the final prosthesis.

If the impression is of prepared abutments it is poured in dental stone, sectioned to produce individual dies.

Occlusal registration

It is recommend that the casts for single-tooth cases should be mounted on a semi-adjustable articulator. This will require a face-bow transfer for mounting the maxillary cast; where there is a sufficient number of occluding teeth the casts may be mounted in the intercuspal relationship.

Laboratory cast-fixture level

Producing custom laboratory-made abutments

After the construction of a master cast, the abutments can be custom made in the laboratory, usually by waxing and casting onto a gold alloy platform.

Precision fit and customized abutment support are dual advantages. While maintaining a premachined fit to the implant head, the technician is still able to customize the contours of the abutment to support the final prosthesis.

Custom laboratory abutments may also be produced in titanium. After construction of a master cast these can be formed in the laboratory, usually by waxing to the ideal contour. The wax-ups are then placed on a scanning machine, the abutment scanned, and the data sent to a specialized centre where the final version is produced (Fig. 8.27).

Computer-generated abutments

After the construction of a master cast, this is placed in a scanner and electronic records are automatically taken of the implant position and angulation relative to the desired restoration. Using computer software the ideal abutment shape can be generated and viewed in three dimensions. The position of the gingival margin can be superimposed on the image. The data is then sent to a specialized centre where the abutment is produced. These abutments have the advantage that their design is carried out using specialized software.

The disadvantage of this method is that it has no three-dimensional orientation with the opposing teeth or adjacent teeth.

It is possible to make computer-generated abutments in either titanium or a ceramic, which are considered more biocompatible materials.

Preparation of the definitive prosthesis on a preformed machined abutment

Gold cylinders are placed on the laboratory analogues and conventional waxing procedures are performed to a full contour wax-up with consideration for the type of veneering material that will be used. This will enable the technician to develop the appropriate occlusal contacts and occlusal scheme. It is recommended that wherever possible a mutually protected occlusion should be provided. That is a scheme in which there are stable occlusal contacts in the posterior part of the mouth in ICP, and where possible no working or non-working contacts on the implant-retained prosthesis.

Canine guidance, if present on the natural teeth, should be provided on the implant-stabilized prosthesis. If canine guidance needs to be provided by the implant, wherever possible this should be as shallow as possible, while providing a similar appearance to the opposite side of the arch.

In replacing an anterior tooth there should be light occlusal contacts in the intercuspal position, while in protrusive movements these should be smooth, and similar to those on the remaining anterior teeth (Figs 8.28, 8.29).

Metal-bonded porcelain is the material of choice for a posterior single-tooth implant crown. Following careful reduction of the wax pattern, this is directly sprued, invested and, utilizing standard lost-wax techniques, cast in a gold bonding alloy. It may then be reseated on the master cast for fit verification.

The final veneering with porcelain follows standard laboratory techniques. All ceramic crowns may be made for anterior crowns.

Preparation of the definitive prosthesis on prepared abutments

These follow similar techniques to conventional crown techniques, using a full-contour wax-up, cutback, spruing and investing and casting in gold bonding alloy.

Fitting the completed restoration

(Figs 8.30, 8.31)

On the day of fitting the completed restoration, the temporary prosthesis should be removed. The new crowns may then be seated with finger pressure. Discomfort is usually due to pressure on the gingival

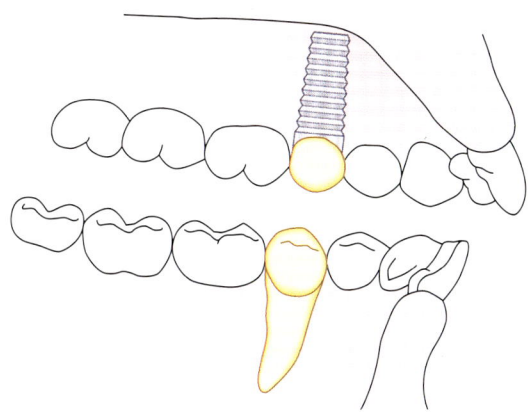

Fig. 8.28 When designing an implant crown opposing a natural dentition, light contact in the intercuspal position is preferred while maintaining heavy contact between the adjacent natural dentition.

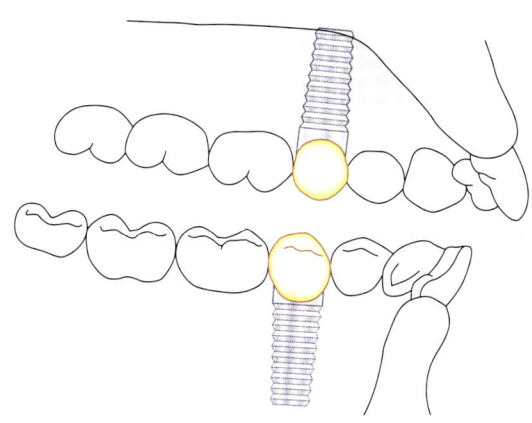

Fig. 8.29 If implant crowns oppose implant crowns, it is preferred that there is little or no contact of these crowns when the patient is in the intercuspal position.

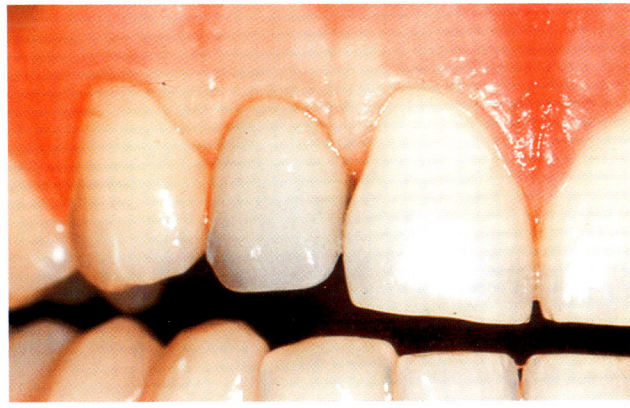

Fig. 8.30 Initial blanching of the soft tissues upon insertion of the porcelain-fused-to-metal crown on 12.

tissue, and may necessitate the administration of a local anaesthetic. The contact points are checked with dental floss as for conventional crowns. Occlusal contacts should be checked prior to cementation and should follow the occlusal pattern on the master cast.

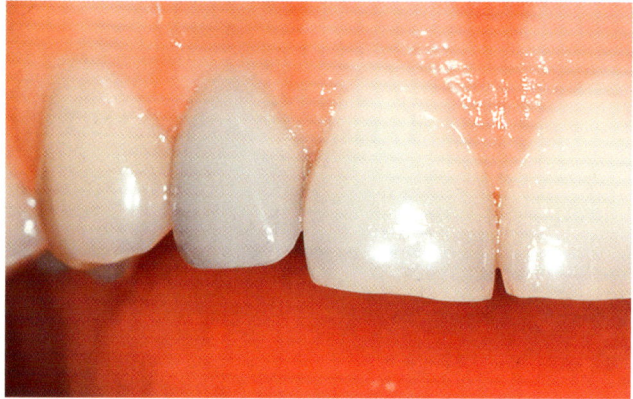

Fig. 8.31 One-week review of 12 showing healthy soft tissue.

There should be light contacts as the patient goes gently into the intercuspal position. The crowns should then be checked for lateral, working, non-working and protrusive movements. The location of the implant crown in the arch will determine what type of contacts are present, e.g. posterior teeth should have no non-working contacts. Anterior teeth would be expected to have contacts in the ICP and shallow anterior guidance similar to that on the adjacent anterior teeth. If the canine has been replaced, then canine disclusion should exist in a similar manner to that on the opposite canine.

Cementation with temporary cement may be prudent when placing the final restoration. This will give time for the soft tissues to adapt, while simplifying removal and modification of the implant crown if required. In cases where abutments have been used the abutment screws should be tightened to the manufacturer's recommended values before the final cementation (Figs 8.32, 8.33).

Following cementation a long-cone periapical radiograph is taken to:

- verify the seating of the restoration;
- check that no excess cement is present;
- act as a record of marginal bone height for comparison with follow-up radiographs (Fig. 8.34).

Two-week review

It is suggested that the single-tooth prosthesis be reviewed after 2 weeks. The status of the soft tissues should be checked and the occlusion examined (Fig. 8.35). Patients who have evidence of parafunctional activity should have a nocturnal occlusal guard to protect the prosthesis.

Where the prosthesis is screw retained and the screws remain tight, a temporary seal can be placed directly over the screw and the hole sealed with a more permanent composite resin restoration. If the screws have loosened then they should be retightened and checked 1 week later. Persistent loosening is often indicative of a poorly fitting prosthesis, uneven occlusal contacts or off-axis loading of the implant.

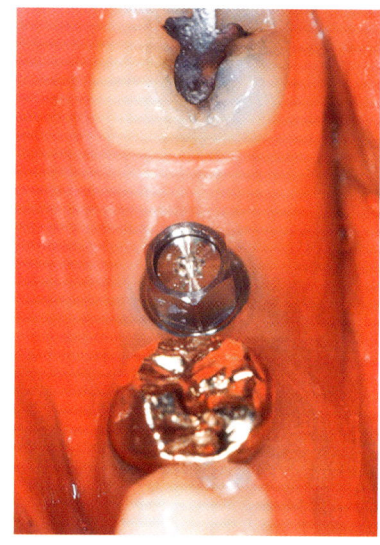

Fig. 8.32 Manufactured 'CeraOne' abutment replacing 46.

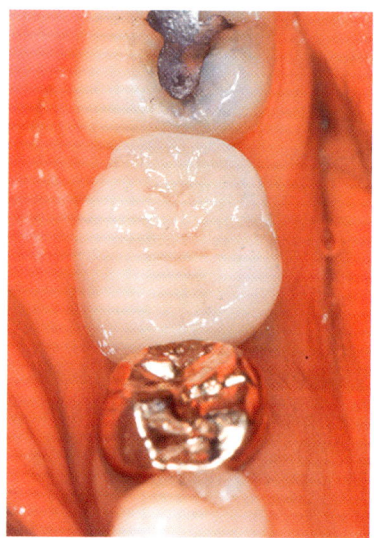

Fig. 8.33 Final crown cemented on 'CeraOne' abutment replacing 46.

Box 8.5 A final radiograph is taken to:

- Verify seating of the final restoration
- Check for excess cement
- Record a base line marginal bone height

Danger signs at a review appointment

The following is a list of the possible damage that may occur to single-tooth implant-retained prostheses.

- cement failure (Fig. 8.36);
- loosening of abutment screws (Fig. 8.37);
- fracture of veneering material, ceramic or resin;
- fracture of abutment screws;
- increased bone loss around an implant;
- fracture of the implant.

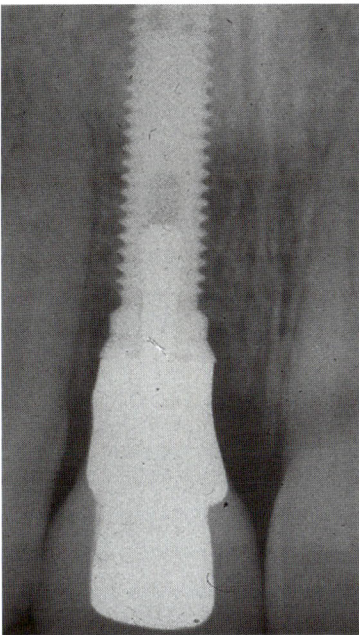

Fig. 8.34 Baseline radiograph after cementation of a crown on 11.

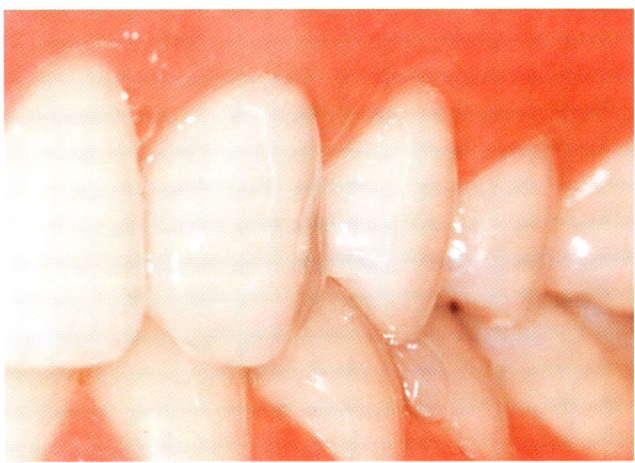

Fig. 8.35 Porcelain crown replacing 23 cemented on a single-tooth implant.

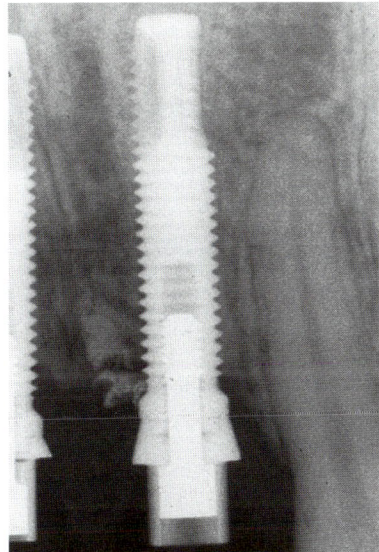

Fig. 8.36 Radiograph showing excess cement in the soft tissues.

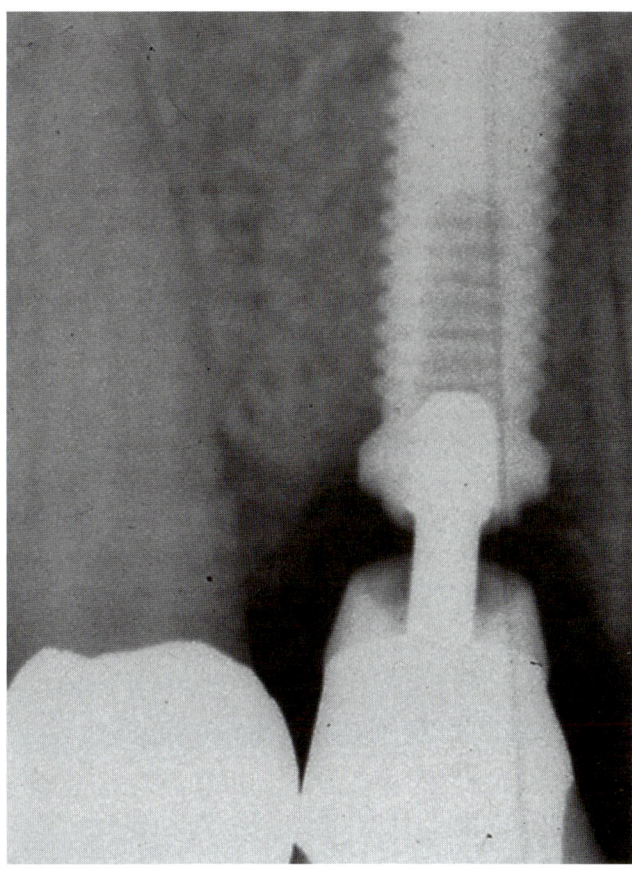

Fig. 8.37 Radiograph showing loosening of an abutment screw due to failure to tighten it correctly.

If any of the above has occurred, a careful diagnosis should be made of the cause. Repeated failure to diagnosis the problem will lead ultimately to failure of the prosthesis or implant.

The most common causes of these problems are:

- occlusal overload: careful review of all occlusal contacts in all patterns of mandibular movement and their refinement may be needed;
- failure to use a prescribed nocturnal occlusal guard;
- faulty construction;
- off-axis loading of an implant.

Evaluation of marginal bone levels

Long-cone periapical radiographs recorded on an annual basis will demonstrate changes in marginal bone heights in the radiographic plane. Most implant systems appear to be associated with a small amount of bone loss in the first year after insertion, after which loss of marginal bone height becomes minimal. If an implant is associated with an increase of bone loss then this may be a sign of overloading, and a careful review of the occlusion will be required. Increased bone loss can also arise as a result of infection.

Oral hygiene

As with patients with a natural dentition, the patient with an implant-retained prosthesis should follow a strict oral hygiene programme. This can be achieved by routine tooth brushing and flossing. Standard methods may be used around the prosthesis. Electric toothbrushes can be recommended and are not contraindicated.

Ultrasonic instruments should not be used around implant-retained prostheses. After the removal of hard deposits, the prosthesis and abutments may be selectively polished with a rubber prophylaxis cup. Aluminium oxide polishing paste is recommended to avoid unnecessary scratching of the titanium abutments and the prosthetic superstructure.

FURTHER READING

Gibbard L L, Zarb G 2002 A 5-year prospective study of implant-supported single-tooth replacements. J Can Dent Assoc 68(2): 110–6

Haas R, Polak C, Furhauser R, Mailath-Pokorny G, Dortbudak O, Watzek G 2002 A long-term follow-up of 76 Brånemark single-tooth implants. Clin Oral Implants Res 13(1):38–43

Levine R A, Clem D, Beagle J et al 2002 Multicenter retrospective analysis of the solid-screw ITI implant for posterior single-tooth replacements. Int J Oral Maxillofac Implants 17(4): 550–6

Romeo E, Chiapasco M, Ghisolfi M, Vogel G 2002 Long-term clinical effectiveness of oral implants in the treatment of partial edentulism. Seven-year life table analysis of a prospective study with ITI dental implants system used for single-tooth restorations. Clin Oral Implants Res. 13(2): 133–43

Other applications

INTRODUCTION

The contribution of implants to oral and maxillofacial rehabilitation is constantly increasing as a result of the changes in the design of implants themselves, and in the use of this type of treatment in patients with a wider range of problems (Box 9.1).

INTRA-ORAL APPLICATIONS

Two obvious examples reflect improvement in the provision of intra-oral prostheses.

Before the introduction of dental implants, the challenge of treating a grossly resorbed edentulous maxilla was handled by prosthodontists. They employed complex impression procedures or, in the last resort, used springs to secure stability for the complete denture. A variety of procedures have been used since then to augment the deficient bone volume, and to permit the use of adequately long implants in sufficient numbers to resist the loads applied to the prosthesis. These include inlay grafting of the maxillary antrum, onlay grafting of the basal bone and segmental osteotomy. Most recently the zygoma itself has been chosen to provide an additional site, into which specially designed implant bodies of increased length can be positioned to integrate with naturally present bone stock. A combination of dental and zygomatic

implants is usually necessary to permit effective restoration with a removable overdenture prosthesis (Fig. 9.1).

Immediate loading

The immediate loading of dental implants was practised for many years prior to the emergence of the Brånemark implant system, which employed the principle of a two-stage approach in which the implants were placed submucosally while healing and integration occurred, after which they were loaded following surgical exposure. It subsequently became evident that there were advantages in a one-stage technique in which the implants were loaded from the time of insertion. These were principally as follows:

- a second surgical stage was avoided, with a consequent reduction in morbidity and cost;
- a more permanent restoration could be placed sooner.

Set against this were concerns that a higher failure rate might result; however, shorter-term results in selected cases suggest that this might not be a problem. It is recommended that at present a two-stage technique be employed, except where there are overriding advantages in the single-stage approach. If this is contemplated, then it should preferably be employed

---

Box 9.1 Other applications for osseointegrated implants

INTRA-ORAL

- Immediate implantation of anterior mandible ('teeth in a day')
- Assisting orthodontics
- Rehabilitation of the resected mandible
- Rehabilitation of the resected maxilla

INTRA-ORAL AND FACIAL SKELETON

- Zygomatic implantation for atrophic maxilla

EXTRA-ORAL/FACIAL

- Ear, eye, nose prostheses
- Bone-anchored hearing aid
- Linked or stabilized prostheses for maxillofacial rehabilitation

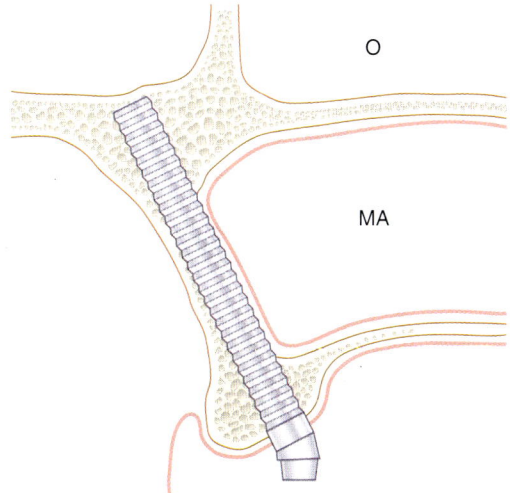

Fig. 9.1 Diagram showing a zygomatic implant engaging the palate and zygomatic bones of the skull lateral to the maxillary antrum and the orbit.

only where the clinical situation is favourable to implant success.

The term 'immediate loading' is not currently defined. Strictly speaking it should only apply when the implant is subject to occlusal loads straight after insertion. In practice the term is also used for implants that penetrate the mucosa from the time of insertion, but have a superstructure placed significantly sooner than occurs with delayed loading. This technique is sometimes referred to as delayed immediate loading.

Three particular situations can be identified:

- the partially dentate case, where a single tooth or temporary bridge is placed at the time of implant insertion;
- the edentulous patient, where a temporary denture is used with the implants;
- the Brånemark System® Novum technique, in which preformed components enable a fixed bridge to be used on the day of implant insertion.

A single tooth or short bridge can be fabricated for placement on an implant or series of implants using conventional restorative techniques. Where a laboratory-made prosthesis is required, then an impression of the opposing dental arch, a jaw registration and a face-bow record can be made some time prior to implant placement. Following implant insertion a working impression including the implant head may be recorded, and the resultant cast mounted using the previous records. A temporary prosthesis may then be made for insertion shortly afterwards.

Where implants are to be used for stabilizing a complete denture and the patient already has such a prosthesis, then this may be reinserted over the freshly placed implants, which should have healing abutments placed on them. The denture is then eased over the implants and modified locally with a temporary lining material.

The Brånemark System® Novum technique makes use of preformed components to enable a fixed bridge to be fitted in the mandible in one day. Very careful case selection is required to ensure that there will be no unforeseen difficulties in the construction of the bridge. Occlusal discrepancies, lack of space and unusual jaw relationships caution against the use of the technique. The lower jaw should conform to the outline of the surgical template, and may require trimming over the ridge crest to ensure this. The template is then mounted on the jaw using screws inserted into the mandible through preformed holes. The implant sites are then prepared using the template, and the implants inserted in the predetermined positions. A preformed superstructure is next mounted on the implants and used to record the jaw relationship corresponding to RCP. This can then be mounted on an articulator, opposing a previously prepared cast representing the upper arch, and the superstructure completed. Finally this is placed on the implants, using an interposing silicone membrane to cover the surgical wound in the mucosa.

Orthodontic applications

The resistance of dental implants to movement by the application of orthodontic forces has led to their use as anchorage for fixed orthodontic therapy, and special implant designs are now used for this. They are commonly inserted in the palate in the midline suture and removed following orthodontic therapy. Their advantage is the provision of stable fixation for fixed orthodontic therapy, which may otherwise be of less certain outcome. They can also function as effective anchorage for osseo-distraction techniques.

An alternative approach in the partially dentate patient who is to be subsequently treated with implant-stabilized prostheses is to insert the implants in the final desired positions and then use them as anchorage for orthodontic appliances to align the related teeth. This is especially helpful in patients with large numbers of congenitally missing teeth, where suitable anchorage for orthodontic therapy may be otherwise unavailable.

How may implants assist restoration of the resected mandible?

Partial rim resection or a full-thickness defect of the mandible has a major impact upon the masticatory function and quite often the appearance of the patient. Appropriate recovery may demand a bone graft to provide continuity to the jaw, and the result will be dependant on restoring part of the dental arch with a fixed prosthesis stabilized by dental implants. The equivalent result is rarely if ever achieved with a conventional denture, which lacks the support, stability and retention provided by dental implants. The demands posed by limited comfort, together with the exceptional tolerance and acquired skill, usually cause the patient to discontinue wearing a denture, however carefully designed and constructed. This is especially so where most or all teeth have been lost from the jaw.

Successful implantation requires the mandible to have a sufficient volume of good-quality bone, appropriately sited in relation to the maxilla.

Extensive rim resection or complete discontinuity will require the jaw to be augmented with an autogenous graft (Fig. 9.2). Without continuity, inappropriate

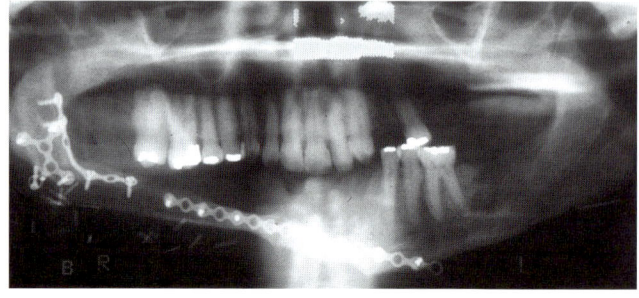

Fig. 9.2 A resected mandible has been reconstructed with corticocancellous bone grafts.

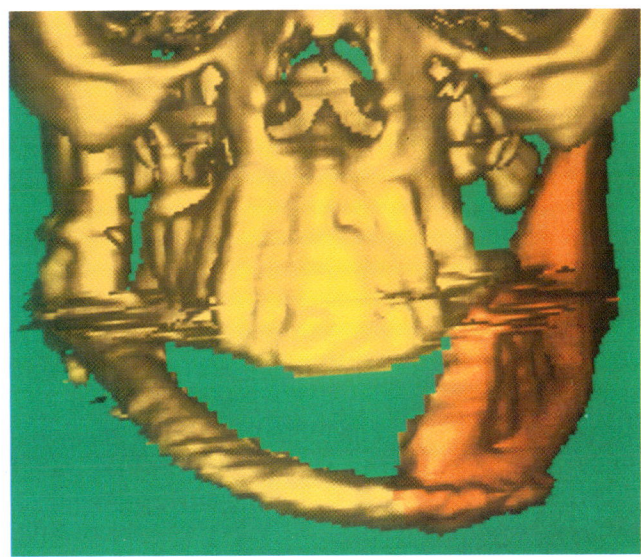

Fig. 9.3 A computer image reconstructed from a CT scan, showing malocclusion arising from the graft of excessive length and inadequate height.

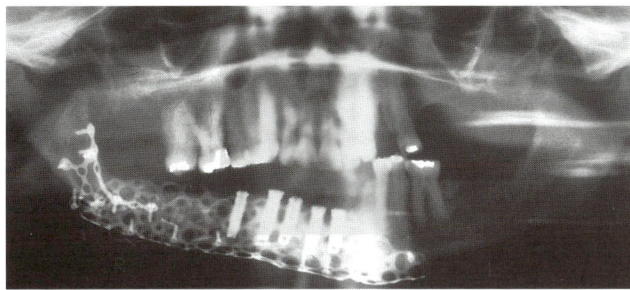

Fig. 9.4 The mandible has been enhanced sufficiently by shortening and the use of cancellous iliac bone enclosed by a preformed titanium mesh tray. Dental implants now support a fixed prosthesis.

Box 9.3 Assessment of resected/reconstructed mandibles

- Does the jaw articulate satisfactorily with the skull without limited gape, deviation on closing and impaired dental occlusion?
- Do the tongue, lips and cheeks function satisfactorily during deglutition, chewing and speaking?
- Is there access to the site of resection, unimpaired by the tissue contraction/graft?
- Is there sufficient bone, appropriately aligned with the maxillary/dental arch?

---

articulation with the skull impairs function, resulting in deviation and malocclusion. Also, loss of the lower border of the mandible alters the facial profile, resulting in disfigurement. Modern treatment uses either a free vascularized flap (e.g. radial), linked block grafts or a corticocancellous graft carried in a swaged titanium tray. Wherever possible the condyle is retained on the defect side. From the perspective of future implantation preoperative planning with CT scanning, computer data analysis and stereolithographic modelling are likely to assist in the creation of the desired volume for the reconstructed mandible. This enables corticocancellous bone to be enclosed within a custom-made swaged titanium tray (Fig. 9.3). Use of block grafts is usually more appropriate for cases of rim resection where alignment with the maxillary arch is easily identified.

The quality of bone used for implantation is particularly affected by irradiation. Although the prospects for continued osseointegration of dental implants are said to be improved by hyperbaric oxygen therapy (HBO) before and after their insertion, current recent advice is to insert implants before or immediately after irradiation, when the effects upon healing are least unfavourable, or to wait 18 months, when the effect is complete.

The siting of dental implants is crucial to the design of the prostheses (Box 9.2). Where possible, maximum use should be made of the residual anterior mandible where optimum integration and survival are achieved. Both clinical and radiological assessment following surgical reconstruction are often needed to determine the availability of appropriate bone and exclude unsuitable sites (Fig. 9.4).

The emergence of abutments through mobile, thin soft tissue at sites judged to be accessible for cleaning and free of movement of the investing tissues of the lip and tongue is of importance.

Failure to acknowledge these two requirements may well result in repeated infections of the peri-abutment tissue, and complaints of bleeding and soreness. This is likely to occur where a repair with a thick skin graft has not been revised, and scar contraction has resulted in restricted mobility of the tongue or lip, and limited gape.

Very careful evaluation of the probable space available for the prosthesis is also important in choosing the appropriate number of implants, and in considering cantilevering of the arch (Box 9.3).

With the aid of carefully articulated study casts it is also possible to relate the proposed arch form, occlusal plane and required interdigitation of the teeth to the maxillary arch and to the investing tissues. All too often the prosthodontist may see severe limitations on the possible sites for inserting the implants. After partial glossectomy the tongue may be reduced and limited in movement, or bulky, with restricted access to the surface of the jaw.

Box 9.2 Siting of dental implants in resected mandibles

- In sufficient good-quality bone
- Allowing emergence of abutments through accessible, immobile soft tissue
- Appropriate to the prosthetic space
- Offering support to the planned arch in occlusion

In either situation speech and movement of food may be severely restricted. The extent of the prosthesis may need to be limited by lack of space or an inability to align the arch with available bone. It should not be forgotten that the procedures for constructing the prosthesis (recording impressions, securing components, etc.) might be exceedingly difficult to carry out where space is restricted.

Choice of prosthesis

Preference is usually for treatment with a fixed prosthesis. This must be based on careful consideration of the likely function resulting from an appropriate occlusion, a suitable form matched to the prosthetic space and favourable loading of the implants.

However, it may be wise where possible problems are foreseen to plan to provide an overdenture stabilized by a linkage to a bar retained on four well-spaced implants in the anterior mandible. Difficulties can arise where there is doubt about the patient's capacity to manipulate food with its accumulation around the prostheses, or with an inability to position it between the opposing arches or during swallowing. The latter is possible where a major glossectomy requires the residual tongue to be squeezed against the vault, which is only possible with overclosure of the mandible. Secondly, poor dexterity may limit the ability to produce good oral hygiene – removal of the prostheses makes this much easier. Finally, it is important to consider what effect may arise from occlusion between a fixed prosthesis and an opposing complete upper denture. Anterior loading may create instability and damage to the denture-supporting tissues of the edentulous maxilla.

Maxillary defects

Defects of the facial skeleton can arise as a result of developmental anomalies, surgery or trauma. Where possible, these are often best managed by surgical correction; however, this is not always feasible or capable of providing a satisfactory outcome. In these circumstances, patients may be best helped using a removable obturator. These have been employed in prosthetic dentistry for a long time, and can dramatically improve the quality of the patient's life. Unfortunately, it can be very difficult or impossible to produce an adequate degree of stability and many ingenious techniques have been developed to manage this. They include linking the obturator to the natural teeth with direct retainers such as clasps or precision attachments, maximizing its extension over less displaceable tissues, linking sectional components together with magnets or precision attachments so as to produce a relatively immobile device and the use of traditional aids to retention such as springs and adhesives. In cases of extensive resection of the maxilla, including exenteration of the orbit a flexible conventional obturator design may be used to secure sufficient stability.

The development of osseointegrated dental implants, and those specifically intended for insertion into the facial skeleton, has made it possible to improve obturator stability dramatically. The principles of the use of these implants are similar to those for regular dental use. They are based on designing an appropriate prosthesis, identifying the most suitable locations for stabilizing components, and then using this information to select the most appropriate sites for implant placement. Following major tissue loss, the number of these that are potentially available for implant placement may be relatively limited. Where feasible, the edentulous alveolar ridges are particularly suitable. Other sites that have been used include the zygomatic buttress, the bony orbital rim, the dorsal aspect of the maxilla where it articulates with the pterygoid plates and, occasionally, the palatal processes of the maxilla. Where the cortex is thin, special short implant bodies may be used, although this can prejudice the final outcome.

Where a suitable bony site is overlaid by very mobile soft tissues, resection of the submucosal layer, leading to a region of mucosa that is tightly bound to the underlying bone, can ease maintenance and minimize soft-tissue irritation and inflammation.

Obturators may be linked to implants using either magnets or precision attachments. The former have the advantages of a variable path of insertion and can be used where the long axes of the implant bodies are markedly divergent. They also minimize horizontal forces on the implants and are simple for the patient to use, particularly where the patient has reduced manual dexterity. The disadvantages of magnets relate to possible problems of corrosion, their inability to act over longer separations, and the exponential reduction in retention as the components are separated. This can create particular problems if the magnet and keeper are not correctly aligned.

The alternative approach is to use precision attachments (such as studs) placed on individual implants or clips, on a gold alloy bar, which joins them together. The latter has the advantage of increasing the choices of locating the retainers, and transmitting forces between the different implants. It can suffer from problems of alignment if the long axes of the implants are divergent. If that is the case then it may not be possible to insert the bar. Similarly, where the implants are relatively close and at divergent angles, then the placing of a superstructure and its retaining screws may prove to be impossible. Individual retainers placed on each implant are simpler to provide, but are not exempt from the need to have largely parallel implants. Where precision attachments are used to link the obturator to the implants, there can be difficulties in accommodating both parts of the attachment due to lack of room. Similarly the anatomy of the site may dictate a path of insertion of the prosthesis that is at variance with the alignment of the attachments. Great care therefore needs to be taken with the planning stage of the process.

Treatment stages

The most important part of providing treatment with an implant-stabilized obturator is the planning stage, when the feasibility of implant insertion and optimum placement are being assessed. Malpositioned implants may prove ineffective and create significant difficulties in their management. This stage may require the construction of a trial appliance and surgeon's guide. Once placed, the implants are restored using broadly similar techniques to those described elsewhere in this book, and a typical sequence would be as follows:

- Primary impressions, recording the implant locations with suitable copings.

- Working impressions: where the defect is small these can be recorded using standard techniques. Where it is very large some operators prefer to record the final working impression using an elastomeric wash impression on the base of the trial prosthesis.

- Jaw registration, including a record of the obturator space so as to achieve optimum facial contour.

- Trial prostheses to confirm the final functional effect. – Design of the retention system.

- Placement of the abutments and retainers. Recording of impressions in the obturator base plate to locate the retainers. This may be done with an elastomeric impression material and transfer copings, or by picking up the retainer with a light cured or autopolymerizing resin.

- Insertion of the completed prosthesis.

The dimensions of the prosthesis, locations of the implant bodies, potential difficulties with access, and the presence of large undercut areas into which impression material can flow and become impacted, present major challenges to the prosthodontist. These can be managed using traditional techniques such as sectional impression trays, multi-part impressions and the packing with paraffin gauze of regions of little direct interest.

Problems

Treatment with implant-stabilized obturators is as prone to problems as any other complex prosthetic treatment. The use of integrated implants does, however, introduce greater complexity, which can present challenges both for the operator and the patient. The reader is referred to the standard texts on the use of oral obturators for management of problems related to their fabrication and clinical use. This section, however, outlines those implant-based problems which may be encountered.

Treatment planning

The number of sites into which implants may be successfully inserted in the maxilla is often very restricted, both in terms of location and the angulations of the implants that have to be used. Furthermore, these often have to be very short and can place some restrictions on the loads which they might be expected to bear.

Inappropriate angulations can make it difficult or sometimes impossible to place linked superstructures or to secure the abutments and gold screws.

Problems that may arise postoperatively are very similar to those that can occur with implants placed in more traditional locations.

Failure of osseointegration

This is a risk with the procedure, wherever an implant is placed; however, the devices used to stabilize obturators are more likely to be subjected to unfavourable loads, particularly in terms of angulation, and to be housed in low-volume, poor-quality bone. This can be particularly troublesome where the patient has recently had radiotherapy, a not uncommon occurrence in such patients.

Cleaning

The need to ensure a high standard of oral hygiene is equally applicable around implants stabilizing an obturator, as those used to secure a dental prosthesis. There can be added difficulties related to access, and it is important to ensure that the superstructure design facilitates oral hygiene and that the patient has been fully instructed in these procedures.

In carefully selected situations appropriately designed and fabricated implant-stabilized obturators can provide a dramatic increase in the quality of a patient's life.

Zygomatic implants

Introduction

While the original Brånemark implant was designed as a tooth analogue to be placed partly or totally within the remnants of the alveolar processes, integration can equally occur in other locations. This potential has been used to help patients for whom conventional implant placement is restricted. The zygomatic implant represents one such development and is intended for use in the upper jaw, where there is inadequate alveolar bone for placing sufficient dental implants. The device is much longer than a standard design, typically 30–50 mm, and is inserted from the palatal aspect of the residual alveolar ridge to lie below the mucosal lining of the lateral wall of the maxillary sinus. It extends into the zygomatic process of the maxilla, thus potentially providing good primary stabilization.

Indications

The zygomatic implant should not be considered as a first line of approach when treating the edentulous maxilla or one with missing molar teeth, but rather as a procedure that may be potentially of value in a small number of cases. The possible application of the technique should be evaluated using the same principles as have been considered in earlier chapters. These include the nature of the problem resulting from tooth loss, alternative management strategies and the appropriateness of dental implants. Both systemic and local factors will come into play when making this decision. In the case of the latter, access can be a major problem due to the length of the implants. Two particular situations can arise, relating to the edentulous and partially dentate maxilla.

Where there is adequate bone anteriorly, and it is desired to provide implant stabilization posteriorly, the zygomatic implant may be indicated to avoid the need for grafting in this region. Similarly, where grafting is indicated around the arch it may be possible to limit this to the anterior maxilla by using zygomatic fixtures posteriorly.

Where the patient has retained their anterior teeth but has distal edentulous regions associated with extensive bone resorption, there may be a case for the use of zygomatic implants. These can then reduce the problems of managing the distal extension saddle, in combination with natural tooth abutments.

Patient assessment

In addition to the usual criteria, it is important that the patient has clinically symptom-free sinuses and that there are no infections in the soft or hard tissues at the intended implantation site. All necessary dental treatment should have been completed prior to implant placement, including any periodontal therapy required to ensure oral health.

Radiographic examination of the potential implant site is important and may include the following techniques:

- Intra-oral radiographs. These can help to exclude pathology in the ridge crest.

- Panoramic radiographs. These assist in the identification of anatomical structures and may help to exclude pathological changes in the jaws.

- Lateral cephalograms. These will help to evaluate jaw dimensions and the anteroposterior relationship between the upper and lower jaws.

- Tomograms. These can be invaluable when assessing the potential bony envelope for the implant, particularly those based on computed axial tomography. This technique enables more accurate visualization and measurement of the bony envelope in the potential implant sites.

Surgical stage

Implant placement can be challenging owing to the problems with access, the anatomy of the surgical site and the considerable length of the implant body. The handling of the instruments can be hazardous because of their great length and the difficulty in accessing the insertion site. It is important to ensure that components are fully secured, that a drill guard is used to prevent soft-tissue damage and that lateral pressure is not

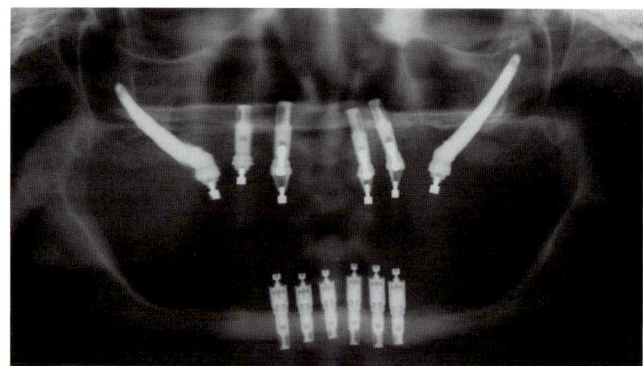

Fig. 9.5 Partial restoration of the maxillary arch has been achieved with dental implants. The posterior sites in the premolar and first molar areas are restored with zygomatic implants.

applied to the drill, which may cause it to fracture as well as creating an oversized osteotomy site. Access is gained using an incision of the type employed for creating a Le Fort I osteotomy, with wide exposure of the bony site. A small window is then cut in the lateral wall of maxillary sinus close to the crest on the inferior border of the zygomatic process. This permits access to the maxillary antrum, so that the soft-tissue lining can be elevated without tearing, thus permitting the implant to lie on the lateral bony wall and in a submucosal location. The osteotomy is then prepared using a progressive range of drills and taking great care over the orientation of the hole and its depth, so as to avoid damage to the floor of the bony orbit. Once the site has been prepared the implant can be inserted using conventional techniques. If difficulties are encountered in placing the implant, it may be necessary to enlarge the osteotomy site, since the use of excessive force to insert the implant body can fracture it.

The head of the implant usually lies palatal to the residual alveolar ridge and is oriented laterally. The manufacturers therefore incorporated in the design an angled head, which permits the use of abutments with their long axes approximately normal to the occlusal plane (Fig. 9.5).

Restoration

Zygomatic implants are rarely restored on their own, since they are unsuitable for supporting isolated bridgework and can create difficulties if used solely to stabilize an overdenture, as this will tend to rotate around the abutments. While it is important to try to locate the head of the implant as close to the crest of the residual alveolar ridge as possible, inevitably this tends to lie on its palatal aspect (Fig. 9.6). This complicates the placing of fixed restorations with a normal occlusal scheme, as considerable buccal cantilevering may be necessary. Hence most restorations are designed as maxillary overdentures with bars linking anterior dental implant abutments or natural tooth crowns to the zygomatic abutments on each side of the jaw.

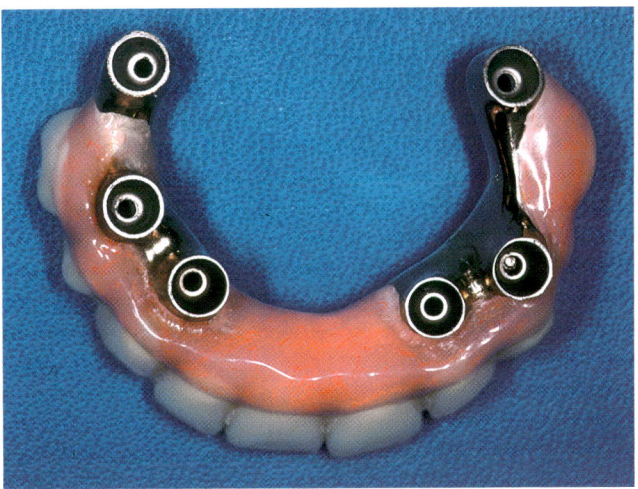

Fig. 9.6 The fixed maxillary prosthesis has been constructed with a cast alloy framework enclosing gold cylinders supporting a resin-based dental arch.

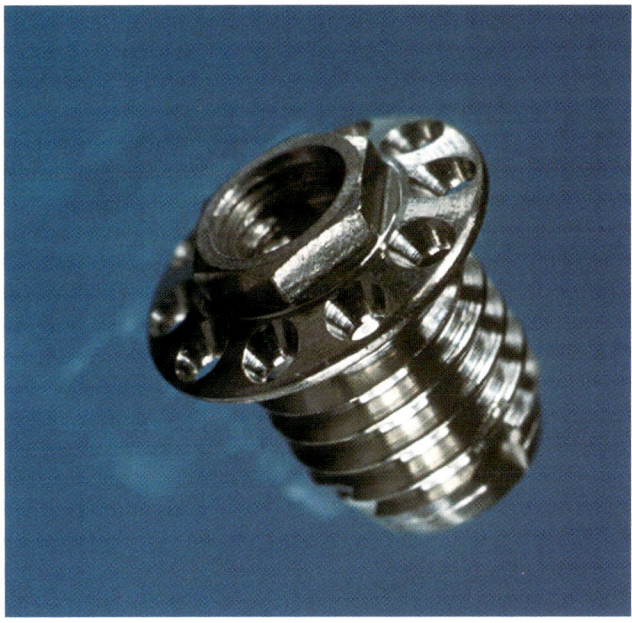

Fig. 9.7 A flanged implant body manufactured for use in the skull.

Box 9.4 Zygomatic implants

WHAT ARE THEY?
- Long (30–50 mm) standard design implant bodies
- Inserted into the zygomatic process of the maxilla through the palatal aspect of the residual alveolar ridge

WHEN MIGHT THEY BE USED?
- Potentially of value in a small number of cases
- Can be indicated in edentulous and partially dentate maxillae
- Rarely used on their own, typically combined with other implants/natural teeth
- May enable implantation without bone grafting
- Used with fixed/removable superstructure in the edentulous case
- Can assist in managing the distal extension saddle

PATIENT ASSESSMENT
- Same basic criteria as for conventional implants
- Special consideration needed due to potential problems with:
  - Access
  - Anatomy of the surgical site
  - Length of the implant body
  - Location: the head of the implant usually lies palatal to the residual alveolar ridge and is oriented laterally

WHAT PROBLEMS MAY BE ENCOUNTERED WHEN USING THEM?
- Same problems as for conventional implants
- Length, location and orientation pose further potential difficulties

---

Problems

Zygomatic implants (Box 9.4) are subject to the same problems that can arise with the more conventional designs; however, their extreme lengths and location adjacent to the maxillary sinus can create specific problems during insertion, as well as when placing restorations. The implants are more difficult to handle owing to their great length and are not immune from failure. It is particularly important to ensure that following implant placement the soft-tissue wound is closed in layers to minimize the risk of breakdown and implant exposure. This can be particularly serious given the location of the implant. Where failure of osseointegration occurs the implant should be removed. If it has fractured then the apical portion, if secure, should remain buried.

REHABILITATION OF EXTRA-ORAL DEFECTS

Replacement of missing facial tissues with a prosthesis, rather than complete repair with plastic surgery, is often appropriate in severe cases of facial deformity arising congenitally, or following trauma or the removal of a tumour. Its effectiveness in restoring the appearance and confidence of the patient has depended on the artistic skills of the maxillofacial technician in creating a lifelike replacement and on the use of mechanical aids such as tissue adhesives and spectacle frames to stabilize it in position.

Now, with the design of implants suitable for insertion into the skull, and new processes of imaging and fabrication, much greater certainty exists in planning treatment, with more predictable results for the patient (Fig. 9.7).

These, and other situations that will be discussed, are dependent on the concerted efforts of a team in order to achieve a satisfactory level of function and a cosmetic outcome acceptable to each individual patient. This commonly includes the expertise of a plastic surgeon, ENT surgeon, ophthalmic surgeon, audiological physician, psychiatrist and make-up artist.

Facial prostheses

Facial prostheses that disguise disfigurement resulting from the loss or absence of the eye, nose, ear and lip/cheek can obtain significant stability from specially designed skull implants. In extreme cases, where the defect involves dental, extra-oral and facial tissues, a combination of dental and skull implants positioned in accessible bony sites may be used to support and stabilize a combination of prostheses (e.g. fixed mandibular prosthesis, removable maxillary overdenture or an intra-oral and facial prosthesis).

The skull implant is designed to engage the limited depth of available bone and make wider contact over an increased surface area. This is achieved with a body of 3–4 mm depth and 3.75 mm diameter plus a perforated flange engaging a recess prepared in the outer cortical plate of the skull. Percutaneous abutments are secured to the top of the implant body with an abutment screw. Depending on the loads to which the implants may be subjected, and the risks of displacement, retention may be gained for the facial prosthesis from clips acting on a bar set between several gold cylinders or from magnets and keepers on individual implants. Hence an ear prosthesis is usually retained by a bar between two implants and an eye prosthesis covering an exenterated orbit may be stabilized by two or three independent magnets. Another factor influencing this choice is the amount of available space between the surface of the prosthesis and the stabilizing components (Figs 9.8, 9.9).

Selection of implant sites is achieved by careful clinical and radiographic examination within the area where implants may be located for prosthetic purposes. However, it is important to appreciate that both prospective and retrospective studies of rehabilitation using implants have demonstrated different outcomes, with osseo-integration sometimes failing, previously irradiated bone demonstrating lower success. Greatest survival has been recorded for implants supporting an ear prosthesis. Less is achieved in the supra-orbital ridge and least in sites supporting a nasal prosthesis. It is important, therefore, to be aware of the dose and timing of previous radiotherapy and the possibility of placing more implants to counteract loss.

The design and construction of facial prostheses

Careful consideration of the medical history, the findings of the clinical examination and radiological assessment, together with an evaluation of study casts of the face and diagnostic wax-ups, are essential in making an acceptable treatment plan (Box 9.5). Most recently, advances in data processing have made it possible to plan some procedures on a computer and prepare accurate models of the defective tissues and the prostheses that will replace them. This is particularly appropriate where there exists a unilateral defect, as it is possible to electronically replicate the image of the sound side and position a reflection of

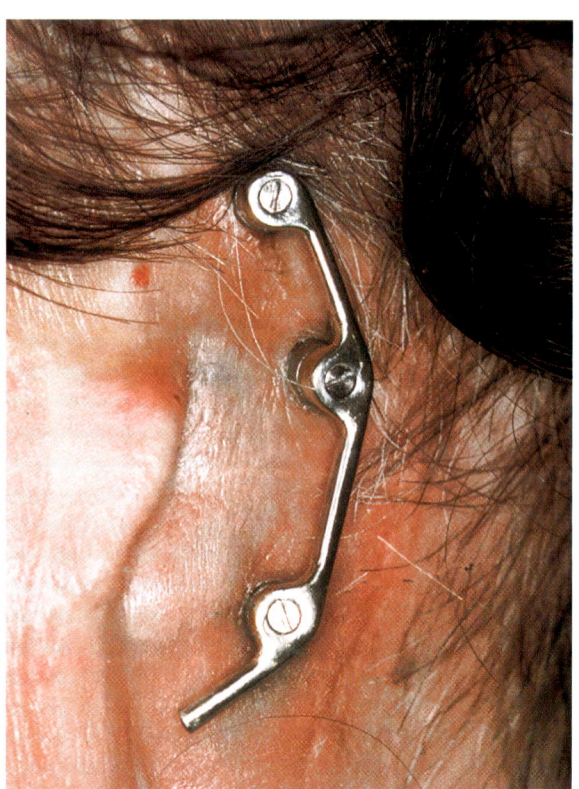

Fig. 9.8 Percutaneous abutments support cylinders linked by a bar.

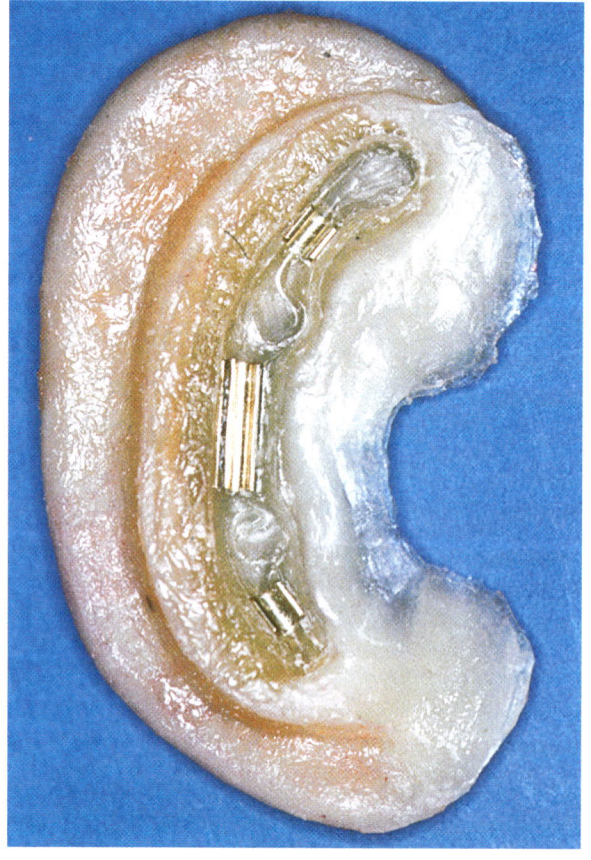

Fig. 9.9 The ear prosthesis is retained by clips on the bar.

Box 9.5 Treatment planning for facial prostheses

CLINICAL APPRAISAL OF DEFECTIVE TISSUE AREA

- Estimation of useful implant sites to provide retention/ support for the prosthesis
- Consideration of surface contours identifying redundant tissue and penetration by the abutments of unfavourable skin or mucosa
- Determination of the desirable form and border shape of the prosthesis

RADIOGRAPHIC EXAMINATION

- CT scan to determine suitable sites for implantation

LABORATORY ASSESSMENT

- Download data to analyse the computer image of defect site/selected normal facial tissues
- Construct rapid process model of defect and model of exactly fitting prosthesis
- Construct computer-generated template for locating implant sites or
- Produce diagnostic laboratory model for preparation of trial prosthesis
- Prepare preliminary prosthesis, mark implant sites

SURGICAL PREPARATION

- Select likely number, type, position, angulation and relation of implants
- Select one- or two- stage procedure
- Select likely abutments:
  - Penetration of skin ensuring fixed, hair-free site or creating thin grafted site
  - Penetration of mucosa creating thin immobile cuffs within prosthetic space or
  - Replacing skin graft
- Confirm fit of surgical template/mark on facial planes

PROSTHESIS DESIGN

- Determine perimeter in relation to fixed or mobile tissue and external form
- Choose retention mechanism; separate or linked abutments using bar, magnets or precision attachment
- Identify space for ventilation
- Consider characteristics (colouration, eyebrows, moustache, hairstyle, spectacles)
- Confirm alignment with normal facial tissues (e.g. eye level, ear prominence)

this shape over the defect. The resultant data can be then used to produce a prosthesis by rapid process modelling. An ear prosthesis, for example, may now exactly replicate the form of the unaffected ear and fit precisely against the tissues on the face while gaining retention from implants positioned in the most appropriate bone.

Despite these improvements it is essential that the patient is made aware that (1) modern artificial silicone polymers require replacement on a regular, frequent basis because of the degradation of colour pigments and that (2) immaculate hygiene is essential around the percutaneous abutment to avoid infection. Also, the cosmetic result remains dependent on the skill and artistic appreciation of the maxillofacial technician in the team.

Evidence from the medical history will show both the period the patient has experienced facial deformity and any operative procedures to overcome it, as well as other functional deficits associated with the loss of local tissue or attributable to other conditions. Examples include speech impediments arising from surgical excision of an oral tumour, or deafness attributable to a congenital syndrome, such as hemifacial microsomia, in which the external ear is microtic. In cases of tumour excision it is crucial to be aware of the levels of irradiation to which residual tissues have been subjected and the projected expectation of recurrence. Increased risks of implant failure and the necessity of additional operative procedures may adversely affect patients and their confidence in rehabilitation. Hence a period of conventional management without implants may be appropriate.

Local examination of the site should identify the extent of the deformity and whether or not the margin of the prosthesis is likely to be associated with discoloured or mobile skin. A poor colour match, or facial movements that cause gaping between the prosthesis and the face, will become obvious. It is also important for the team to appreciate that where thick flaps may have been advantageous in load bearing for traditional prostheses the sites of implant penetration should be thin and well bound down to the periosteum to minimize infection spreading into the skin surrounding the abutment. Obviously the border of the prosthesis should merge with natural skin creases and the skin beneath most of the prosthesis should be free of contact to permit ventilation and avoid the risk of bacterial contamination, which is encouraged by sweating.

While a diagnostic impression may be recorded of the local site, it is often necessary to record the whole face (perhaps including some of the hair of the scalp) in order to evaluate the deformity and to prepare a diagnostic wax-up. With this in position certain key features can be determined at a further clinical examination:

- Will there be sufficient space between the skin surface and the prosthesis to accommodate the implant abutments and retaining components without adversely affecting the appearance or bulk of the prosthesis?

- Is there excessive residual tissue or hair-bearing skin conflicting with the desirable positions of the implants or prosthesis?

- Does the tissue loss/absence result in significant facial asymmetry that will require a compromise in the position or bulk of the prosthesis in order to harmonize with the existing structures?

- Is it necessary to mark certain facial landmarks on the diagnostic cast and wax-up (e.g., level and position of the pupil of the artificial eye, orientation of alatragal line and sagittal plane of the skull for a nasal prosthesis)?

Early consideration must be given to the spacing and alignment of the implants so that subsequent impressions can be recorded and to ensure sufficient access for securing components.

Data from CT scans of the face and skull are particularly beneficial in determining the available quantity and quality of bone suitable for implantation, and for the preparation of models of the skull and facial bones as well as for preparing surgical guides for siting implants. In the preparation of an ear prosthesis, for example, contiguous axial slices 1–2 mm apart about the level of the mastoid process would be recorded and reformatted as images, which may be displayed on a computer using appropriate software. Variations in skull thickness below 3 mm and the presence of mastoid air cells can be located and avoided since such sites offer insufficient resistance to implant loading (Fig. 9.10).

Once predictable implant sites have been chosen MRI or optical surface (laser) scanning is a useful alternative in modelling templates and prostheses that fit the face, without the risks of irradiation by repeating CT scans.

As a result of both clinical and scanning assessments the team should be confident in predicting the precise positions for implants, as well as determining the shape of the intended prosthesis and methods of retaining it. Issues concerning the colouration and characterization of the prosthesis (e.g., the inclusion of hair, the position of a suitable artificial globe of the eye) should be decided by the maxillofacial technician before the first surgical operation.

Surgical placement of skull implants

Percutaneous implant placement is conducted using a full aseptic technique and invariably general anaesthesia. In the majority of cases clinical inspection of the site and the careful placement of a prepared facial template are essential to the correct location of the implants. The ideal sites are marked through the skin onto the cranial bone before the site is liberally infiltrated with a local anaesthetic. When dealing with hair-bearing tissue it is desirable to mark the leading edge of the hairline (assuming it is not to be modified) before shaving the area preoperatively, as hair is bacteriologically dirty. It is also desirable to consider whether the abutment is likely to penetrate such tissue since it will require excision and replacement with a free skin graft at the second surgical stage.

A curved incision 1–2 cm to the side of the sites is made to the periosteum and a flap is mobilized. The dye pricked through can be seen staining the sites in the periosteum. Sharp dissection of this tissue then exposes key landmarks, for example the superior temporal line, mastoid process and descent into the external auditory meatus at the supramental spine (when preparing the site of an ear prosthesis).

Sequential use of cutting tools, commencing with a rose-head burr, identifies the bony texture and need for subsequent tapping of the canal prepared by the twist drill. In many situations a self-tapping implant is appropriate both for the 3–4 mm canal and the skull surface, following the application of the countersink (Fig. 9.11).

Penetration to the dura is appropriate but further penetration, even the involvement of a venous sinus, requires the use of a muscle plug. The decision whether to carry out a two-stage procedure by first applying a cover screw or to use a single stage that involves adding the appropriate abutment depends on two factors: the

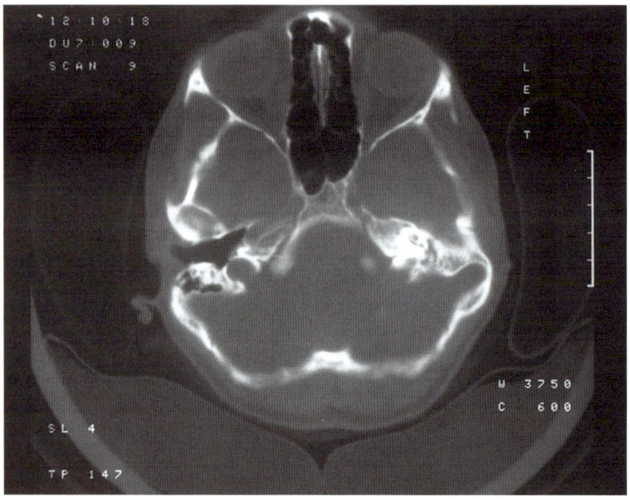

Fig. 9.10 Reconstruction from the CT scan identifies, in an axial slice, the limited thickness of the mastoid bone on the defect side of the skull, where the ear is affected by hemifacial micosomia.

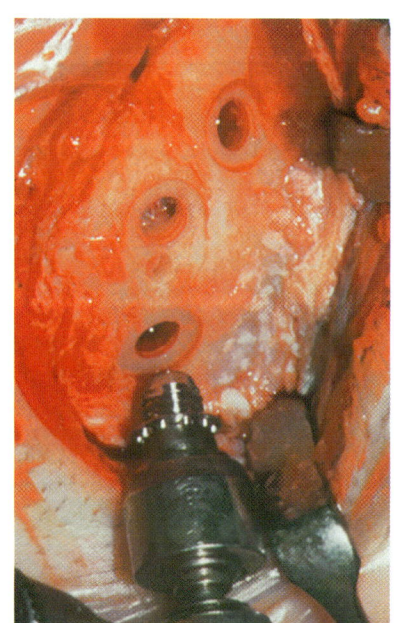

Fig. 9.11 Inserting a skull implant into the prepared site.

thickness and quality of the bone offering stability to the implant, and the need to revise the skin at the implant sites due to hair-bearing tissue or excessive bulk of soft-tissue remnants. The periosteal layer is closed with 5/0 glycolic acid sutures and the skin with 6/0 nylon. Whether a single- or two- stage procedure is adopted it is essential to remove soft tissue between the periosteum and skin for approximately 2 cm around each implant, to ensure that the skin cuff is closely adapted and tightly bound down to the periosteum. This offers no movement and so reduces the risk of inflammation in the cuff. This is not uncommon if the patient fails to sustain an excellent standard of cleaning around the abutment.

Prosthesis construction

The procedure adopted for securing a diagnostic impression may also be used for securing a working impression, whereby the implants are related to the surrounding tissue. In the case of a small area, a special tray is prepared with access holes for transfer impression copings. These are screwed to abutments which protrude approximately 2 mm above the skin. Hair should be coated with petroleum jelly before the wash of polyether or addition cured silicone material is applied to the tray. It is also desirable to mark the tray with those landmarks that will assist in orienting the case to other facial structures, e.g. the Frankfort plane. The advantage of using a well-designed, close-fitting tray is that of securing some tissue displacement at the intended prosthetic margin when, for example, the mouth is open and the facial contour is distorted by the movement of the ascending ramus.

After removal of the impression, replica abutments are secured to the impression copings and a cast is poured in dental stone. Where patients exhibit unilateral absence of facial structures it is an advantage to record an MRI or laser scan. Data downloaded to the computer and to a stereolithographic machine will allow mirror imaging and the preparation of models of the defective site, as well as of an exactly fitting prosthesis replicating the normal tissues (Figs 9.12–9.16).

In extensive tissue loss the entire face is encircled with a collar and sealed at the margin to avoid the escape of impression material. The eyebrows, lashes and hair are coated with petroleum jelly and the airway is established with tubes protruding from the nares before a fluid alginate mix is poured onto the face. Where there is access to the mouth the prosthetic obturator should be in position supporting the facial tissues. Before removal the impression material requires to be backed with impression plaster to avoid distortion. Where a framework is planned to stabilize the prosthesis, cylinders are positioned on the abutments and bars are soldered between them, in the laboratory. It is essential to check the precise fit of the framework clinically before adapting the trial prostheses to receive sleeves or clips and the acrylic resin substructure, which encloses them. An appropriately designed

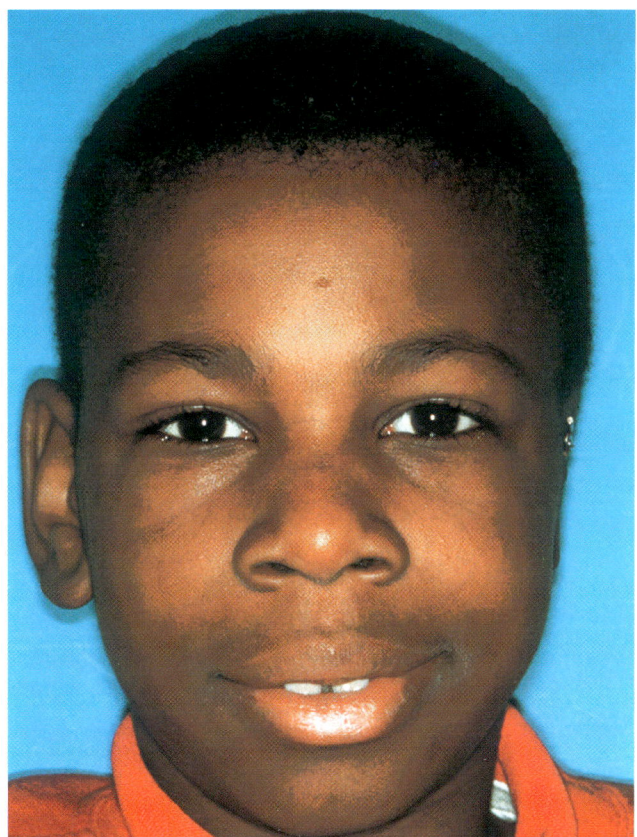

Fig. 9.12 The patient has been born with hemifacial microsomia including a missing external ear (anotia).

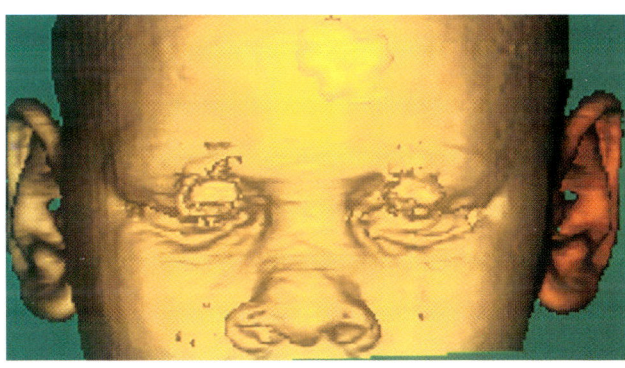

Fig. 9.13 A computer image from an MRI scan may be manipulated to include a mirror image of the normal ear in a planned position on the defective side of the face.

sectional mould is required when investing the prostheses since it should be retained for future use when replacing the flexible silicone prostheses.

The mould is packed with a room-temperature-curing silicone elastomer (e.g. Silastic™, Cosmesil™) in the presence of the patient. These materials allow the incorporation of appropriate pigments to achieve a close representation of the skin tones. They have good dimensional stability and high tear resistance. The acrylic resin shell enclosing the clips is lightly roughened and cleansed with acetone before being primed. Mechanical undercuts may be used where rough handling is anticipated to avoid detachment of the silicone prosthesis from the acrylic core.

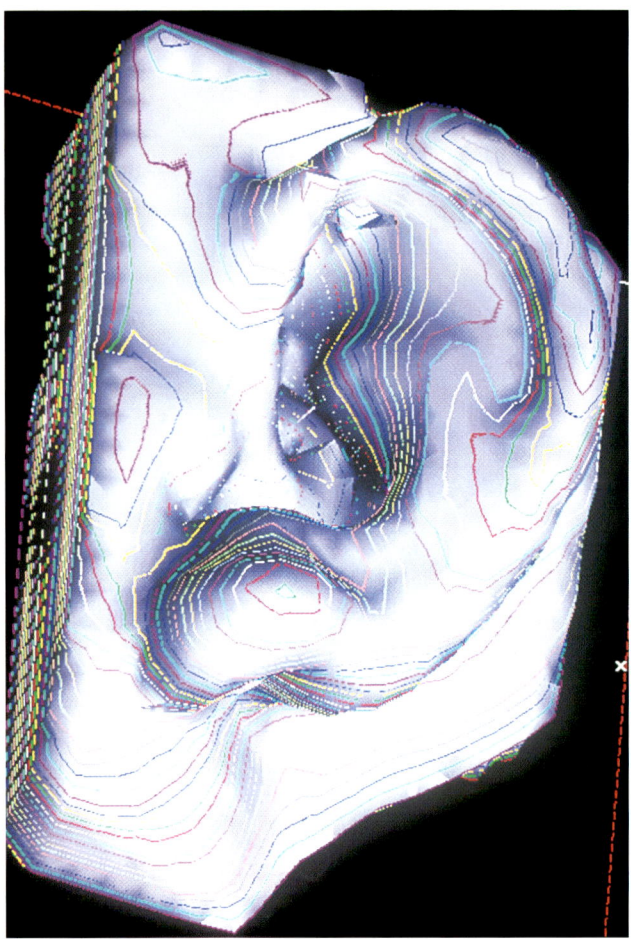

Fig. 9.14 This image from the computer shows a slice file prepared for rapid proces modelling.

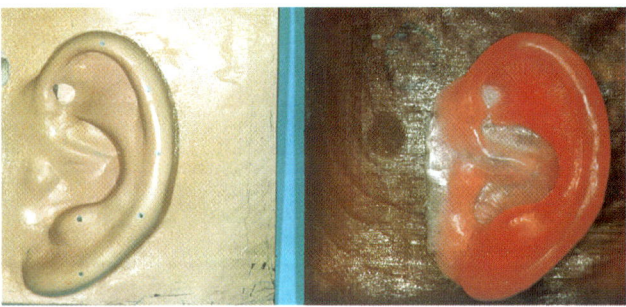

Fig. 9.15 Rapid process models can be prepared of the prosthesis fitted to the face and of the defect side for a precisely fitting wax replica.

Regular monitoring is essential to ensure the prosthesis remains secure and functional. It is important to monitor the cleansing of the implant abutments, as it is not always easy for the patient to visualize the result. Assistance from a relative or friend should confirm that debris/secretions are removed using a bactericidal soap and that the cuffs are free of oedema or erythema.

Local infection may require professional guidance in the use of an antifungal, antibacterial steroidal cream, e.g. Tera-cortril ointment. The patient may require carefully supervised instruction in placing the prosthesis when it is newly made or worn for the first time. They should also be advised that colour changes may occur

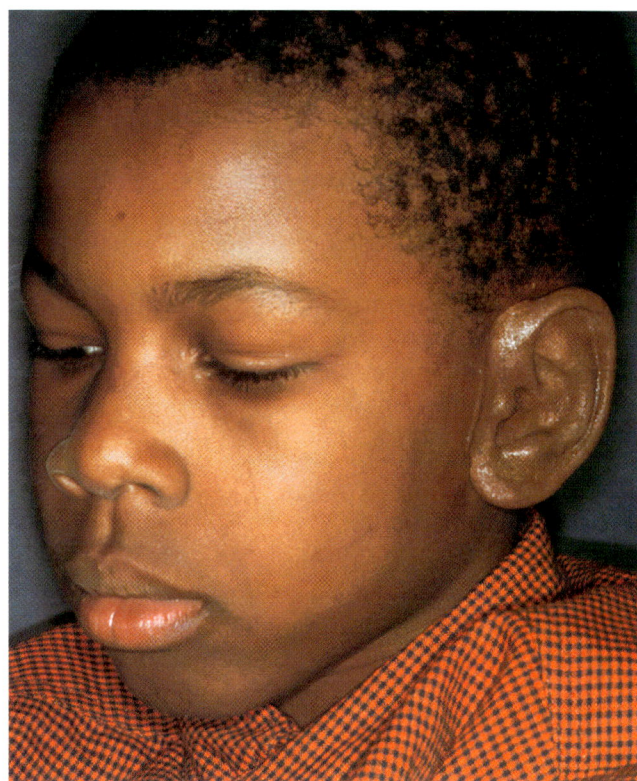

Fig. 9.16 Rehabilitation achieved with the implant-retained silicone prosthesis.

rapidly when the elastomer is exposed to bright sunlight, seawater or industrial atmosphere and smoke. It is possible to colour the material extrinsically but replacement may be necessary after 18 months to 2 years.

Key issues

Key issues arise in positioning implants and securing effective function for some prostheses:

- Implants must be positioned in accessible sites, which enable abutments to be screwed into position and where conflict does not exist with the desired shape of the prosthesis. This is exemplified by an orbital prosthesis where there must be room to position the artificial globe correctly, including the centring of the pupil of the eye. While some masking can be achieved by tinted lenses in spectacle frames, this must not be relied upon to achieve an acceptable result (Figs 9.17, 9.18).

- The level and form of the tissue margin around a facial defect are often crucial to avoiding leakage. A nasal prosthesis may, even when fully implant stabilized by a supporting frame, require both an inferior exterior and interior lip to prevent the escape of mucus.

- It is particularly important to be aware that a diminished sensation in facial tissues may allow the patient to wear a prosthesis that is traumatizing the tissues. Recall is essential within 1–4 weeks of fitting a new or remade facial prosthesis to exclude unnoticed damage.

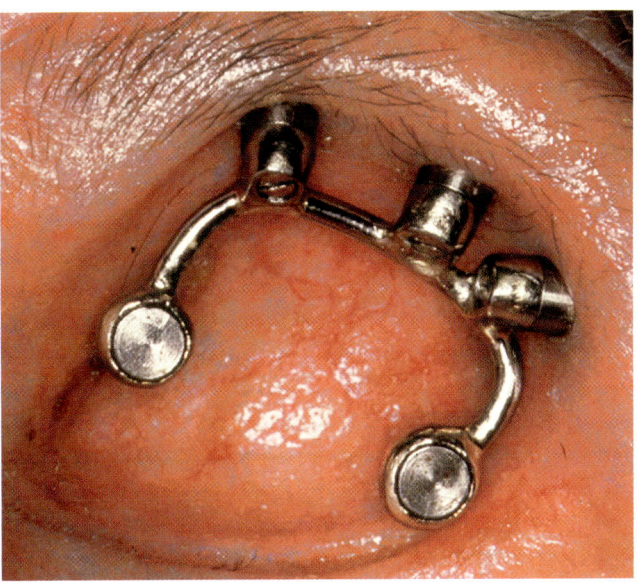

Fig. 9.17 Skull implants positioned in the orbital rim, support a bar carrying magnets for retention of a facial prosthesis.

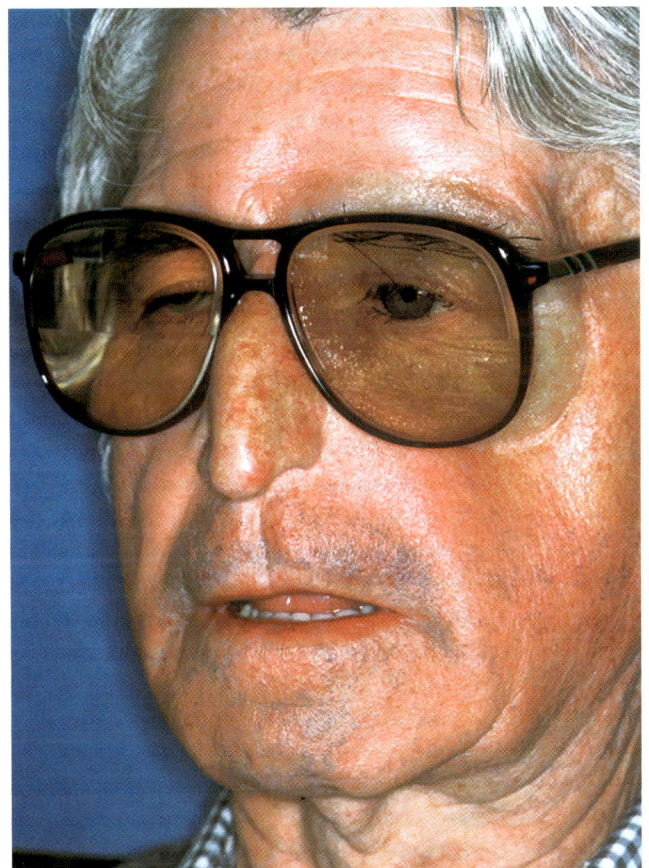

Fig. 9.18 The orbital facial prosthesis is retained by keepers. The spectacles mask the perimeter.

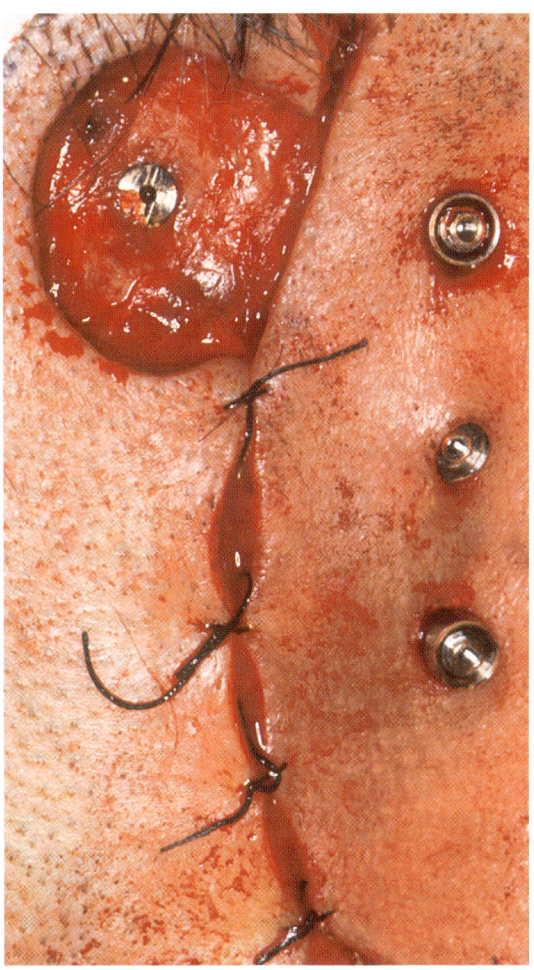

Fig. 9.19 The skin has been penetrated by four abutments. The thick, hair-bearing skin has been replaced by a free graft to create thin, tightly bound tissue around the abutment, which is to be used for a bone-anchored hearing aid (BAHA).

Bone anchored hearing aids

Bone-anchored hearing aids (BAHAs) connected to implants in the mastoid bone of the skull receive direct stimulation and bypass that normally produced in the middle ear. This aid is one alternative to resolving the problem of hearing loss, others being traditional air-conducting hearing aids, cochlear implants and surgical procedures such as stapedectomy.

Connection to the implant is simply achieved by the patient inserting the BAHA linkage into a specialized abutment that is screw retained on the top of the skull implant. A single implant is located within the hairline of the patient, sufficiently posterior to the external ear to avoid direct content with the helix. The surgical procedure of implantation is the same as that described for retaining an auricular prosthesis and many patients benefit from both, e.g. those with hemifacial microsomia (Figs 9.19, 9.20).

The provision of a BAHA assists patients who have the following problems with hearing:

- bilateral hearing loss;
- discharging ears, preventing wearing of air-conducting aids;
- congenital malformation (atresia) of the outer or middle ear.

Those with otosclerosis may have two alternative treatments: stapedectomy and hearing aid rehabilitation. Air-conducting aids are unsuitable when the patient complains of poor sound quality, discomfort, insecu-

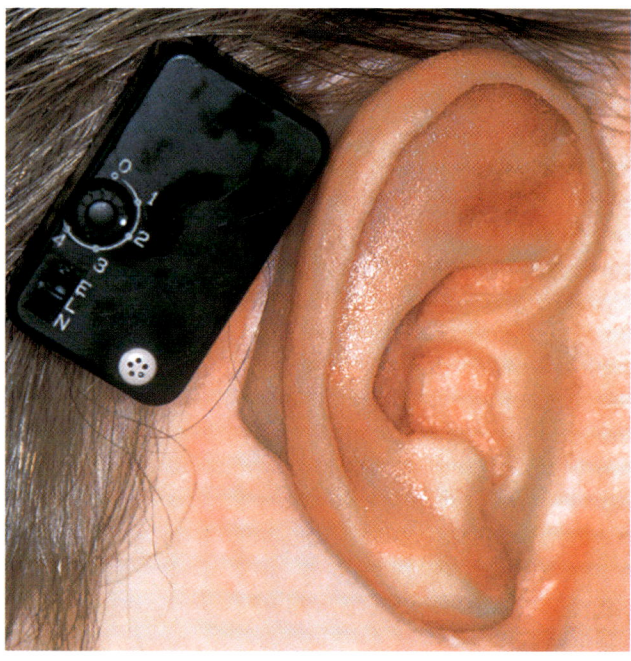

Fig. 9.20 The ear prosthesis and BAHA are slightly separated.

Box 9.6 Indications and contraindications of BAHAs

INDICATIONS FOR PATIENTS
- Bilateral hearing loss
- Astresia of external/middle ear
- Discharging ears

CONTRAINDICATIONS
- Poor hearing thresholds
- Unilateral otosclerosis
- Mild impairment

They are not considered suitable for patients with very poor hearing thresholds, with unilateral otosclerosis/unilateral normal hearing or where impairment is slight (Box 9.6). There are different patterns of BAHA: the standard, superbass worn with an additional body-worn amplifier and a bicross with additional microphone and teleloop facilities.

Studies conclude that measurable tests of advantages of significant improvements over other hearing aids are not conclusive, but those provided with BAHAs report significant subjective gains in sound quality, comfort and appearance. (Half of the patients in one study also found an improvement in coping with background noise.)

rity and poor aesthetics that enhance the sense of disability.

BAHAs have the advantage of no risk of damaging hearing or creation of vertigo and trismus. Also the implant may be simply removed.

FURTHER READING

Brånemark P I, Tolman D E 1998 Osseointegration in cranio-facial reconstruction. Quintessence Publishing Company Inc. Chicago

Cooper L F, Rahan A, Moriarty J, Chaffee N, Sacco D 2002 Immediate mandibular rehabilitation with endosseous implants: simultaneous extraction, implant placement and loading. Int J Oral Maxillofac Implants 17: 517–525

Coward T J, Watson R M, Wilkinson I C 1999 Fabrication of a wax ear by rapid process modelling using stereolithography. Int J Prosthodont 12: 20–27

Engstrand P, Nannmark U, Mårtensson L, Galéus I, Brånemark P I 2001 Brånemark Novum: prosthodontic and dental laboratory procedures for fabrication of a fixed prosthesis on the day of surgery. Int J Prosthodont 14: 303–309

Ismail S F, Johal A S 2002 The role of implants in orthodontics. J Orthod 29 (3): 239–45

Parel S M, Brånemark P I, Ohrnell L O, Svensson B 2002 Remote implant anchorage for the rehabilitation of maxillary defects. J Prosthet Dent 86 (4): 377–81

Roumanas E D, Freymiller E G, Chang T-L, Agerhoot T, Beumer J 2002 Implant retained prostheses for facial defects: an up to 14 year follow-up report on the survival rates of implants at UCLA. Int J Prosthodont 15: 325–332

Stevenson A R, Austin B W, Ann R 2000 Zygomatic fixtures – the Sydney experience. Australas Coll Dent Surg 15: 337–9

Watson R M, Coward T J, Clark R F, Grindrod S 2001 The contribution of imaging and digitised data to mandibular reconstruction and implant stabilised occlusal rehabilitation; a case report. Brit Dent J 190: 296–300

Wilkes G H, Wolfaardt J F 1994 Osseointegrated alloplastic versus autogenous ear reconstruction: criteria for treatment selection. Plast. Reconstr. Surg 93: 967–979

10 Problems

INTRODUCTION

Any form of dental treatment is not immune from failure; however, where that treatment is complex in conception and execution then problems are more likely to arise. Such treatment may also have more serious implications than simpler procedures in terms of its impact on the patient, difficulty of management and potentially irreversible nature.

Management of problems often has to be reactive, but where possible should be proactive.

PREVENTION

Prevention is much to be preferred in problem management, continues throughout active treatment and subsequent reviews, and starts at the first appointment.

PATIENTS' COMPLAINTS

A patient's request for treatment is driven by their perceptions of an oral problem, which often only partly mirrors the clinical situation. Many patients who seek implant treatment will do so on the basis of information in the popular press and second-hand advice from friends. Typically, they have little concept of the realities of the procedure, its scope and potential hazards. Others may have acquired significant amounts of information via the Internet, but have had difficulty placing it in context, or have done so in a manner that is markedly at variance with their needs. It is the role of the dental team to ensure that the patient understands the nature of their condition, and the options for its management, and to help them to make a decision as to the preferred management strategy. Many problems arise later due to the gap between reality and the patient's expectations, which often reflects a failure on the part of the dental team.

Unrealistic expectations

Simplistic therapy

It is not uncommon for a patient to believe that implant therapy provides a direct analogue of the natural dentition, that it may be accomplished in a short time frame, is immune to the requirements of oral hygiene and may be used in all quadrants. The first appointment is the best opportunity for patient education using face-to-face explanation, supplemented as appropriate to the patient's needs with printed material or audiovisual aids.

Function

Many patients will have unrealistic expectations of the function of their appliances, particularly in terms of the appearance of the final prosthesis. This dangerous preconception can give rise to great dissatisfaction with the outcome, and result in often fruitless attempts to replace or improve the prosthesis and modify the patient's views. The latter are rarely successful. Explanations before the event are usually interpreted as such; afterwards they are often seen as excuses for treatment deficiencies.

Lifestyle benefits

A particularly difficult problem is the patient who, often as a result of psychological problems, has come to believe that implant treatment will resolve other problems in their lives. Such unfortunates frequently have a history of seeking support from a series of health care professionals, typically with an unsatisfactory outcome, and after numerous appointments. Every dental implant unit has a number of such patients for whom, in retrospect, such therapy was ill advised. Prevention involves the taking of a comprehensive history and a detailed exploration of the patient's expectations for the treatment. Explicit or implied outcomes often include improvements in body image, resolution of interpersonal problems, happiness, promotion at work and professional advancement. Attempts to help such patients using implant therapy are very rarely successful, and they are frequently best helped by professionals specializing in the treatment of behavioural problems.

MEDICAL HISTORY

Problems arising as a result of medical conditions are unusual. Chapter 4 (medical, dental and social history) and Chapter 5 (preoperative management) include considerations of those that contraindicate implant therapy or increase the risk of its failure. Where such factors have been ignored, then problems are more likely to ensue. If implant therapy is still deemed appropriate, then it should be as simple and as certain of outcome as possible. Bone grafting, implant placement in poor-quality bone, the use of short implants, complex superstructure designs and those that are difficult to maintain should be avoided.

LOCAL FACTORS

Problems that can be avoided by considering local factors largely relate to failure to consider the space required for implant insertion and restoration, and the relationships between the surgical and prosthodontic space envelopes (Fig. 10.1)

The surgical envelope controls the limits of the dimensions and orientations of the implant bodies, the prosthodontic envelope the extent of the super-structure. Their relationship may also impose limitations on the prosthesis, which can result in excessive cantilevering or the use of severely angled abutments. The space available in the mouth will also restrict access, and in some cases make the insertion of instru-ments and impression trays difficult or impossible. Failure to recognize these factors may preclude implant insertion or restoration.

FAILURE TO CONSIDER ALTERNATIVES

Implant treatment is a valuable addition to the range of procedures available to the restorative dentist; however, it must be viewed as complementary to more routine procedures and not as a substitute for them. Three types of situation typically arise:

- Excessive focus on implant treatment. The use of dental implants where more straightforward techniques would be more effective and efficient, for example managing a problem caused by poor complete dentures by using implant-stabilized prostheses, when new well-designed and constructed dentures would satisfy the patient's needs.

- Excessively focused approach to problem management. This occurs when attempts are made to manage a localized problem in the dental arch, without considering the patient's oral needs in general. For example, by restoring an edentulous space with an implant-stabilized prosthesis while failing to treat caries or periodontal disease elsewhere in the mouth.

- Short-term treatment plans. The potential functional life of a dental implant is not known, but on current evidence is likely to be many decades. Unfortunately, in some patients this greatly exceeds the probable lifespan of their remaining dentition. As a result dental implant treatment, which appeared appropriate when provided, may create management problems later. The patient with missing anterior maxillary teeth and extensive caries or periodontal disease who is treated with an implant-stabilized bridge may become an oral cripple in a few years with an edentulous maxilla and two anterior implants of doubtful functional value.

Box 10.1 Avoiding problems

PREVENTION
- This is always better than cure!

PATIENT-RELATED PROBLEMS
Misconceptions
- *Unrealistic expectations*. The implant therapy will provide far more benefits than are possible
- *Simplistic therapy*. Expectations are of a simple 'fit and forget' procedure carried out in one visit, with no further active involvement by the patient
- *Function*. The implant prosthesis will have the full functionality of the natural teeth
- *Lifestyle benefits*. The patient anticipates that a wide range of personal problems relating to appearance, career and interpersonal relationships will be solved by dental implants

Informed consent
This must be obtained, and be informed

Medical history
There is a range of factors that contraindicate implant treatment or increases the likelihood of failure

Local factors
These reflect potential problems with access, insertion, restoration, appearance, integration and long-term management of oral health

Failure to consider alternatives
Implant therapy is not always the most appropriate treatment; other procedures must be considered when treatment planning and used where appropriate. They may include observation, complete dentures, RPDs, adhesive bridges, conventional bridges and orthodontic therapy

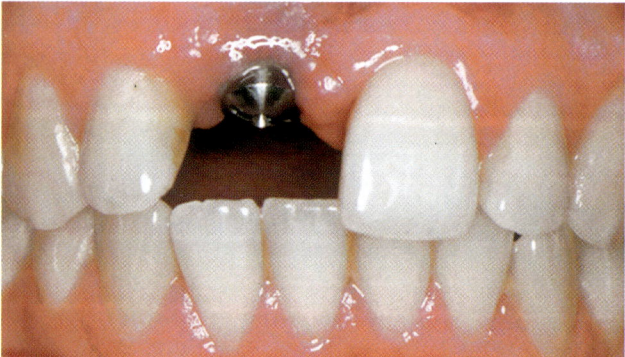

Fig. 10.1 Restoration of this implant with a single crown will be difficult owing to the width of the space to be restored, which is greater than that of 21, and the labial alveolar resorption, which has resulted in the implant being placed more palatal than the root of 21.

TECHNICAL PROBLEMS

Treatment with dental implants is technically demanding, and has functional limitations imposed by the pre-manufactured components. These relate to:

- Appearance. Dental implants frequently impose restrictions on the location and contours of the prosthetic superstructure, owing to their design and the need to make provision for oral hygiene and access for placement of screws.

- Mechanical strength. Implant components are of necessity small and have limited strength, especially when loaded non-axially due to cantilevering, where long components are used, or where there are heavy occlusal loads.

- Bone overload. Excessive occlusal loads may have a deleterious effect on osseointegration, a situation that can arise when the superstructure design causes high stresses in the surrounding bone, or results in high localized masticatory loads. These often relate to excessive cantilevering or inappropriate occlusal schemes (Figs 10.2, 10.3).

SKILL LEVELS

All implant treatment requires an advanced mix of skills from the entire dental team. This is especially the case when carrying out complex procedures in the maxilla, involving for example bone grafting, multiple implants, unfavourable ridge and soft-tissue contours, extensive superstructures and complex occlusal schemes. Clinicians must ensure that they and their team are well versed in the relevant techniques before embarking on implant treatment, if future problems are to be minimized.

A particular problem can arise where treatment is provided by different specialists, for example a surgeon and a restorative dentist. Care must be taken in these circumstances to ensure that both are suitably skilled, and that they communicate effectively at all stages of the treatment planning and provision. Key and often irreversible decisions taken by one member of the team can create significant problems for the overall treatment. A regrettably common scenario is one in which the decision to provide implant treatment, or the choice of implant bodies and their locations, is made by one member of the team in isolation, subsequently placing severe constraints on the feasibility of the procedure and its outcome.

INFORMED CONSENT

A lengthy discussion on informed consent is beyond the scope of this book, and while this should be obtained for any clinical procedure irrespective of its complexity, it is especially important where the treatment and its possible failure may have a major and irreversible impact on the patient. This is often the case with implant treatment, which, because of its

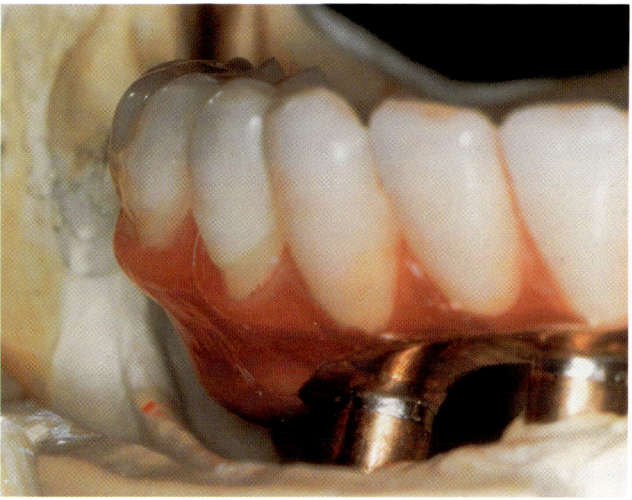

Fig. 10.2 Buccal cantilever on a fixed bridge.

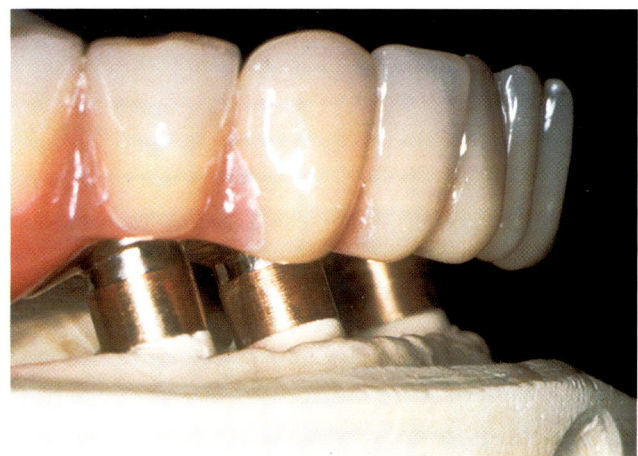

Fig. 10.3 The incisors on this prosthesis are placed significantly labial to the most anterior abutment, partly reflecting the unfavourable positions of the implant bodies. Biting on these teeth will result in torquing of the implants and a greater upwards force on the gold screws in the more distal implants.

unfamiliarity and public image of high-technology glamour, can give rise to totally unrealistic expectations. Patients must be fully aware of the nature of their oral problems, in terms they can understand. The various treatment modalities should be explained, including their principal advantages and disadvantages, and the patient helped to make an informed choice. Such discussions should be noted in the clinical record, together with details of components used. Where treatment is carried out jointly it is important to have a record of key joint decisions and the agreed treatment plan, in order to minimize the occurrence of problems later.

SURGICAL PROBLEMS
STAGE-ONE SURGERY
Haemorrhage

Excessive haemorrhage usually occurs as a result of involving a blood vessel or perforating the bony cortex

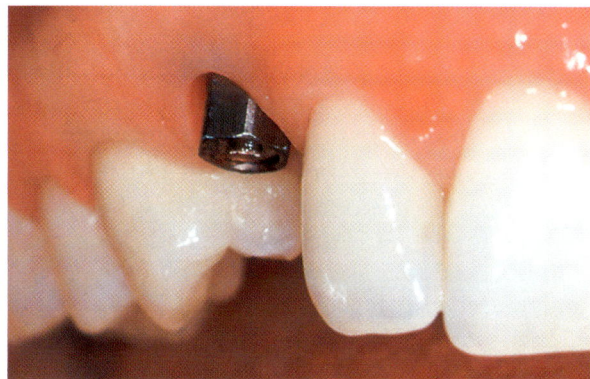

Fig. 10.4 This implant has been placed too far buccally, making it difficult to achieve a natural appearance with the final restoration.

so that the adjacent soft tissues are traumatized. Management is usually straightforward, using standard techniques, provided that a major vessel is not involved. Where this occurs in the mandible distal to the mental foramina the possibility of damage to the mandibular canal must be considered. Prevention of this is based on careful radiographic assessment and surgical technique.

Implant mobility

This can arise where there are problems in obtaining primary stability because of the anatomy and density of the bone, or the implant site has been prepared without due care so that it is oversized. Thorough preoperative assessment, the use of a surgeon's guide and careful surgery can avoid some of these problems. Where they arise they can often be managed by the use of 'oversized' or tapered implants, which a number of manufacturers provide. Failure to secure good primary fixation is associated with increased implant failure.

Implant location

Incorrect positioning of the implant can lead to considerable difficulties during the restorative phase of treatment. It is extremely important that implant locations are planned with the prosthodontist prior to surgery. (Figs 10.4–10.8).

Problems placing cover screw

These usually arise as a result of contamination of the linking recess in the implant body, misalignment of the screw or damage to the screw threads in the implant body. Management is based on avoidance of these causes and thorough cleansing of the recess. Where necessary, the internal thread in the implant body may have to be redefined with the tap provided by the manufacturer, although this is a rare occurrence.

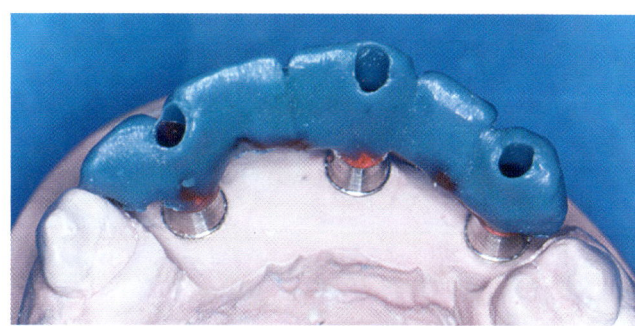

Fig. 10.5 Two of these implants are not coincident with the central axes of the artificial crowns in the laboratory wax-up, resulting in a less than optimal appearance.

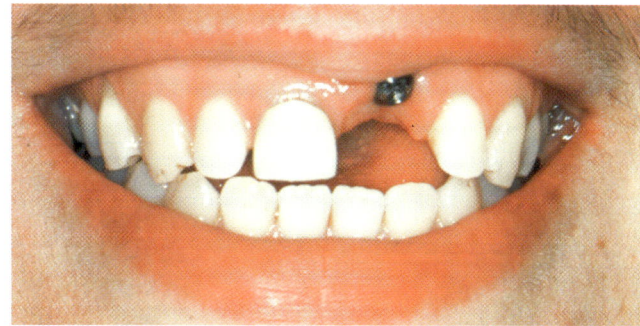

Fig. 10.6 This implant has been placed too far labially and is incorrectly oriented.

Postoperative pain

This is an uncommon complaint and its diagnosis is related to the time of onset. Where it occurs immediately after implant placement, nerve involvement, inflammation and thermal trauma should all be considered. Pain arising later is often related to peri-implant infection, or excessive pressure from the temporary prosthesis, where one is used. Pain immediately following implant placement can usually be managed with mild analgesics; however, if it persists then further investigations are required. In some cases implant removal may be indicated. Pressure from an overdenture can lead to implant failure and must be managed symptomatically as soon as possible. In

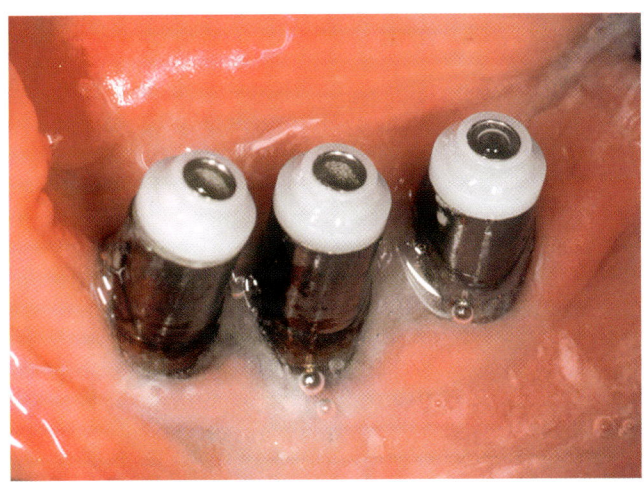

Fig. 10.7 The two implants on the left of the picture have been placed too close to each other, which will create problems when designing the prosthesis and make effective oral hygiene more difficult.

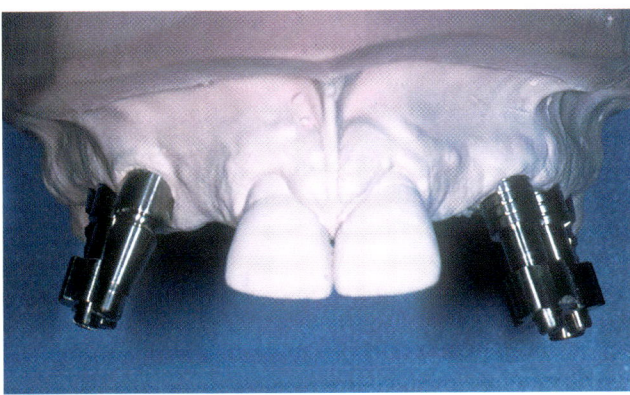

Fig. 10.8 These implants have been placed at excessively divergent angles to the occlusal plane, and restoration will require the use of custom or angulated abutments. As a result the appearance of the prosthesis may be compromised.

addition to the use of mild analgesics, inflammation and discomfort can be relieved by gently rinsing with a hot saline mouth bath.

Paraesthesia

This arises due to trauma to one of the nerves in the region of the implant site. It usually subsides where direct mechanical damage to the neurovascular bundle has not occurred. The longer the delay in recovery the less likely this is to occur. It is more common in the mandible and following extensive surgery in the region, such as repositioning of the interior alveolar nerve. It is best avoided by careful preoperative assessment and surgery.

Infection

Infection following surgery is unusual provided that a careful sterile technique has been used. There is evidence that the use of prophylactic antibiotics can

reduce both this problem and the incidence of early implant failure. Where infection occurs it should be managed symptomatically.

Exposure following placement

Exposure immediately following implant placement is not now considered as serious an issue as previously, however it may prejudice implant success and can indicate excessive local pressure from a temporary denture. It is most likely to occur as a result of poor design of the surgical flap, tension in the flap, or excessive pressure from a temporary prosthesis or its premature insertion. Avoidance of these causes will minimize the problem. Where it arises the patient should be instructed to clean thoroughly around the area, and if a denture is being used, then this should be eased to relieve any excessive pressure.

Box 10.3 Surgical problems

STAGE ONE SURGERY

Haemorrhage
- More major haemorrhage implies damage to a blood vessel

Implant mobility
Problems in obtaining primary stability may reflect bone anatomy and density, or over-preparation of the implant site

Problems placing cover screw
- Has the screw or internal thread on the implant body been damaged?

Postoperative pain
- *Uncommon.* Diagnosis is related to the time of onset
- *Immediately after implant placement.* Nerve involvement, inflammation and thermal trauma?
- *Later.* Peri-implant infection, excessive pressure from temporary prosthesis?

Paraesthesia
- Typically reflects trauma to one of the nerves in the region of the implant site

Infection
- Unusual provided that a careful sterile technique has been used

Exposure following placement
This can prejudice implant success. Its causes are typically:
- Poor flap design or closure
- Local infection
- Trauma, for example from a denture

STAGE-TWO SURGERY
Failure to integrate

This is usually noted as a loose implant and is more likely to occur where factors predisposing to implant failure are present (see Ch. 2, systemic and local factors affecting implant treatment). Since integration is very unlikely to be established around a clinically loose implant at this stage, management requires its removal. An assessment must then be made of the implications, and consideration given to either replacement of the implant, after a healing period, insertion of an implant in an adjacent site, or modification of the treatment plan using a smaller number of fixtures. Where the potential exists for increased implant failure, some clinicians advocate the initial insertion of a generous number of implants so that the original treatment plan can proceed, even if some do not become integrated. This requires adequate space for implant insertion and resources to pay for the additional costs. In this technique it is common, where failures do not occur, for some of the implants to remain buried. These are known colloquially as 'sleepers'.

Problems placing abutment

These frequently arise due to damage to the internal linking features of the implant body during implant placement, particularly if this is a screw, or misalignment of the abutment, producing a crossed thread. Contamination of the internal features of the implant, typically by bone chips, can also cause the problem. If a thorough cleaning of the recess in the implant body does not solve the problem, then, where the joint is screwed, it may be necessary to clean the thread using manufacturer-specific instrumentation. This is a delicate task and subsequently care must be taken to remove all the debris, which frequently includes metal swarf, by thorough irrigation with normal saline.

Pain

Pain at the time of second-stage surgery can arise prior to, during or following the placement of the abutment. Pain prior to placement is indicative of infection, poor integration or mechanical problems related to the temporary prosthesis. These must be resolved before the abutment is placed. It should be noted that pain is not in itself diagnostic of failure of an implant to integrate, and may often be absent in these circumstances. Where infection is present, this must be resolved prior to placement of the abutment. Pain during second-stage surgery is usually indicative of failure to achieve adequate local anaesthesia. Where it occurs immediately after implant abutment placement, it is often indicative of trapping of the oral mucosa between the abutment and the head of the implant body, or inadequate seating of the abutment due to misalignment or trapping of adjacent bone.

This is particularly likely to occur where new bone has been formed over the cover screw, and which has had to be trimmed back prior to the placement of the abutment. Its management requires removal of the abutment, checking of the site and abutment replacement. Pain is also sometimes associated with an inadequately secure abutment, typically where these are held in place by a screwed joint.

Some operators recommend the use of post-placement radiographs to confirm correct alignment of the two components; however, this is best confined to situations where this cannot be confirmed visually or by gentle probing, or where a cemented super-structure is to be placed. In these circumstances misalignment can cause significant problems as such superstructures, especially where they are single crowns, may be impossible to remove without damage. Their management requires removal of the abutment, checking of the site and abutment replacement.

IMPLANT-RELATED PROBLEMS
Biological
Pain

Pain arising some time after implant placement may be associated with mechanical overload, loss of integration, loosening of the joints between the implant body and connecting components, infection and mechanical failure of one of the components. Its diagnosis is based on examination, which may require removal of the implant superstructure and partial dismantling of some of the joints. This can be difficult or impossible where cement retention is employed, without damaging components irretrievably, but is usually readily carried out where screwed joints are

---

Box 10.4 Surgical problems

STAGE TWO SURGERY

Failure to integrate

- Usually noted as a loose implant, more likely when factors which predispose to implant failure are present

Problems in placing an abutment: possible causes

- Damage to the internal linking features of the implant body during implant placement
- Crossed threads
- Contamination of the internal linking features of the implant
- Bone overgrowth

Pain: possible causes

- Prior to abutment placement: infection, poor integration, pressure from temporary prosthesis
- Shortly after abutment placement: trapped mucosa, inadequate seating of the abutment, loose abutment

used. The management of the various possible causes is described below.

Infection

Infection may arise as a result of poor oral hygiene or the impaction of a foreign body, such as a small seed, in the cuff between the soft tissues and the abutment. Calculus on the abutment can be a significant problem. Attention to oral hygiene, syringing of the pockets around the abutments using a chlorhexidine solution, and cleaning of the abutments where necessary, using plastic scalers, usually result in a significant improvement in the condition. Sometimes it is necessary to remove the abutment to aid in irrigation of the site or scaling of the abutment. Where the adjacent soft tissues are inflamed, care must be taken when removing the abutment, since they readily collapse into the space that it occupied. This can make its replacement difficult, particularly if the abutment is removed for more than a few minutes.

Peri-implant mucositis

This is a condition characterized by inflammation of the soft tissues adjacent to the implant but excluding involvement of the peri-implant bone. This is a more serious situation and is called peri-implantitis.

The characteristics of the condition include increased probing depths, inflammation, swelling, ready bleeding on probing and tenderness. It is associated with mechanical irritation and bacterial proliferation in the peri-implant sulcus. Oral hygiene is therefore important, especially as many implant patients will have lost their own teeth through failures in this regard. The condition can also arise as a result of mechanical irritation, particularly the presence of calculus and other foreign bodies within the peri-implant sulcus (Figs 10.9–10.11), as well as a poor fit between the abutment and the implant body. Similar difficulties can arise with a cemented superstructure where surplus cement has not been removed. Where

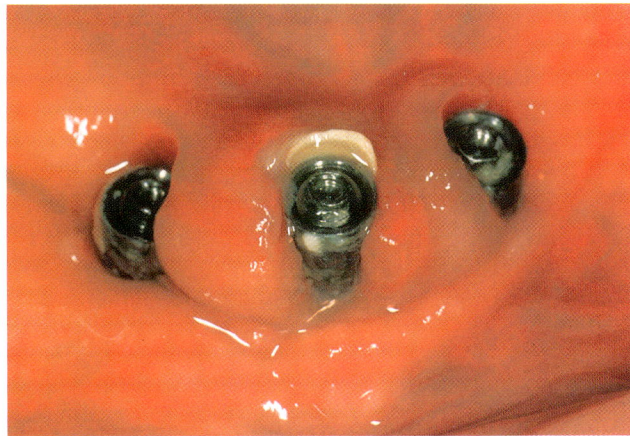

Fig. 10.10 Patient shown in Figure 10.9 with the bar removed. The extent of the soft-tissue swelling is evident.

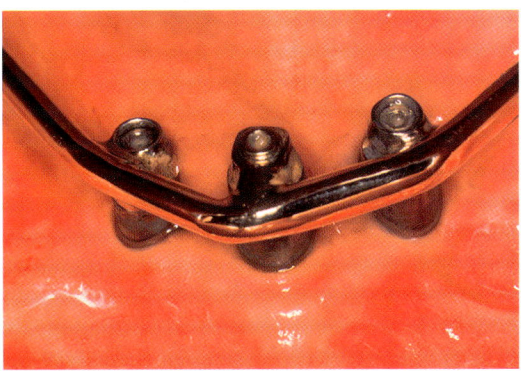

Fig. 10.11 The patient shown in the previous two illustrations seen at 3-month review. The removal of the calculus deposits and improved, although not optimal, oral hygiene have resulted in a significant improvement in soft-tissue health.

the shoulder of the implant body is significantly below the level of the oral mucosa the removal of all cement can be particularly troublesome.

Treatment of peri-implantitis is based on removal of the cause, prevention of its recurrence and symptomatic treatment of the inflamed tissues. This typically involves scaling the abutment using plastic scalers, irrigation of the sulcus and advice on home care. Occasionally the condition can prove somewhat intractable and in these circumstances it can be advantageous to take the implant out of function for a short period. This is dependent on the system being assembled with screwed joints. It can only be carried out where there is an adequate number of implants, in the case of a fixed superstructure, or the patient is prepared to tolerate using a less secure removable prosthesis for a short period where a superstructure is of that design. The technique involves removing the abutment, excising a small wedge of soft tissue, placing a cover screw over the implant body and closing the wound with sutures. Resolution of the inflammation usually occurs quite rapidly and the abutment, after suitable cleaning, may be replaced.

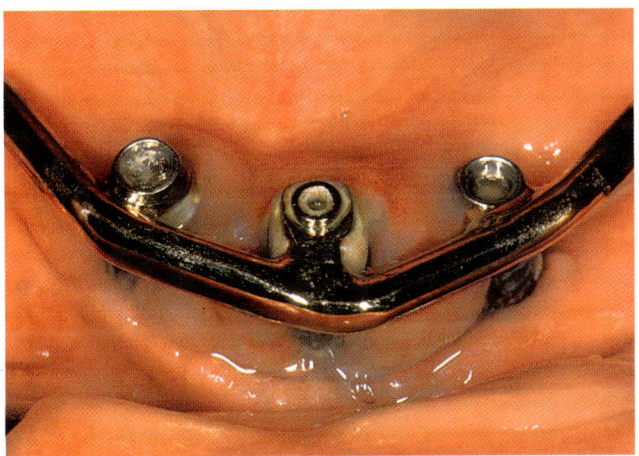

Fig. 10.9 Poor oral hygiene. This patient has a large calculus deposit on the middle abutment, which has caused inflammation of the adjacent soft tissues.

Peri-implantitis

Peri-implantitis is a more severe condition, which involves loss of bone–implant contact due to infection of the connective tissues adjacent to the implant.

The condition can result in pain around the implant; however, due to the often chronic nature of the problem, this is unusual, and diagnosis is usually by means of clinical examination, including probing of the peri-implant sulcus. This will be deepened where bone loss has occurred in the crestal region, typically all around the implant body, a finding which will also be evident on radiographic examination.

Peri-implantitis can have both general and local causes, and is more likely to occur in patients with systemic factors that predispose to implant failure, typically those who smoke tobacco and patients with poorly controlled diabetes. Local predisposing factors include poor plaque control, bacterial colonization of the peri-implant sulcus, mechanical irritation and mechanical overload of the implant–bone interface. Peri-implantitis is associated with bacterial invasion, particularly by periodontal pathogens. These have been identified in the peri-implant sulcus in partially dentate patients with periodontal disease and it is postulated that they have arisen from existing periodontal pockets. Such bacteria can also be found around implants with peri-implantitis in edentulous patients. The link between ongoing periodontal disease and peri-implantitis is unclear; however, it is recommended that implants should not be used in patients with ongoing periodontal disease.

Where the systemic factors are amenable to control then management of these should be started as soon as the condition is diagnosed. Local management, however, is particularly important, and must be instigated as soon as possible to minimize risk of the loss of the implant. Examination should include an assessment of masticatory loads, plaque control, the presence of any foreign bodies around the implant and fit of the implant components between each other. There is currently some debate over the relative relevance of infection and mechanical overload in peri-implantitis; in practice both factors are likely to play some part. The latter is hinted at by the use of implant support for extensive superstructures, excessive cantilevering, and a history of loosened screws and fractured components.

Removal of mechanical and bacterial causes may bring the condition under control in its very early stages; however, where there has been significant tissue loss it may be necessary to expose the bony crest by reflecting a soft-tissue flap and clean the implant and abutment, using standard periodontal techniques. A variety of cleansing agents has been used, and there are reports of attempts to correct a bony defect with natural or synthetic materials, and coverage with various membranes. The reported outcome of these manoeuvres has been variable.

It is recognized that this condition tends to occur in some patients where several implants may be affected, the so-called 'cluster phenomenon'. A history of such a problem cautions against the placement of further implant bodies without careful consideration of the potential outcome. Nevertheless, where an individual implant has been lost, replacement using conventional techniques after an interval to allow for healing is often successful.

Thread exposure

This occurs where implants have been placed too superficially, allowance has not been made for the buccal curvature of the alveolus or marginal bone loss has been greater than anticipated. This can also arise if the bone is excessively heated during site preparation.

Exposed threads do not in themselves predispose to an increased risk of implant failure but can appear unsightly, since it is often difficult to disguise them, especially in the anterior maxilla. Where this is a problem, a short flange may be provided, or consideration be given to soft-tissue grafting to cover the defect. This is not always successful, and can create problems with breakdown of the soft tissues and with plaque control. Management by prevention is to be preferred, and when problems are anticipated careful planning on a diagnostic cast should be carried out. This can also occur after several years of successful implant function, in some cases with little apparent detriment.

Loss of integration

Given that the term osseointegration does not imply a particular amount of bone–implant contact, but rather that this is maintained in a viable bony environment under functional loads over an extended period, it is not feasible to define a given bone level and density around the implant as characterizing osseointegration or its lack. Nevertheless, changes over time are very significant, and the maintenance of bone–implant contact and loss of crestal bone at a slow rate are defining characteristics of implant success, and their absence presages failure. It is common to speak of loss of integration in association with the radiographic or clinical diagnosis of loss of crestal bone; however, where this process can be brought under control, the implant can remain functional for many years. Loss of integration in the sense that there is no longer sufficient bone–implant contact to maintain functionality is the terminal outcome of that process. It may be diagnosed radiographically as well as by looseness of the implant; however, it is not unknown for it to be first evident when removing a healing abutment and finding that both this and the implant body remain linked, with the latter rotating out of the bone.

Total loss of integration is usually recognized clinically by looseness of the implant or the ability to rotate it out of the bone. It is sometimes, but not always, associated with pain, which is more likely to occur when the implant is loaded; however, some patients also describe sensations of tenderness or altered sensation around the implant. The condition may be diagnosed radiographically where it has been present for some time, so that the changes in bone architecture have become sufficient to be detectable in this manner. Loss of bone–implant contact in the crestal region is usually diagnosed by routine radiography or probing of the sulcus around the abutment.

Once an implant is no longer integrated then the only effective treatment is to remove it. A new implant may be placed in an adjacent site or alternatively in a similar location after healing has occurred. Before doing so it is important to attempt to identify the reason for the original failure; however, this is not always evident. Interim treatment will depend upon the superstructure design and number of implants remaining. If there are sufficient implants, and the patient is using a fixed superstructure, it may be possible to use the prosthesis with a reduced number of abutments; a final decision will depend upon the number, length and location of the implants, the nature of the surrounding bone and the occlusal loads. If the patient is using a removable prosthesis with ball attachments, they can usually manage the denture for an interim period with reduced stabilization. If a bar retainer has been employed, then it is only rarely that this will function with a reduced number of abutments, since fewer implants will tend to have been used with this type of design. In these circumstances the bar should be removed and given to the patient for safe keeping, while healing caps may be placed on the implants. If necessary the denture may be modified with a tissue-conditioning material; however, this is not always necessary, needs more regular maintenance and may be troublesome to remove. The longer-term treatment will depend on whether it is decided to replace the implant that has been lost and construct a new prosthesis, or to accept its failure and produce a new or modified prosthesis.

Biomechanical

Fractures

Screws

The principle of a screwed joint is that as the screw is tightened it is put into tension due to its elastic deformation and that of the clamped components, and thus compresses the joint. This force is known as preload, and maintains the integrity of the joint provided that the forces which tend to separate the components are less than the preload. Forces above this will open the joint and, if they exceed the plastic limit of the screw, cause its permanent deformation and loss of joint integrity. This will result in excessive movement of the components and increased risk of screw fracture (Fig. 10.12). Excessive tightening of the screw will similarly cause plastic deformation of the screw, leading to a potentially weaker joint, followed by fracture. Undertightening, however, will result in

---

Box 10.5 Implant-related problems

BIOLOGICAL

Pain
- Possible causes; some time after abutment placement: mechanical overload, loss of integration, loosening of the joints in the system, infection, mechanical failure

Infection (peri-implant mucositis, peri-implantitis)
- Possible causes: systemic factors; local factors: poor oral hygiene, impacted foreign body, calculus deposits

Threads exposure
- Associated with superficial implant placement, marginal bone resorption and thermal trauma
- If unsightly may need covering surgically or with a flange

Loss of integration
- Minor: identify and if possible remove cause
- Major: identify cause, remove implant body. Consider replacement

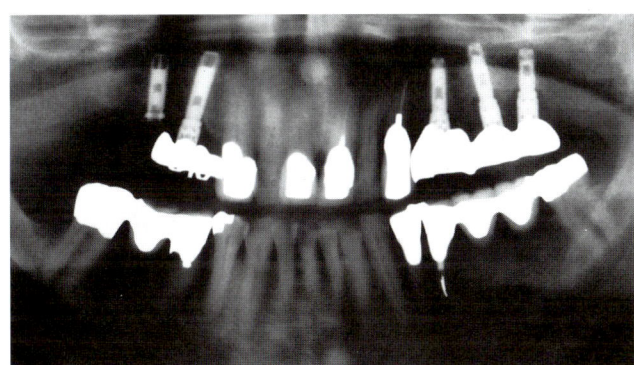

Fig. 10.12 This patient has fractured the abutment screw in the implant in the 16 region, as well as the bridge that it partly supported.

---

the joint being more likely to be opened in function. Screw heads are prone to damage if mishandled and care should be taken to fully seat the screwdriver before applying any torque (Fig. 10.13).

Preload in a screwed joint tends to fall following tightening, and this can be due to several factors, including plastic deformation of the mating screw surfaces, torsional recovery of the screw, cyclical loading, plastic deformation of the joined components and overload of the joint. Where the components do not fit accurately, much of the preload will be used in approximating them. In these circumstances a smaller separating force will open the joint, putting the screw at increased risk of fracture.

Components should therefore fit as accurately as possible and screws be tightened to the optimum torque, which is why many manufacturers produce torque wrenches of various designs, both mechanical and electromechanical.

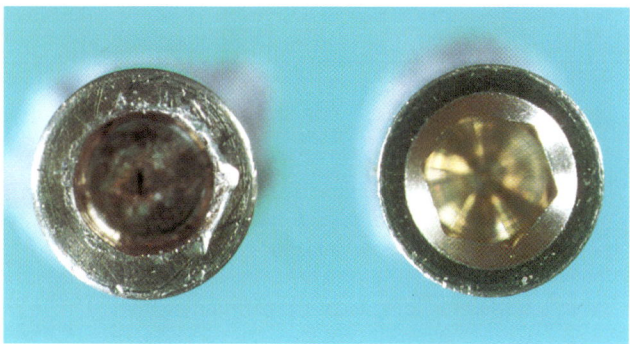

Fig. 10.13 The hexagonal sockeets of gold screws can be easily damaged by careless handling, especially with powered instrumentation.

Screws may fracture for many reasons, and often several in combination. Principal amongst these are:

- *Overtightening.* This can occur where screws are tightened manually, or an incorrectly set torque wrench has been used.

- *Poorly aligned components.* As described above, these reduce the potential of the screw to resist separating forces.

- *Overload.* Non-axial loading of a screwed joint reduces its fatigue strength, and occurs due to cantilevering effects. These can range between the lateral off-axis locations of load-bearing cusps to extensive distal cantilevers. In both situations joint failure is more likely. The loading pattern will, however, be partly determined by the configuration of the superstructure.

- *Fatigue failure.* This arises as a result of cyclical loading.

Management

Screw fracture can have dramatic effects on the implants and their superstructures, and patients must be advised to report any suspicion of abnormal movement or sensation as soon as possible. Patients who continue to use an implant-stabilized superstructure after one or more screws have fractured inevitably place higher loads on the remaining components, which may be distorted or fractured as a result.

The first action must be to remove the superstructure and identify the scope of the damage. Following this, the fractured screw should be removed and its housing assessed for damage. Fractured gold screws can usually be readily removed, since they tend to break immediately below the head, and the top portion of the screw can therefore be grasped in a pair of fine mosquito forceps once the superstructure has been removed.

Fractured abutment screws are more difficult to remove where they have broken within the implant body; however, where a component of the screw remains accessible it can be removed as for a gold screw. If the screw has fractured within a recessed component, it is often possible to remove it by wedging a tapered fissure bur inside its central hole and using a torque driver handpiece in reverse to remove the screw. When doing this, it is important to ensure that the bur grips the inside of the screw, which will otherwise be damaged if allowed to rotate freely. If the screw has fractured within the implant body there are two options, depending upon its length and that of the implant body. The first, and preferable, is to remove the screw. This can sometimes be accomplished by gently rotating it with a sharp straight probe, or alternatively using a proprietary screw retrieval kit (Figs 10.14, 10.15). This comprises an

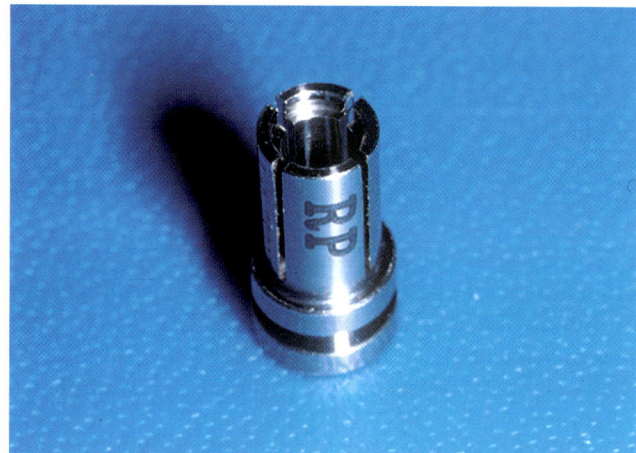

Fig. 10.14 Locating collar for use with a screw retrieval kit. This is placed over the top of the implant body to locate the rotating instruments used for removal of fractured screws.

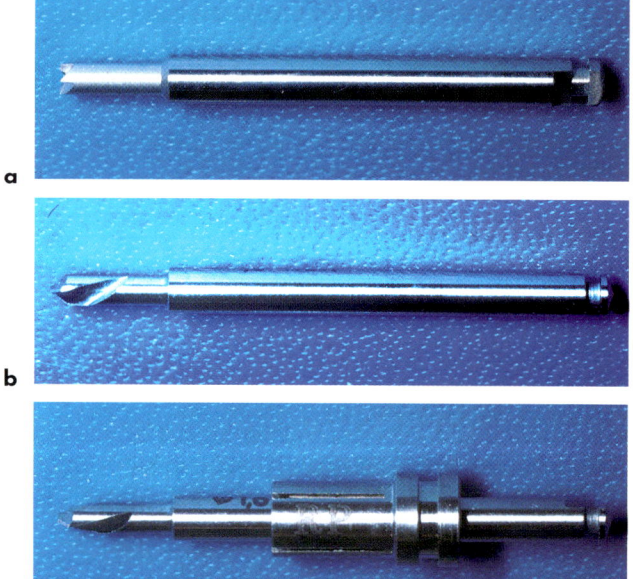

Fig. 10.15 Instruments used for managing broken abutment screws. **a** Toothed removal tool, which is inserted into the central hole of the TMA, pressed against the end of the fractured screw and rotated in reverse to extract it. **b** Reverse-cutting drill, which is used to drill out a fractured abutment screw. Following this it is sometimes necessary to clean the thread with a tap, which should be rotated by hand. **c** Shows the drill mounted in the alignment sleeve, which is seen in Figure 10.14.

alignment tool and extracting bit, which is similar in principle to an end-cutting bur but has teeth that engage in the top of the screw. It is extremely important when removing screws to avoid damaging the threaded portion of the implant body, as this will prevent removal of the screw. Where a screw cannot be removed in this fashion, it is possible to drill it out using a proprietary kit. This is similar to the screw retrieval device but uses a spear drill to remove the fractured screw. This is rotated anticlockwise and it can take a considerable time to remove a screw. Care is extremely important if the threaded inner aspect of the implant body is not to be damaged. Should screw removal be impracticable, then in some circumstances it is possible to rotate it down further within the implant body, leaving room to place a further screw. Once the screw has been removed or driven deeper into the implant body, it may be necessary to re-form the thread within the implant, which may be accomplished with the manufacturer's screw tap.

Once the screw has been removed, the remaining components should be checked for damage and, if possible, replaced using new screws.

The next phase in the management of the problem is to identify the cause of the fracture and where possible remove it, otherwise the problem is likely to recur. Typical causes are excessive loading, particularly where long cantilevers have been used either distally or buccally, poor-fitting superstructures and overtightening of a screw. Patients who use high masticatory forces, or who have a bruxing habit, are also likely to fracture their implant superstructures or components. Appropriate patient advice and modification of the masticatory scheme may help to overcome the problem. Where the superstructure design is thought to be the cause, for example by being excessively cantilevered, it is sometimes possible to modify this to reduce the problem. This is best carried out in the laboratory, and will be restricted if porcelain facings have been used or the framework requires extensive changes. In these circumstances a new prosthesis will be required.

Box 10.6 Implant-related problems

BIOMECHANICAL

Fractured screws

- Related to overload, poorly aligned components, poor component fit, and excessive or inadequate tightening torque
- Management: identify cause and correct. Fractured screws can be removed with varying degrees of ease

Fractured implant body

- Rare, associated with high occlusal loads, external trauma and significant horizontal bone loss
- Manage by removal or, if deep and asymptomatic, leave buried

Implant body

Fracture of the implant body is very unusual and almost invariably occurs as a result of high occlusal loads or external forces, as for example in a road traffic accident. The only available options in these circumstances are either to remove the implant body or, where the remaining components are deep within the tissues, to leave it buried. This is the preferred option where the potential risks of removing the remaining component outweigh the benefits obtained. Chief amongst these are significant loss of alveolar bone and potential damage to adjacent structures; however, a remaining component will usually preclude insertion of a further implant body in that region.

PROSTHESIS PROBLEMS
Fixed
Biomechanical

Prosthesis fracture

Fracture of a fixed implant superstructure can involve either loss of a porcelain or acrylic resin facing, or fracture of the metal substructure itself. Fracture of porcelain facings can occur as a result of high occlusal loads or poor design, such that the interface between the ceramic and the underlying framework is placed in shear. Porcelain may also fracture where the framework is insufficiently rigid or so large that it flexes in function to such an extent that the porcelain/metal interface fails. Similar problems may arise with an acrylic resin facing, although this material has a much lower modulus of elasticity than porcelain and is therefore unlikely to fracture as a result of substructure flexure. It does not, however, perform well in thin sections and care must be taken over framework design to maximize its retention. Management of this problem is best carried out by removing the cause, where possible, and repairing the prosthesis. In some cases it will be necessary to make a new superstructure.

Fracture of the substructure, which is usually cast in gold alloy or welded from titanium, usually arises as a result of poor design or construction, or excessive functional loads (Figs 10.16–10.18). These can result from habit, bruxism, inappropriate occlusal schemes or extensive cantilevering. Poor design and construction features include excessive thinning, porous castings, badly soldered or welded joints and excessive cantilevering. It is a problem best managed by avoidance of the causes, since once it has occurred the prosthesis almost invariably requires replacement.

Tooth fracture

Fracture of teeth can occur on both fixed and removable prostheses, and may be caused by:

- excessive loads;
- fatigue failure;
- substructure flexure;

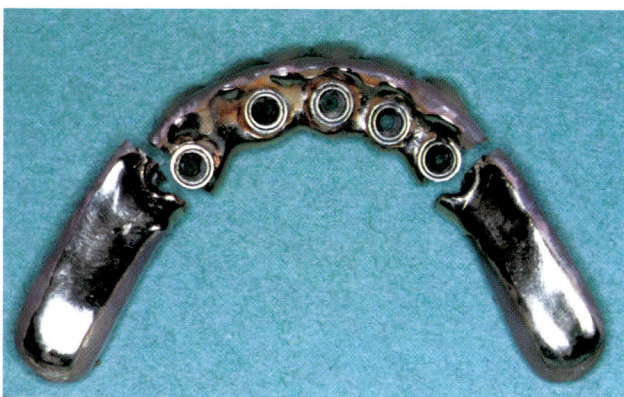

Fig. 10.16 A fractured mandibular fixed prosthesis. Possible causes include mechanical overload, and design and fabrication errors.

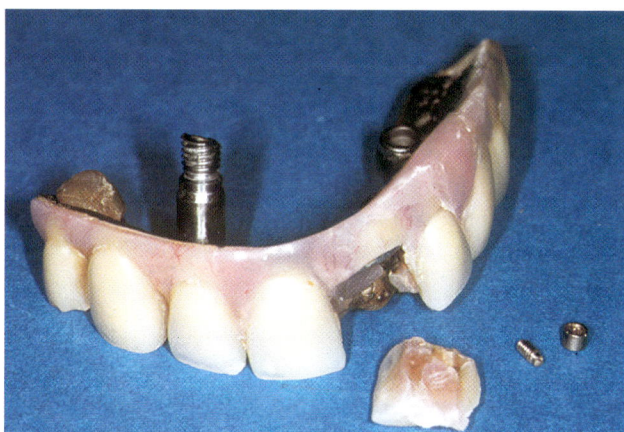

Fig. 10.17 The patient for whom this was made had a history of bruxism and has overloaded their implant-supported prosthesis with consequent fractures of a gold screw, labial facing and implant body.

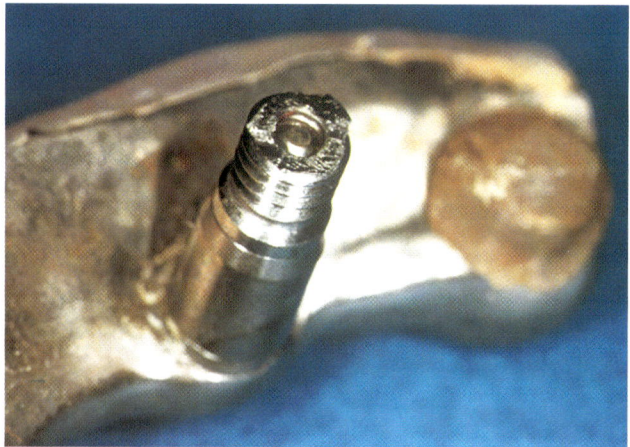

Fig. 10.18 Close-up view of the fractured implant body shown in Figure 10.13.

- poor bonding between the tooth and framework or base;
- inadequate design or construction.

Excessive loads

These can arise from occlusal schemes that place high loads on individual teeth, for example canine guidance. They are also associated with tooth clenching and grinding habits, and are managed by modified design of the occlusion and strengthening of the teeth or their occlusal or palatal coverage with metal where they are made of porcelain or a polymer.

Fatigue failure

This by definition occurs after extended use, especially where loads are unduly high, and is best avoided by designs that minimize the loads on individual teeth.

Substructure flexure

This reflects inadequate design or failure to recognize the patient who is likely to use high occlusal loads. It results in high shear stresses at the interface between the tooth and the substructure, which is therefore more likely to fail.

Bond failure

Poor bonding between the tooth and the framework or base results from inadequate construction, whether it be the bonding of porcelain to an alloy or a polymeric tooth to the underlying acrylic resin.

As with other problems tooth fracture is best managed by avoidance. Where this is not practicable then repairs are usually possible, especially with polymeric teeth. The replacement of porcelain is much more expensive as it requires often extensive refiring. At the same time the cause should be identified and if possible removed or reduced. Nevertheless there are situations where the prosthesis needs to be replaced.

Loosening of implant body

This has been considered in the section relating to loss of integration.

Functional problems

Appearance

Appearance problems related to fixed-implant superstructures are more common in the upper jaw. They are inherently related to the difficulties of placing teeth in the positions of their natural predecessors, which usually gives the most attractive appearance, while linking them to implants that have to be placed in a resorbed jaw. The lost tissue can be replicated using acrylic resin, or occasionally porcelain, although this has to be shaped so as to enable oral hygiene to be maintained around the abutments. This places considerable constraints on the design of the superstructure, which can compromise its appearance. Where it is desired for the crowns to have the appearance of arising from the edentulous ridge, the disparity in the preferred positions of the crown and implant body may be difficult or impossible to disguise effectively, resulting in an unnatural appearance. Bone-grafting procedures can be used to modify the ridge contour;

however, as a result of the unpredictable outcome, the results are not always ideal.

Other problems can arise as a result of inappropriate soft-tissue contours, and in particular the lack of replicates for the interdental papillae, producing the so-called 'black triangle' appearance. Soft tissues can be the contoured at the second stage of surgery or subsequently; however, it is difficult to achieve a satisfactory result if there is an excessive gap between the implants.

Management of this problem can be particularly vexatious, and is best avoided by appropriate patient advice prior to implant treatment. Where the appearance of the final superstructure is in any doubt, the patient should be provided with a trial prosthesis to demonstrate its likely appearance. This can take the form of a trial or a temporary denture. Once implant bodies have been placed, the flexibility in design of the superstructure is considerably reduced, although much can be achieved with the newer designs of abutments, including those that may be custom modified to provide a particular shape and emergence profile.

Sometimes it is necessary to produce a new super-structure; however, the location of the implant bodies and occlusal scheme, together with the lips, may place considerable restraints on what can be achieved.

Problems relating to tooth mould, shade and contour are no different from those encountered in conventional fixed prosthodontics and are similarly managed.

Speech

Speech problems can arise as a result of changes in the labiopalatal positioning of the anterior teeth and the level of the occlusal plane. Where the patient has a fixed superstructure with a normal profile as it emerges from the soft tissues, then many of these problems are usually quite quickly overcome by adaptation, and the patient should be encouraged to practise reading aloud to develop the necessary skills. These may have been lost or maladapted as a result of accommodation to a previous, and poorly designed, removable prosthesis.

Where the superstructure has a gap between its framework and the underlying mucosa, problems can arise as a result of the escape of air or saliva, which can influence the speech as well as being embarrassing. This area is also often difficult to clean. Some patients learn to adapt to this situation, while others need to make use of a removable component to obturate the defect. This may consist of an elastomeric bung, which is placed palatally, or a removable acrylic labial flange. It is important when planning implant treatment to inform the patient in advance if it is thought that speech problems are likely to occur. This is particularly the case where teeth are to be markedly repositioned, or the superstructure design is to include spaces between the framework and mucosa to facilitate oral hygiene.

Mastication

Masticatory problems when using implant-stabilized bridges are unusual, owing to the stability of the device, and largely reflect non-implant-related features, such as the occlusal scheme and nature of the opposing dentition. These can be managed using standard prosthodontic techniques. Cheek biting sometimes occurs due to the failure to place maxillary teeth sufficiently buccally, since they may need significant lateral cantilevering where the alveolar ridge has been severely resorbed, and as a result the implant bodies are markedly palatal to the optimum position of the dental arch. Difficulties sometimes also arise where the superstructure has limited distal extension due to problems in placing implants in these regions. Patients must be warned of such potential problems when planning treatment.

Removable prostheses
Biomechanical problems
Fracture

Fracture of the retainers for an implant-stabilized removable prosthesis can occur in a similar fashion to that for a fixed prosthesis; however, the effects are usually less catastrophic and more readily managed.

Box 10.7 Prosthesis problems: fixed

BIOMECHANICAL

Prosthesis fracture

- Common causes are inadequate design, construction faults, high occlusal forces, and bond and fatigue failure
- Tooth fracture. This may be promoted by a deterioration in the occlusion

Loossening of implant body

- This may be related to overload and/or poor primary stability in poor-quality bone

FUNCTIONAL PROBLEMS

Appearance

- Problems often reflect bone resorption and the resultant disparity in the relationship of the implant to the prosthesis
- Soft-tissue contours can be difficult to reconstruct, for example as a result of local resorption of alveolar bone

Speech

- Associated with changed contours and dead space below fixed prostheses required for oral hygiene

Mastication

- Masticatory problems are unusual but can arise with occlusal wear when using implant-stabilized fixed prostheses

Broken retaining clips can be replaced in the denture either in the clinic or laboratory. In the former situation this may be done with self-curing acrylic resin or a light-cured resin. This has the advantage of better control, but necessitates access for a light source. Care must be taken to ensure that the locating resin does not engage undercuts on the retainers or the denture will become fixed and need cutting free with a bur.

Laboratory relocation of retainers provides more control; however, it is necessary to transfer the relationship of the implant-mounted retainer to the removable prosthesis. Where a bar design is employed, this may be conveniently done by recording a rebase impression for the denture with the bar in place (Figs 10.19–10.22). If this is retained using long screws or guide pins, which penetrate appropriately located holes drilled in the denture base, these may be unscrewed and the impression removed with the bar in situ. The technician can then make a master cast using abutment analogues, rebase the denture and locate the replacement clips. Where ball attachments are used, it is usually feasible to record a rebasing impression in an elastomeric material. A laboratory analogue of the retainer can then be placed in the impression and a master cast poured, on which the denture can be rebased and a new female attachment located.

Prosthesis fracture

Implant-stabilized overdentures tend to be subjected to greater loads than conventional prostheses, since they have much more effective stabilization. As a result, fractures resulting from masticatory overloads are more common, particularly where the opposing dentition consists largely of natural teeth. These include fracture of both the denture base and the artificial teeth, difficulties which are not unique to implant-stabilized prostheses. Fractures of the denture can also arise due to rocking around the retainers where suitable spacers have not been used to minimize this problem. Since many implant-stabilized

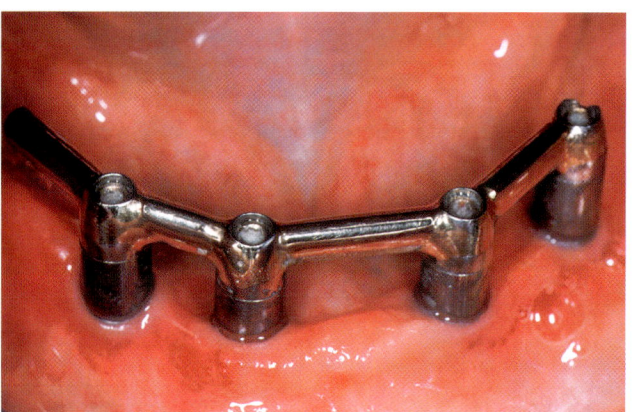

Fig. 10.19 The left distal cantilever on this bar retainer has fractured at the soldered joint with the gold cylinder. It may be repaired using a pick-up impression technique in the overdenture, which would be rebased as part of the procedure.

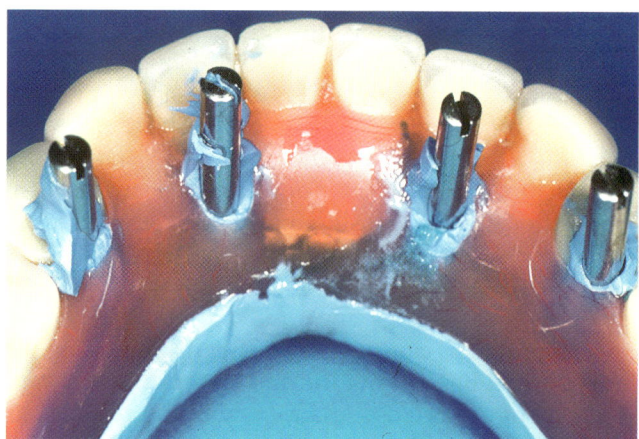

Fig. 10.21 The completed impression. This is used to produce a master cast on which the bar can be repaired and the denture rebased.

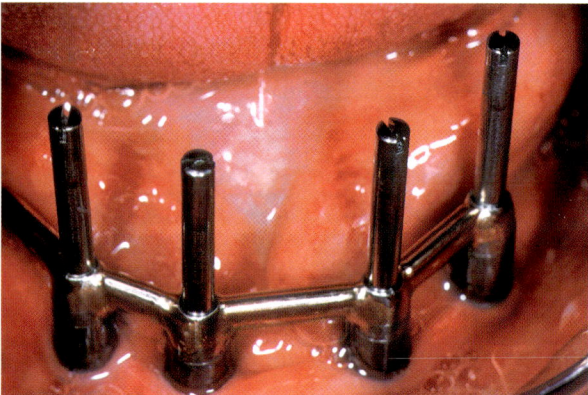

Fig. 10.20 The pick-up impression technique. The gold screws have been replaced with guide pins, undercuts removed from the fitting surface of the denture and holes drilled through the base to allow it to be seated over the pins. A light-bodied elastomeric impression material is then used to record the denture-bearing area, abutments and gold bar. Once the impression material has set the pins are unscrewed and the complete assembly is removed from the mouth.

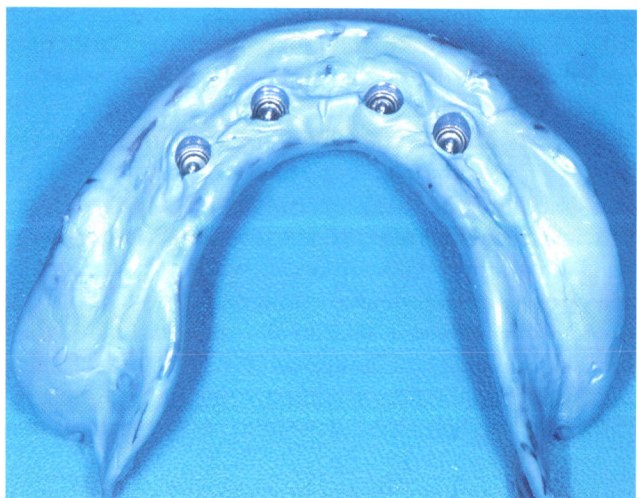

Fig. 10.22 The mucosal surface of the impression. The bar and gold cylinders provide an accurate record of the positions of the abutments and their relationships to the adjacent tissues.

mandibular overdentures have mechanical characteristics similar to a Kennedy Class I partial denture, resorption of the alveolar ridge distally can result in a tendency of the denture to tip anteroposteriorly. This causes rocking around the distal abutments, and can result in fracture of the denture base. Where problems arise as a result of differential support of the prosthesis, this should be controlled as much as possible using selective displacement of the soft tissues in the non-implanted regions. The spacers that many manufacturers provide with their retainers should also be used in the laboratory to minimize rotation around the retaining abutments.

Looseness

Looseness of an implant-stabilized overdenture is an unusual complaint, provided that suitable retainers have been employed both in terms of their distribution and mechanical design. It is important when diagnosing this problem to separate difficulties that arise during mastication from those that occur during speech or when the patient is at rest. Looseness during mastication is usually associated with differential displacement of the support for different regions of the denture, particularly where one region is supported by implants, and the remainder by the soft tissues. The difficulty can also arise due to cantilevering of the dental arch labial or buccal to the axis of rototation running through adjacent implant abutments. Masticatory loads, particularly during eccentric positions of the mandible, will then tend to cause the prosthesis to rotate around the retainers closest to the dental arch. This can be reduced by constructing an occlusal scheme with balanced articulation, as is commonly used with conventional complete dentures. Minimizing the cantilevering of the arch, and ensuring that there is mechanical retention of the denture located so as to resist tipping, can also prove beneficial. These design features are best incorporated into a new denture, and while it is sometimes possible to modify the occlusion to reduce the problem, in many circumstances it is necessary to remake the prosthesis. Repositioning the teeth can be difficult if their locations are dictated by the natural dentition or aesthetic requirements.

Looseness associated with speech, or when the patient is at rest, is indicative of inadequate retention or overextension of the denture periphery. The cause of the latter can usually be managed using conventional prosthodontic techniques, while inadequate retention may reflect poor prosthesis design, the use of an inappropriate retainer or the distortion of a component. This can be managed by adjustment or replacement. A not uncommon difficulty is for a patient to complain of the distal part of the mandibular denture being loose as it rotates around anterior retainers. This can often be managed by reducing displacing forces. While the use of implants distally can usually control the problem, this is often not feasible and recourse must then be made to cantilevering retainers distal to the most posterior implants in the arch. This is usually carried out in a bar retainer; however, excessive cantilevering can result in fracture of the bar or cold cylinder, or repeated loosening of the retaining screws. Cantilevers longer than 10 mm from the centre of the most distal implant are therefore not generally recommended.

Excessive retention

Occasionally, patients complain of excessive retention of their implant-stabilized prostheses. This can make it difficult to remove the dentures, particularly in the lower jaw, or where the patient has reduced manual dexterity or muscle strength. Adjustment of the retainers, or indeed the removal of some of them, can often control this, while patients may benefit from the modification of the flanges of the denture in inconspicuous locations so as to improve the grip that can be obtained.

Functional problems

Appearance

Implant-stabilized complete and partial dentures are capable of producing a very natural appearance, since there is usually greater flexibility in the choice and positions of the teeth and the ability to replicate the natural contours of the supporting tissues. Problems can arise where implants are inappropriately located, as a result of anatomical constraints, surgical errors, or failure to construct and use diagnostic prostheses and a surgeon's guide. Difficulties can also arise where patients do not understand that their new implant-stabilized prostheses will essentially be complete or partial dentures, although with enhanced stability and usually significantly reduced bulk. Difficulties may also arise, as when treating patients with conventional complete dentures, where they or their families decide that the appearance produced by the new dentures is not after all satisfactory, despite having approved this at the trial denture stage.

Once dentures have been completed it is difficult to extensively modify their appearance, and it may be necessary to remake them. As with many problems, avoidance is better than cure and it is essential before implant treatment commences that the patient understands what this will entail and the limitations that will be imposed on the outcome.

Speech

Problems with speech when using implant-stabilized removable prostheses are less common than with fixed ones, since the contours can be made more extensive and any gaps covered by gumwork, as there is no need to provide access for oral hygiene. When difficulties arise they usually relate to changes in tooth position over those to which the patient is accustomed, and can often be overcome by training. Occasionally, it is necessary to recontour the polished surfaces, and this may be conveniently done in the first instance at the chairside, either by trimming or by using a light-cured resin to enhance the contours until a suitable shape has been achieved. Subsequently this material can be made more permanent by replacement with heat-cured acrylic resin.

Mastication

Masticatory problems are unusual. Anteriorly they are usually related to tooth positions, which, if inappropriate, can lead to problems with tipping of the prosthesis or lip biting. Posteriorly they are typically caused by errors in the level of the occlusal plane, a lack of freeway space or buccolingual positioning of the teeth. A mandibular occlusal plane that is too high makes it difficult for the tongue to move the food bolus between the teeth. Lack of freeway space can also create problems with tooth separation and again bolus positioning, while errors in relative buccolingual positioning of the posterior teeth can be a cause of cheek biting.

Box 10.8 Prosthesis problems: removable

BIOMECHANICAL

Fracture

- Many causes, as for fixed prostheses
- Components of retention systems may fracture, or become detached from prosthesis

Prosthesis fracture

Looseness

- Looseness is an uncommon complaint
- Manage by diagnosing cause and removing it where possible. Peripheral errors, occlusal faults, incorrect tooth positioning and incorrect design, fracture or wear of retainers can all cause looseness

Excessive retention

- Occasionally, patients complain of excessive retention. Manage by adjusting/removing retainers. Check that the patient can grip their denture

FUNCTIONAL PROBLEMS

Appearance

- Implant-stabilized removable prostheses have a similar ability to improve appearance to conventional dentures
- Problems can arise where implants are inappropriately located

Speech

- Problems with speech when using implant-stabilized removable prostheses are less common than with fixed ones, since the contours can be made more extensive

Mastication

- Masticatory problems are unusual. They often reflect errors in tooth positioning or the occlusion

---

MAINTENANCE
Introduction

The maintenance of dental implant treatment and the management of problems are inextricably linked; however, they have been separated in this chapter for convenience although in a clinical situation one will tend to run into the other. Maintenance is concerned with correction of normal wear and routine measures to minimize the risk of catastrophic failure. For these reasons regular monitoring should follow the completion of treatment. It involves the bone–implant interface, the surrounding soft tissues, and the implant and its associated components and superstructure. This, in particular, has similar maintenance requirements to a conventional fixed or removable prosthesis, while the implant and associated components and related tissues are structures unique to dental implantology, whose maintenance is important for long-term success.

While it is currently considered that it is impossible to have successful implant treatment without the creation and maintenance of an osseointegrated interface, that in itself does not secure success. Nevertheless, once a patient has been satisfactorily treated using this technique, the maintenance of that interface is paramount to the long-term outcome. Maintenance will therefore involve routine checks on the integrity of osseointegration and the avoidance of any conditions that might threaten it. These are both mechanical and biological.

Clinical methods for confirming osseointegration are currently very limited and dependent on recognizing the signs and symptoms of its loss, or of evidence that this might occur. This is based principally upon the following:

- Radiographic appearance. This only provides an image in one plane but is used routinely to assess bone levels around an implant. Where they are receding crestally at a greater rate than 0.1 mm per year after the first year then this is considered to indicate a lack of success. Radiographs can also indicate lack of bone–implant contact, and more extensive bone loss.

- Probing depths. These indicate the height of the crestal bone–implant contact and changes will reflect loss of its extent. Probing is not without its hazards and if injudicious may lead to damage to the bone–implant interface. A probing depth of 3–4 mm is often found and is not diagnostic of loss of bone–implant contact at the ridge crest.

- Implant mobility. While tapping an implant will indicate whether it is still rigidly linked to the bone, the method gives no indication of the extent of bone–implant contact and cannot be used to make measurements. Its value is therefore very limited, although an implant that has lost integration is usually very evident. Techniques have been developed for examining the vibration frequency of an individual implant; however, this is not yet a straightforward diagnostic tool.

The immediate biological environment of the implant includes both the soft and hard tissues, the principal threat to which is infection, which can result in inflammation and a reduction in the extent of the osseointegrated interface. From the maintenance viewpoint such problems are principally related to plaque control, although other systemic and local factors, especially mechanical, can also play a part.

Failure to maintain healthy tissues around an implant can result in peri-implant mucositis and peri-implantitis. Looseness of the abutment is also often associated with soft-tissue inflammation and can cause significant swelling. Routine examinations of the tissues around the implants are therefore required to confirm that these conditions are not present, that suitable home care routines are being maintained (Fig. 10.23) and that normal wear of the prosthesis is not causing potential problems. The soft tissues should be checked using routine periodontal procedures to assess the levels of plaque control, inflammation and changes in peri-implant 'pocket' depths. Changes in these can reflect not only loss of crestal attachment but also swelling of the soft tissues.

Assessment of bone levels and density around the implants may also be made using long cone periapical radiographs, employing a paralleling technique. The frequency with which radiographic examinations should be carried out will vary from patient to patient and with the length of time for which the implants have been present. It is usual to monitor these at relatively frequent intervals in the period immediately after placement of the superstructure. Experience has shown that changes in the tissues around implants are most likely to occur in the period immediately following their insertion and therefore for the first 2 years following implant placement it is prudent to monitor bone levels and tissue health at intervals of initially 6 and later 12 months. Thereafter, the

frequency of inspection can be reduced if it is found that the patient can maintain satisfactory levels of oral hygiene and there is no evidence of an excessive rate of bone loss around the implants. Routine reviews may then occur at intervals of 1 year, although it is important to advise patients to seek professional advice should any untoward event occur. Where there are problems with plaque control or evidence of harmful tissue changes then a more intensive review strategy will be needed. While it could be argued that more frequent radiographic examinations would detect early stages of bone loss, this procedure is not without its hazards. Once a healthy and stable relationship has been established between the implant and surrounding tissues, significant changes in bone levels are so uncommon as to make radiographic examination at 6-monthly intervals of questionable value. Frequency will depend on individual circumstances but intervals of 2 years are usually appropriate.

Soft tissues

It is important to maintain soft-tissue health around implants, since it is possible that inflammation of those adjacent to the device may subsequently proceed to peri-implantitis, although the evidence for this currently is not robust. Furthermore, inflamed tissues can be painful, exacerbate the difficulties of oral hygiene, produce an unsightly appearance and result in deepened 'pockets' around the implants, which are more difficult to clean. It should also be borne in mind that many patients who have lost all or significant numbers of their teeth have done so as a result of poor plaque control. Oral hygiene has a significant role to play in helping to maintain soft-tissue health in all implant patients. Where this is inadequate the patient's role can often be usefully supplemented with support from a dental hygienist. There are two principal dimensions to plaque control: mechanical, including superstructure design, and chemical.

Plaque control

Mechanical

Mechanical removal of plaque from implant superstructures is an essential component of implant maintenance. Its success commences at the planning stage when an assessment must be made of the patient's manual dexterity and the superstructure designed so as to facilitate cleaning. Where access is difficult due to lack of space, excessively extensive fixed flanges, narrow embrasures and undercut areas then plaque will tend to accumulate. This can result in inflammation of the adjacent tissues and increased risk of implant failure.

Inherent in the process of prosthesis design is the choice as to whether to use a fixed or removable superstructure, since the latter can by definition be much

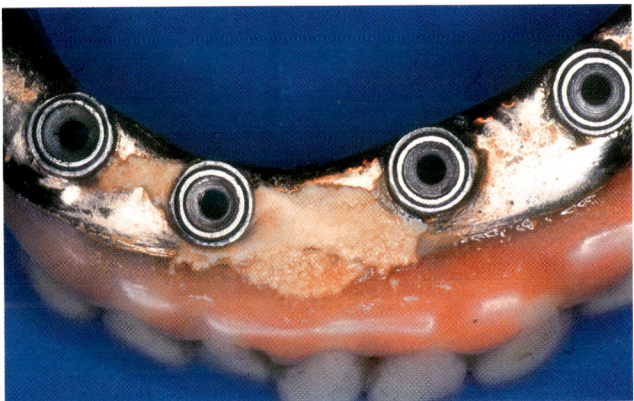

Fig. 10.23 Poor oral hygiene. Calculus deposits such as these can be troublesome in some patients and require the prosthesis to be removed for effective cleaning. If mechanical processes are used then protective caps should be placed on the gold cylinders.

more readily cleansed, while the retainers that remain in the mouth are also easier to clean than applies around most fixed superstructures. Nevertheless, each clinical situation is unique and it is essential that time is spent with the patient, assessing their oral hygiene needs, advising them and demonstrating cleaning with the most appropriate mechanical aids and techniques at the time of prosthesis insertion, and in the early months afterwards. Some can manage with the traditional dental brush; however, many others need to use interspace brushes of various designs, the majority of which were originally developed for periodontal applications. The further group of mechanical aids is a range of dental flosses, some of which have stiffened ends, which can be threaded between the implant superstructure and the mucosa around the abutments so as to aid cleaning. These are manufactured in a range of dimensions with stiffened ends to facilitate threading. It is prudent during the fabrication of a fixed superstructure to confirm in the laboratory that aids of this type can be used before the prosthesis is completed. If access is difficult in the laboratory, it will be doubly so in the mouth.

Where hard deposits have formed on the superstructure professional cleaning is necessary. Care must be taken to avoid damage to the abutment surface, which will merely exacerbate further accumulations of plaque and calculus. A range of fibre-reinforced plastic scalers is available to help with this task. In some cases this is most readily achieved by removing the superstructure and abutments, and cleaning them in the laboratory, on the bench top, for which an acidic denture cleanser can prove effective. Conventional scalers and rotating instruments should not be used for removing calculus, since they can damage the surface of the connecting components.

Chemical

Chemical control of plaque is a valuable addition to the range of techniques, and is particularly useful in the period immediately following second-stage surgery, when the tissues may be too sensitive for mechanical cleansing of the implant components. Chlorhexidine solution is particularly effective, but its use can lead to staining of the superstructure, particularly where acrylic resin components are employed. It is not recommended for long-term use, when mechanical techniques should be employed.

Swelling

Swelling of the soft tissues adjacent to an implant often represents an acute problem, which is described above. A less common difficulty is the enlargement of soft tissues under retention bars, which can prove difficult to manage and tends to recur following its excision. It has been suggested that this is caused by poor plaque control, although the evidence for this is weak.

Superstructure

Fixed

Tooth wear

Wear of occlusal surfaces is a phenomenon well recognized in dentistry, whether it occurs on natural teeth or their artificial replacements. Its causes are multiple and relate to the material from which the surface has been made, masticatory frequency and loads, dietary habits and chemical damage.

There is a view that it is preferable to construct an implant superstructure with surfaces made from acrylic resin, since this material is relatively resilient and will tend to cushion the effects of occlusal loads. It is argued that loss of osseointegration is less likely to occur as a result of mechanical trauma, although there is little evidence to support this view. Nevertheless, since the majority of implant superstructures are much more readily replaced than those used to restore natural teeth, it has been considered that a sacrificial occlusal surface may be preferable to one that places the implant–host interface at risk. The alternatives are to use porcelain or gold alloy. The former is aesthetically satisfactory; however, there can sometimes be difficulties in using it where there are space restrictions, and the material has to be employed in an excessively thin section. Gold alloy has much to commend it as an occlusal surface from the viewpoint of wear, but not all patients consider its appearance to be attractive. The choice of an occlusal surface will be governed partly by these factors and partly by the nature of the opposing dentition. Where the patient is edentulous in both jaws it is usual to employ acrylic occlusal surfaces; however, where the patient is partially dentate and the superstructure forms part of a dental arch or opposes the natural teeth, then this material can be less satisfactory due to its relatively rapid wear. Patients with implant-stabilized prostheses can usually generate significantly higher forces on their teeth than occurs with conventional removable devices, and as a result tooth wear can in some cases be very rapid. This occurs particularly where softer artificial teeth are used and it is preferable to use the more expensive heavily cross-linked resin teeth, some of which contain wear-resistant fillers.

Where an occlusal surface is excessively worn, it will need to be replaced. As a temporary measure, where acrylic teeth have been employed, this can be carried out at the chairside using self-curing or light-polymerized resin. Correction in a laboratory will provide a better result and would be mandatory for porcelain or gold alloy occlusal surfaces. In the case of complete dentures it is often appropriate to combine this with rebasing the prostheses. Where a fixed superstructure has been employed the replacement of the occlusal surfaces is more complex. Two techniques may be used: one where the master casts are still available, and the other where they are not.

In the former situation all that is required is to record

an impression of the opposing dentition, using either reversible hydrocolloid or an elastomer. A registration may then be made of the jaw relationship at the desired anteroposterior position of the mandible. This can be produced using any of the standard restorative techniques, including wax wafers, elastomeric registration materials and bite registration pastes in combination with gauze bibs. It is important, however, to ensure that the tendency of the patient to protrude the mandible as a result of tooth wear does not result in an incorrect record. Depending on the availability of master casts, a face-bow record may also be needed. The desired shade for the replacement teeth is also recorded and the superstructure and other records are returned to the laboratory. Note should also be made of any changes that are required in the vertical dimension of occlusion.

In the laboratory the fixed prosthesis to be refurbished is mounted on the master cast in the articulator. The opposing cast is then mounted using the clinical record, and the articulator adjusted to provide the desired increase in occlusal vertical dimension. The teeth may then be stripped off the fixed superstructure and replaced using standard techniques. Where a significant change is to be made some operators prefer to have a retrial stage before finishing the prosthesis.

At this stage the patient is unable to use the prosthesis while it is being refurbished. Recourse must therefore be made either to a temporary fixed prosthesis or partial denture. In the latter case it will be necessary to place healing caps over the tops of the abutments.

Removable superstructures

Maintenance of these is usually confined to rebasing the denture, and/or replacement of the teeth, and adjusting or replacing retainers.

Replacement of the teeth involves similar procedures to those described for fixed superstructures, while rebasing an implant-stabilized complete denture is similar to the procedure used with conventional complete dentures. The technique is, however, more demanding and varies slightly between upper and lower jaws and with the type of retainer.

The basic principle of the procedure is to record an impression of the underlying soft tissues, and their relationships with the implants and the denture. This may be done using the following techniques.

The retention bar

This is the preferred technique if a bar is present and fits satisfactorily, since it provides what are effectively linked impression copings. The bar needs to be retained in the laboratory while the denture is rebased.

Impression copings

If the bar does not fit well and a new one is to be made then impression copings are used. The disadvantages of the technique are that copings are required and the denture may need extensive trimming to accommodate them. The technique is essentially the same as when recording working impressions, and where possible non-tapered, screw-retained copings are used so as to ensure optimum accuracy.

Impression of retainers in situ

Where the implants carry individual retainers, typically male components, an overall elastomeric impression will record them and their positions very accurately. It is thus possible to place laboratory analogues in the impression and pour a working cast on which the denture may be rebased and the new female components located.

It must be remembered that the impression will not only record the changes in the soft-tissue contours since the denture was made, but also modify the relationship between these and the occlusal plane of the denture. This effect is minimized by the location provided by the implants, but nevertheless gross occlusal errors can be produced if care is not taken.

Procedure

Undercuts must be removed from the fitting surface of the denture so as to enable its removal from the working cast. This does not apply around a retaining bar or individual retainers.

Select the transfer system. If a bar is being used then the gold screws must be replaced with longer screws (guide pins) and the denture perforated so as to enable the denture to be seated. If the screws are not parallel then surprisingly large holes may be needed.

If impression copings are to be used it is preferable to use the non-tapered type, which is retained within the impression, as this improves the accuracy of the technique. The impression copings should be placed on the implant abutments and the denture then adjusted so that it can be fully seated. As when recording the impression of the bar, it will be necessary to perforate the denture to permit it to be fully seated and have access to the screws that retain the impression copings.

Where an impression is to be recorded of the individual retainers mounted on each implant, the denture can remain intact, apart from the removal of undercuts. An impression may then be recorded of the retainers directly. Some manufacturers provide impression copings for this procedure, which may alternatively be used, although it may then be necessary to modify the denture so that it can be fully seated with adequate clearance around the copings.

The denture is then painted with a suitable adhesive and loaded with an elastomeric impression material. Many operators find an addition-cured silicone suitable for this purpose. It can be helpful to inject a light-bodied impression material around the implant bar, impression copings or individual retainers so as to minimize the trapping of air, which can reduce the accuracy of the technique by allowing the component to move within the impression.

Once the impression material has set, any retaining screws should be removed and the denture is then removed from the mouth and checked. Provided that it is satisfactory it may then be sent to the laboratory for processing. A helpful technique for minimizing occlusal errors is to replace the denture without screwing any included retainers or copings into place, and then make a jaw relationship record against the opposing dentition using a suitable technique. An impression of the opposing occlusal surface is also required, unless this is provided by a removable denture, that can be sent to the laboratory. These records enable the technician to mount the denture that is being rebased on an articulator, together with a representation of the opposing occlusal surface, and then make any necessary adjustments prior to returning the finished work to the clinic.

While the denture is being rebased the patient may need to use a spare denture, which may require temporary modification with a temporary lining material. To prevent damage to the abutments or their contamination with food debris, they should be covered with healing caps.

In the laboratory the denture is rebased using standard techniques, incorporating any necessary attachments into the prosthesis during the process. Where a bar is being used this will be mounted on the master cast, with the undercuts below the bar blocked out with plaster.

The denture is then returned to the patient and checked in the normal manner, when any necessary adjustments may be made. This includes modifications to the retainers to increase or reduce their force as required clinically. When doing this care must be taken to follow the manufacturer's instructions for such adjustments.

Screws

Screws should normally need little maintenance; however, it is prudent where feasible to check their tightness with a torque driver shortly after placement of the prosthesis, since they can become loose as a result of embedment relaxation or excessive external loads. Once this has occurred, then the screw is more likely to fail. Should the screws be loose on checking, they should be reviewed 1 month later to confirm that all is well. If they repeatedly loosen then the prosthesis will have to be modified or remade. Possible causes of loosening are:

- Poor superstructure fit. This results in the majority of the pre-tension being dissipated in closing the joint, which is then easily separated.

- Interaction between joints. Errors of fit on implants on either side of a joint result in its initially being closed and then placed in tension as the screws on the adjacent implants are tightened.

- Excessive off-axis loads. These can result from lateral or distal cantilevering.

Where the repeated loosening is caused by poor fit then the superstructure may need to be remade or modified by sectioning and resoldering. Problems related to excessive cantilevering can often be managed by adjustment.

It is prudent to seal the hole immediately above a screw with an elastomer, when space permits, as this is easily removed as compared with hard materials, which can be difficult to dislodge from the head of a prosthetic screw with an internal recessed socket. The top of the hole, however, should be sealed with a more permanent tooth-coloured material, usually a composite resin or light-polymerized methacrylate.

Box 10.9 Maintenance

BONE LEVELS AND DENSITY

Monitor

- *Radiography*. Two-dimensional
- *Probing depths*. Use and interpret with care
- *Implant mobility*. Currently of limited routine clinical value for assessing prognosis; marked mobility is diagnostic of failure

SOFT TISSUES

Monitor status

Control health with plaque control

- Mechanical
- Chemical

SUPERSTRUCTURE

Fixed

- Tooth wear. Can be troublesome, monitor and refurbish

Removable superstructures

- *Tooth wear*. Refurbish
- *Retainer wear*. Replace
- *Fitting surface changes*. Rebase prosthesis

Screws

- *Loosening*. May be due to poor superstructure fit, interaction between joints, excessive off-axis loads

Cemented joints

- Normally require no maintenance. Inflammation in the adjacent soft tissues may reflect poor fit or excess cement
- Loosening, similar causes to screwed joints plus cement failure

Cemented joints

Cemented joints normally require no maintenance, although inflammation in the adjacent soft tissues requires investigation to confirm that the fit of the joint is satisfactory and that there is no excess cement adjacent to the components. Loosening has similar causes to that of screwed joints; however, it can also reflect failure of the cement, possibly as a result of incorrect technique.

FURTHER READING

Esposito M, Hirsch J M, Lekholm U, Thomsen P 1998 Biological factors contributing to failures of osseointegrated oral implants. (I). Success criteria and epidemiology. Eur J Oral Sci 106(1):527–51

Esposito M, Hirsch J M, Lekholm U, Thomsen P 1998 Biological factors contributing to failures of osseointegrated oral implants. (II). Etiopathogenesis. Eur J Oral Sci 106(3): 721–64

Quirynen M, De Soete M, van Steenberghe D 2002 Infectious risks for oral implants: a review of the literature. Clin. Oral Implants Res 13:1–19

Appendix
Self-assessment questions

This Appendix contains a number of questions on Dental Implantology together with suggested frameworks for answering them. Most answers are amenable to a range of responses, and these should be viewed as potential approaches, rather than definitive answers. The detail which would be incorporated in them would depend on the level of the examination, and the time which was available. We have defined neither.

Where the material for a suggested framework may be readily gleaned from the text we have indicated this rather than repeating it in this Appendix.

1. When might you consider treating an edentulous patient using dental implants?

What is the question about?

This question is concerned with those factors which would lead you to consider implant treatment in an edentulous patient. It has parallels with a question about the advantages of implant treatment in the edentulous patient, and is essentially asking; which complete denture problems are amenable to implant treatment?

Basis of answer: when the patient has problems with their dentures, which may be amenable to implant management.

Answer plan

Introduction

Set the scene – be brief.
  Indicate very briefly the plan which you will follow:

- What are the patient's perceptions of their complaint and what are their expectations of treatment?
- Define the problem by history and examination. What is its time-scale, is it getting worse?
- Is the problem related to the upper or lower denture, or both? Problems with the lower are more common.

Body of answer (See also Chapter 6)

Problems which may be amenable to implant treatment:

Looseness. Related to:

- The anatomy of the region, poor denture bearing areas, anatomical features such as highly displaceable tissues, severely resorbed ridges.
- Poor denture control skills.

Pain. Related to:

- Problems in the denture bearing areas such as thin mucosa, uneven alveolar bone.

Problems where implant treatment should be considered only after conventional procedures have been carried out to a good standard and failed to resolve problems:

- Pain and looseness related to poor denture design and construction.
- Dissatisfaction with appearance when wearing dentures, due to stability problems.
- Problems with chewing.
- Unrealistic expectations of treatment outcomes on the part of the patient.

Resource related factors:

- Team skills, are they adequate?
- Financial resources to fund treatment

Closing section

Future management:

- New dentures.
- Review.
- Consider implant treatment.
- Assessment of systemic and local factors.
- Special investigations.

2. When might you consider treating a partially dentate patient using dental implants?

What is the question about?

This question has similar characteristics to the previous one, however the range of treatment alternatives is potentially much wider and there is unlikely to be enough time to discuss them all in detail. Some sub-division of the sections will make the material more manageable. Essentially the examiners are asking about treatment alternatives and when would implant procedures be the preferred option. A suitable matrix would be to consider the main treatment options and then apply these briefly to the principal scenarios of a single missing anterior tooth, and posterior bounded and free-end saddles (FES).

Basis of answer: when the patient requires tooth replacement, which may most effectively meet their needs using an implant-stabilized prosthesis?

Answer plan

Introduction

- Set the scene – be brief.
- What are the patient's perceptions of their complaint and what are their expectations of treatment?
- Define the problem by history and examination.
- Recognize the need for overall management of oral health, not the focused replacement of missing teeth.

Body of answer (See also Chapters 3 & 4)

Treatment Alternatives.
List, and for each provide a brief resumé of their main advantages and disadvantages (See Chapters 3 & 4).

- Observation.
- Removable partial denture.
- Adhesive bridgework.
- Conventional bridgework.
- Orthodontic management.
- Implant treatment.

Treatment problems
For each of these indicate main features and treatments of choice.

The anterior single missing tooth
Main factors to consider:

- Appearance, lip line, alveolar contour.
- Alveolar resorption.
- Problems with spacing of the natural teeth.
- Occlusal considerations.

Implants are particularly suited to situations where natural abutments are sound, natural teeth are spaced, there is adequate bone for implant insertion, the teeth have a good prognosis, and there are no teeth missing posteriorly.

Posterior saddles
Main factors to consider:

- The need to replace missing teeth.
- Surgical and prosthodontic envelopes.
- Occlusal considerations.
- The status of the natural abutment teeth.
- A requirement for a fixed prosthesis in a free-end edentulous span.
- Management of a loose free-end saddle RPD (FES).

Implants are particularly suited to situations where technical criteria for treatment are met, restoration with an adhesive or conventional bridge is contraindicated, the remaining natural teeth have a good prognosis, and there is a need for a fixed prosthesis or stabilization of an RPD free-end saddle (FES situations).

Closing section
Summary statement. Key points:

- Comprehensive approach to oral care.
- Thorough clinical examination.
- Consider all alternatives.
- Implant-based treatment has considerable benefits in suitable patients.

3. What factors may contribute to a decision to extract a natural tooth in order to place a dental implant at the same site?

What is the question about?

This question is concerned essentially with the advantages and disadvantages of retaining a tooth or replacing it with an implant. No other treatment alternatives are offered and therefore the answer can be relatively narrow in coverage, but will need a greater depth of knowledge than the previous two. Do not stray into peripheral areas such as other forms of treatment.

Basis of answer: which alternative will have a better function and/or prognosis?

Answer plan

Introduction

Set the scene – one sentence.

Indicate the importance of a thorough history and examination of the patient.

Split the answer into systemic and local factors, further subdivided into indications and contraindications.

Body of answer (See also Chapters 3 & 4)

Systemic factors:

- These are largely based around contraindications, as there are few systemic indications, apart from positive motivation and the demands of some occupations.
- Contra-indications to implant treatment include poor motivation, inability to co-operate, health factors, poor residual life expectancy, activities or disorders which increase the risk of trauma to the mouth, and some habits such as tobacco smoking.

Local factors:

- What is the status of the remainder of the dental arch?
- How would localized implant treatment relate to the long-term management of other oral problems?
- Prognosis of the tooth. If this is good, why should it be replaced?
- If the tooth is unsaveable does it need replacement?
- Poorly controlled periodontal disease; should the tooth be replaced before extensive bone destruction occurs?
- Surgical envelope; is insertion in a suitable site feasible?
- Prosthodontic envelope; is restoration feasible?
- Status of the host tissues?
- Unsuitability of other forms of treatment for replacing the tooth.

Closing section

Summary statement. Key points:

- Comprehensive approach to oral care.
- Thorough clinical examination.
- Value of implant-based treatment.

4. What are the relative advantages and disadvantages of screw- and cement-retained implant superstructures?

What is the question about?

This question essentially requires an 'advantages and disadvantages' type of answer, the matrix for which is to produce a series of headings with a short paragraph about each. Spread the answer evenly, though with more emphasis on the more important issues. The answer is also dependent on specialized knowledge. Less repetition will result if the two techniques are compared under each heading.

Basis of answer: a series of statements, with some exploration of issues.

Answer plan

Introduction

Briefly set the scene.
  Indicate how you will approach the question.

Body of answer (See Chapter 2)

Headings will include fit, cement excess, angulation changes, retrievability, strength, complexity, appearance, seal between components, and potential effects on the occlusion.

Closing section

Summary statement. Key points:

- Both techniques widely used.
- Neither technique resolves all issues.
- Select on basis of knowledge of advantages and disadvantages and clinical objectives.

5. What problems can arise following treatment with dental implants? Indicate how they may be managed.

What is the question about?

This is basically a test of knowledge and the ability to organize a large body of information. Make sure that you have identified all the key points, arrange them in a logical sequence, and divide your available time between them. Note that you are asked to indicate, not discuss, the management of the problems. Problems could be assembled on a timeline basis, or alternatively by location such as implants, bone, soft tissues. The question also does not define the start point, stating, 'following treatment with dental implants'. It would therefore be sensible to define your interpretation in the introduction: following insertion of the implant bodies, stage II surgery or superstructure placement?

Basis of answer: A series of statements indicating problems grouped in a logical sequence.

Answer plan

Introduction

Briefly set the scene.
  Define the start point.
  Indicate how you will approach the question.

Body of answer (See Chapter 10)

A series of headings. Divide problems along a timeline or location basis and then into systemic and local factors.

Closing section

Summary statement. Key points:

- Importance of avoiding problems before they arise.
- Management of problem based on identifying cause, removing it where possible, and correcting the outcome if feasible.

6. What systemic factors may contraindicate treatment with dental implants?

What is the question about?

This is basically a similar type of question to No. 5. It is again a test of knowledge and the ability to organize a large body of information. Make sure that you have identified all the key points, arrange them in a logical sequence, and divide your available time between them. Depending on the time available you may have the opportunity to discuss some of the more controversial issues such as smoking habits.

Basis of answer: A series of statements indicating contraindications, grouped in a logical sequence.

Answer plan

Introduction

Briefly set the scene.
   Indicate how you will approach the question.

Body of answer (See Chapters 3 & 4)

A series of headings. Divide problems logically, and do not spend excessive time on any one topic, although the more important will require greater coverage than the least significant.

Closing section

Summary statement. Key points:

- Importance of taking an overall view of the patient's treatment.
- Systemic factors very important, however some now less significant than previously thought.

7. What local factors may contraindicate treatment with dental implants?

What is the question about?

This is basically similar to question 6, and the same general approach applies. Remember to consider both the partially dentate and edentulous patient. Do not focus solely on the technical issues of implant placement and restoration, but include broader local factors, such as the long-term prognosis of the remaining teeth, existing oral disease, the status of any prostheses.

Basis of answer: A series of statements indicating contraindications, grouped in a logical sequence.

Answer plan

Introduction

Briefly set the scene.
   Indicate how you will approach the question.

Body of answer (See Chapters 3 & 4)

A series of headings. Divide problems logically, and do not spend excessive time on any one topic, although the more important will require greater coverage than the least significant.

Closing section

Summary statement. Key points:

- Importance of basing treatment on overall oral care, rather than focusing solely on implant treatment.
- The importance of careful assessment prior to commencing treatment.

8. Indicate the techniques which may be used to replace all four maxillary incisors in an otherwise intact dentition. When would treatment with dental implants be indicated?

What is the question about?

This is basically similar to question 2. Key features are the requirement to indicate techniques rather than discuss them, and that the dentition is otherwise intact. A significant component of the answer will be the indications for implant treatment. Remember that implants can be used to stabilize both fixed and removable prostheses.

Basis of answer: Two major sections, the first listing the alternative techniques, the second exploring the indications for implant treatment, which has both systemic and local dimensions.

Answer plan

Introduction

Briefly set the scene.

Indicate, but do not explore, the importance of systemic and local factors, and the reasons for tooth loss.

Indicate how you will approach the question.

Body of answer (See Chapters 7 & 9)

Principal treatment alternatives:

- Observation.
- Removable partial denture.
- Adhesive bridge.
- Conventional bridge.

When would implant treatment be considered?

- Systemic Factors:
  - absence of contra-indications;
  - occupation;
  - resource availability (financial and team skills).
- Local factors:
  - technically feasible;
  - surgical envelope;
  - prosthodontic envelope;
  - lip line when smiling;
  - access;
  - superior treatment outcome;
  - bone preservation;
  - security;
  - management of spaced dentition;
  - appearance.

Closing section

Summary statement. Key points:

- Importance of basing treatment on overall oral care.
- Significance of both systemic and local factors.
- The importance of considering all alternatives before commencing treatment.

9. What procedures may be used to ensure that dental implants are optimally placed?

What is the question about?

This is not solely a question about radiography or surgeons' guides, but includes treatment planning and team working. It is therefore concerned with prosthesis design, clinical and radiographic assessment of the patient, surgeons' guides and surgical technique. The answer could therefore have sections addressing each of these areas.

Basis of answer: Key features on a timeline running from treatment planning to implant placement.

Answer plan

Introduction

Briefly set the scene.

Indicate the importance of designing the prosthesis before planning implant locations.

Indicate how you will approach the question.

Body of answer (See Chapters 4 & 5)

Treatment planning:

- Identification of the desirability of implant treatment.
- Agreement on surgical and prosthodontic feasibility of implant treatment.
- Prosthesis design:
  - edentulous patient;
  - partially dentate patient.
- Radiography:
  - intra-oral views;
  - extra oral views;
  - conventional;
  - tomographic;
  - computerized axial tomography.

Preparation of surgeon's guide.

Surgical technique .

Closing section

Summary statement. Key points:

- Importance of basing implant location on prosthesis design, thorough clinical examination and appropriate special investigations.

10. What problems may be encountered during implant insertion? Discuss their management.

What is the question about?

This is a straightforward question, which tests the candidate's knowledge and ability to organize a significant amount of material in a restricted time. The problems could be logically based on a timeline, the commencement of which should be defined in the answer. The start of the appointment to place the implants would be a logical choice, and it would also be necessary to define the end point of implant insertion; should stage II surgery be included for example? Problems could be both local and systemic, and include general management issues such as collapse, as well as more local technical issues. It may be preferable to cover the systemic issues in a shorter paragraph and deal mainly with the local problems and their management.

Basis of answer: indicate key systemic and local problems on a timeline running from the start of the appointment to insert implants, and outline their management.

Answer plan

Introduction
Briefly set the scene.
   Indicate how you will approach the question.
   Define time frame.

Body of answer (See Chapter 5)
Systemic problems arising prior to starting surgery:

- Anxiety.
- Anaesthetic problems.
- Collapse.

Local problems arising during surgery:
- Flap management.
- Bone quality, quantity and shape.
- Involvement with other structures.
- Implant insertion:
  – poor primary fixation;
  – difficulty inserting;
  – inability to insert in desired location.
- Haemorrhage.
- Damaged components.
- Wound closure.

Closing section
Summary statement. Key point:

- Importance of prevention in problem management.

---

11. A patient requires extraction of a maxillary central incisor in an otherwise healthy and intact dental arch. What factors would favour its replacement with a dental implant?

What is the question about?

This question is concerned with alternative methods of replacing missing anterior maxillary teeth; although with the emphasis on the advantages of implant therapy. There is also an opportunity to discuss the use of implants immediately after tooth extraction. It would be important to include comments on systemic as well as local factors, and these should include the significance of the reasons for tooth loss. A suitable approach would be to consider systemic and local factors, treatment alternatives, the factors favouring implant therapy, and to comment on the timing of implant placement.

Basis of answer: indicate key systemic factors, underline treatment alternatives, and explore indications for implant treatment, including a comment on immediate insertion of implants.

Answer plan

Introduction
Briefly set the scene.
   Indicate how you will approach the question.

Body of answer (See Chapter 7)
Systemic factors:

- Health, social and occupational factors which might influence treatment decisions.
- Contraindications to implant treatment.

Treatment alternatives:
- Observation.
- Removable partial denture.
- Adhesive bridge.
- Conventional bridge.
- Implant treatment.

Indications for implant treatment:
- Sound abutment teeth.
- Good prognosis for remaining teeth.
- Spacing of the anterior maxillary teeth.
- Feasibility.
- Resources available for this treatment modality.

Closing section

Summary statement. Key point:

- Importance of taking a comprehensive view of treatment.

---

12. Discuss the range of radiographic techniques which may be used in the planning of implant treatment.

What is the question about?

This question asks you to <u>discuss</u> radiographic techniques. It will therefore be necessary not only to list them, but also to explore their relative merits. The techniques could be conveniently subdivided into intra-oral and extra-oral, covering both conventional and tomographic techniques.

Basis of answer: subdivide the techniques as indicated, briefly describe each method and discuss its relative merits.

Answer plan

Introduction

Indicate the value of radiography for treatment planning and diagnosis.

Outline your essay plan.

Body of answer (See Chapters 4 and 5)

Intra-oral techniques:

- Indicate role of long-cone methods and value of alignment devices.
- Applications.
- Advantages and disadvantages, include applicability, and problems relating to radiation dosage.

Extra-oral techniques:

- Conventional.
- Tomographic:
  – rotational and spiral techniques;
  – computerized tomography.
- Describe the techniques, be brief.
- Applications.
- Advantages and disadvantages.

Closing section

Summary statement. Indicate the value of radiography in implant treatment and the importance of familiarity with the various techniques so as to be able to select the most suitable.

Index